TRAUMA-INFORMED FORENSIC PRACTICE

Trauma-Informed Forensic Practice argues for placing trauma-informed practice and thinking at the heart of forensic services. It is written by forensic practitioners and service users from prison and forensic mental health, youth justice, and social care settings.

It provides a compassionate theoretical framework for understanding the links between trauma and offending. It also gives practical guidance on working with issues that are particularly associated with a history of trauma in forensic settings, such as self-harm and substance use, as well as on working with groups who are particularly vulnerable to trauma, such as those with intellectual disabilities and military veterans. Finally, it considers organisational aspects of delivering trauma-informed care, not just for service users but for the staff who work in challenging and dangerous forensic environments.

The book is the first of its kind to address such a broad range of issues and settings. It is aimed at forensic practitioners who wish to develop their own trauma-informed practice or trauma-responsive services. It also provides an accessible introduction to trauma-informed forensic practice for undergraduate and postgraduate students.

Phil Willmot is a Consultant Forensic and Clinical Psychologist and Joint Lead Psychologist for the Men's Personality Disorder Service at Rampton Hospital. He is also Senior Lecturer in Forensic Psychology at the University of Lincoln, UK.

Lawrence Jones is Head of Psychology at Rampton Hospital. He is a former chair of the Division of Forensic Psychology and has published in a range of areas including therapeutic communities, formulation, "personality disorder", iatrogenic responses to intervention, motivation, offence paralleling behaviour, sexual offending, and trauma- and diversity-informed care.

ISSUES IN FORENSIC PSYCHOLOGY

Series Editors
Richard Shuker
Geraldine Akerman

For more information about this series, please visit: www.routledge.com/Issues-in-Forensic-Psychology/book-series/IFP

TRAUMA-INFORMED FORENSIC PRACTICE

Edited by Phil Willmot and Lawrence Jones

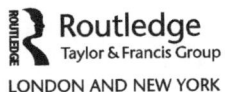

Routledge
Taylor & Francis Group

LONDON AND NEW YORK

Cover image: © Getty images

First published 2022
by Routledge
4 Park Square, Milton Park, Abingdon, Oxon OX14 4RN

and by Routledge
605 Third Avenue, New York, NY 10158

Routledge is an imprint of the Taylor & Francis Group, an informa business

With thanks to Widgit Software for the use of their symbols;
Widgit Symbols © Widgit Software 2002–2021 www.widgit.com

British Library Cataloguing-in-Publication Data
A catalogue record for this book is available from the British Library

Library of Congress Cataloging-in-Publication Data
A catalog record has been requested for this book

ISBN: 978-0-367-63803-0 (hbk)
ISBN: 978-0-367-62691-4 (pbk)
ISBN: 978-1-003-12076-6 (ebk)

DOI: 10.4324/9781003120766

Typeset in Bembo
by Newgen Publishing UK

CONTENTS

Contents

Contents

Contents

ABOUT THE CONTRIBUTORS

Geraldine Akerman is Principal Psychologist at HMP Grendon, Chair of the Division of Forensic Psychology Executive Committee and Trustee of the Safer Living Foundation.

Rachel Beryl is a Forensic Psychologist at the National High Secure Healthcare Service for Women (NHSHSW), Rampton Hospital.

Naomi Callender is a Chartered Forensic Psychologist in the Mental Health Service at Rampton Hospital.

Julie Carlisle is Lead Consultant Clinical Psychologist at Mersey Care NHS Foundation Trust.

Fiona Clark is a Consultant Clinical Psychologist at Broadmoor Hospital.

Peter Clarke is a qualified and Registered Social Worker at Glebe House. He is currently the Chair of the NOTA Policy and Practice Sub-Committee, and Chair of the Royal College of Psychiatry Accreditation Panel for Community of Communities.

John Farnsworth is an Assistant Psychologist and Forensic Psychologist in Training in the Mental Health Service, Rampton Hospital.

Kate Geraghty is a Chartered Forensic Psychologist at Aylesbury Young Offenders Institution.

Nicola S. Gray is a Professor of Clinical & Forensic Psychology at Swansea University. She also works for the NHS in Swansea Bay University Health Board, where she provides a clinical service to the forensic mental health directorate.

Rachel Hicks is an Assistant Psychologist and Forensic Psychologist in Training in the National High Secure Learning Disability Service, Rampton Hospital.

Victoria Hiett-Davies is a Registered Mental Health Nurse who has worked in forensic and non-forensic services with Nottinghamshire Healthcare NHS Foundation Trust and has led on the development and delivery of the Forensic Division's trauma strategy.

Kerensa Hocken is a Registered Forensic Psychologist who has a lead role in her Majesty's Prison and Probation Service psychology services. She is a trustee and co-founder of the Safer Living Foundation (SLF), a charity to prevent sexual abuse.

Jane Jones is a Registered Mental health Nurse and psychotherapist. She is Clinical Lead for ReGroup, working with veterans in the Criminal Justice System, a partnership between Nottinghamshire Healthcare Foundation Trust Offender Health and two veterans' charities Care after Combat and Project Nova.

Nathan Joshua is a former resident in the therapeutic community at HMP Grendon. He is a member of the Prison Reform Trust Prisoner Policy network, the Learning Together Alumni (Cambridge University Institute of Criminology) and the British Convict Criminology Group at the University of Westminster.

Jessica Lewis is a Consultant Clinical Psychologist at the National High Secure Healthcare Service for Women (NHSHSW), Rampton Hospital, joint lead for the NHSHSW Psychology Service and the Clinical Lead for the National Women's Outreach Service.

Emma Longfellow is a Consultant Forensic Psychologist and Psychology lead for the National High Secure Learning Disability Service, Rampton Hospital.

Frank McGuire is a Consultant Clinical Psychologist with Mersey Care NHS Foundation Trust.

Claire Moore is a Consultant Forensic Psychologist and Lead for the Mental Health Service at Rampton.

Estelle Moore is the Trust-Wide Strategic Lead for Psychological Services, West London Mental Health Trust and Head of Psychological Services, Broadmoor Hospital in Berkshire, UK. She is a Chartered Scientist and Consultant Clinical and Forensic Psychologist and Chair of the Psychological Professions Network for London.

Karen Orpwood is a Forensic Clinical Psychologist working in Greater Manchester Mental Health NHS Foundation Trust.

Karen Parish is Clinical Director at Glebe House specialist residential treatment service working with adolescents who display harmful sexual behaviours.

Jennifer Pink is a Psychology Graduate Researcher at Swansea University. Her doctoral research explores psychological pathologies, psychopathy and offending. She is also an Associate Lecturer at the Open University.

Sue Ryan is a Consultant Clinical and Forensic Psychologist working at Merseycare NHS Trust in the Offender Personality Disorder Pathway.

Louise Sainsbury is a Consultant Clinical and Forensic Psychologist and Joint Lead psychologist for the Men's Personality Disorder Service at Rampton Hospital.

Chantal Scaillet is a Consultant Clinical Psychologist and Clinical Lead for a Complex Needs Service in a Young Offenders' Institution.

Yasmin Siddall is a Consultant Forensic Psychologist and Joint Lead Psychologist of the National High Secure Healthcare Service for Women (NHSHSW) at Rampton Hospital.

Nicola Silvester is a Highly Specialist Clinical Psychologist and the Clinical and Strategic Lead for the Children and Young People's Complex Needs Service, an Integrated Care System within Lincolnshire Children's Services.

Michelle Smith is a Chartered Forensic Psychologist and Senior Lecturer at the University of Lincoln, undertaking teaching, research and professional practice consultancy. She is currently the CPD Lead on the BPS Division of Forensic Psychology Committee.

Sarah Todd is the Psychological Lead in the National High Secure Deaf Service (NHSDS) and a Principal Psychologist in the Mental Health Service at Rampton Hospital.

Jon Taylor is a Consultant Forensic Psychologist and Psychotherapist who has worked in range of prison, secure hospital and community forensic settings for almost 30 years.

Elizabeth Utting is Principal Forensic Psychologist and Clinical Lead for Horizon Care and Education, who provide care and schooling for looked after children across England.

Jamie Walton is a Lead Psychologist in HM Prison and Probation Service. He is a Registered Forensic Psychologist and co-author of two accredited offending behaviour programmes.

Tamara Woodall is a Forensic Psychologist currently working in a trauma-informed service within a prison setting. Prior to this, she worked for a therapeutic children's residential service.

SERIES FOREWORD

The previous edition of Issues in Forensic Psychology addressed how forensic therapeutic communities emerged from being outside of the "what works" narrative to having a significant role in influencing the growth in services for people with complex needs. This current edition addresses another area whose presence the editors observe has, for many years, only been acknowledged as "the elephant in the room". The edition reflects the recognition now given to the role that trauma and adversity have in the onset and maintenance of offending and describes the significant developments and growth in trauma-informed approaches. In much the same way as relational working and therapeutic environments explored in earlier editions have arisen from a place of relative obscurity, this edition highlights how trauma and adversity have now come to provide a central position in forensic services.

What this edition provides is a highly relevant and compelling account of how an understanding of trauma and its impact has developed and how this has influenced and improved forensic practice. It suggests that a more inclusive and compassionate understanding of the nature of risk, personal responsibility, and rehabilitation is becoming evident. The editors also acknowledge the importance of avoiding seeing trauma-informed working as holding the status as a new model which should be adopted uncritically. Instead they argue for a more nuanced approach to how trauma-informed work is understood. A theme which emerges in the book is the importance of understanding why and how people respond to trauma and adversity in ways that can be rather different. This is perhaps a real strength of the edition. It provides a well-argued case for why a trauma-informed approach offers such a promising way of understanding work within criminal justice and forensic mental health. It also highlights how an appreciation of the impact of trauma can be used to help understand organisations, support and equip staff and influence how we work with, support, and engage those we are seeking to help. However, the editors also reflect on the risks of unquestioningly adopting any framework, arguing strongly for an individualised and inclusive approach to understanding risk, need, and treatment pathways.

This edition of Issues in Forensic Psychology brings together developments in our understanding of trauma, and how this can help us to work more effectively with those in our care. Despite exercising a cautionary note, however, the book makes a clear case for why an understanding of trauma will improve and enhance practice and how this is now seen in recent developments in practice. This edition is noteworthy in the accounts it draws from experts by experience, and shows how this experience has had the capacity to shape our understanding of trauma, its impact, and its consequences. The text asks challenging questions to organisations in reflecting upon how they may unwittingly create a social climate where structures, relationships, and dynamics can re-traumatise residents. It also explores ways in which social arrangements in institutions can be traumatising for those who work there and offers a framework for how this can be responded to, recognising that working with traumatised people in any setting can itself be traumatising. The book does though contain a message of hope. It advocates how a trauma-informed understanding of offending can lead to a more compassionate and humane approach and how this can instil safe, decent, and effective ways of working within criminal justice and forensic mental health services.

Richard Shuker
Geraldine Akerman
Series Editors

INTRODUCTION

Phil Willmot and Lawrence Jones

Trauma: The Elephant in the Room

The idea that childhood adversity and maltreatment are important antecedents to offending is not new. The idea that people re-enact childhood trauma goes back to the early days of psychoanalysis in the 1890s (Herman, 1992), while Bowlby (1944) identified a pattern of prolonged early separation from primary caregivers in his sample of juvenile offenders. Widom's (1989) cohort study was arguably the first to systematically establish a correlation between being childhood abuse or neglect and increased risk of delinquency and violence.

There are many studies that show higher rates of childhood adversity among offenders than among the rest of the population (Thornberry, Ireland, & Smith, 2001; Widom, 1989). Many practitioners working in the criminal justice or forensic mental health systems will have met service users for whom the links between their own maltreatment and their offending seem abundantly obvious. Even in popular culture, the notion of the offender whose crimes are some sort of reaction to their childhood experiences is a common trope in crime fiction (Bergman, 2014), while movie villains as diverse as Darth Vader and Cruella De Vil are set on their wicked ways by early trauma or adversity.

And yet, despite evidence for a link between childhood adversity and offending, little attention has been paid to it in forensic psychology theory and practice. For example, the UK's National Institute for Health and Clinical Excellence guidelines on antisocial personality disorder (2009) or the mental health of adults in contact with the criminal justice system (2017) make virtually no mention of developmental adversity, and neither does the Risk Needs Responsivity model (Bonta & Andrews, 2016), arguably the most influential model in forensic psychology over the past 20 years. So why is developmental trauma still the "elephant in the room"? We suggest several reasons.

DOI: 10.4324/9781003120766-1

The Relationship Is Not Simple or Obvious

While the link between childhood adversity and offending may seem clear in some individuals, the larger scale picture is less clear. While retrospective studies of childhood adversity among offenders show high rates of adversity, prospective studies of child abuse survivors show that the majority do not go on to offend (Fitton, Yu, & Fazel, 2020). Indeed, studies of trauma in the general population show that childhood maltreatment is sadly the norm rather than the exception. Hillis, Mercy, Amobi, and Kress (2016) estimated that, globally, 70% of children between the ages of two and seventeen had experienced physical, emotional, and/or sexual violence *in the previous year*, while the World Health Organisation (2020) estimates that three in four children aged between two and four regularly suffer physical punishment or psychological violence at the hands of caregivers. The impact of early adversity or maltreatment is likely to be mediated by a wide range of factors including the frequency and intensity of the adversity, its meaning, the attachment, and wider social environments and the presence of other protective or risk factors.

The relationship between childhood maltreatment and offending is further obscured for certain groups, including men and those from ethnic minorities, among whom childhood maltreatment tends to be significantly under-reported. O'Leary and Barber (2008) reported that 36% of women and 74% of men who had survived childhood sexual abuse did not report the abuse at the time, while 25% of women and 45% of men took more than 20 years before they talked about their experiences. In cultures that value modesty and virginity in girls, that stress respect for elders, or that place a taboo on discussing sex, disclosure is likely to be even harder (Fontes & Plummer, 2010). In minority communities, reporting abuse to authorities that are viewed as hostile may be seen as betraying or bringing shame on the whole community. Language problems may also prevent children from immigrant communities from reporting abuse (Fontes and Plummer). Children from minority communities may have good reason to be wary of reporting abuse; Owen and Statham (2009) found that African Caribbean children placed on the child protection register in the UK were more likely to be placed in care, less likely to be returned to their parents and less likely to be adopted from care than children from other ethnic groups. Also, particularly in prison, survivors can go to great lengths to conceal their victimhood, because being identified as a survivor can be dangerous (de Viggiani, 2012).

Trauma Is Difficult to Define

Research into childhood maltreatment generally categorises childhood events into broad categories such as sexual or emotional abuse. However, the meaning, impact, and consequences of a term such as "sexual abuse" is likely to vary enormously depending on a range of factors including the age at which the abuse took place, the identity of and relationship to the perpetrator, the degree of physical or emotional coercion involved, the duration of abuse, the anticipated or actual response of family and the wider community to the abuse, and the individual's cultural position in relation to it.

Medical approaches have tended to define trauma in terms of events. The American Psychiatric Association, for example, defines trauma as an *event* "that involved death or threatened death, actual or threatened serious injury, or threatened sexual violation". On the other hand, authors such as Moskowitz, Heinimaa, and van der Hart (2019) have argued that it is more useful to think of trauma as a biopsychosocial *response* to external events that is mediated by the personal meaning of those events. In this book, most authors use the term trauma as a convenient shorthand to describe a range of experiences that may include physical or emotional neglect, bullying, social deprivation, harassment, and discrimination and which may not fit any of the recognised definitions of trauma. While a definition based on the meaning of events to the individual may be more useful clinically, it points to the complexity or futility of attempting to establish a correlation between trauma, or particular forms of trauma, and offending behaviour.

While there is growing evidence for a broad correlation between trauma and offending, the extremely broad range of what constitutes trauma (or indeed what constitutes offending) as well as individual differences in the meaning of that trauma and how it affects individuals make that broad correlation virtually meaningless. For some individuals the impact of trauma appears to be extremely strong, while for others it does not. However, to quote Elliott, Bjelajac, Fallot, Markoff, and Reed (2005; p.463):

> since providers have no way of distinguishing survivors from non-survivors, best practices are those that treat all [service users] as if they might be trauma survivors, relying on procedures that are most likely to be growth-promoting and least likely to be retraumatizing.

Societal Pressures

There may also be some broader, societal reasons why trauma-informed approaches have not yet been widely adopted in forensic services.

Is it too awful? If you have worked for any length of time in forensic services, chances are that you will have heard, or at least read, accounts of seemingly relentless abuse, neglect, trauma, and adversity that are truly harrowing and overwhelming. If we multiply these individual accounts by the statistics on how widespread such experiences are, both nationally and globally, the picture it presents is of a boundless ocean of suffering that is too overwhelming to contemplate, let alone to intervene in.

Is it too difficult or too expensive? The recovery process for individual survivors of trauma can be complex and expensive and can take years. At a time when, as Allison and Grierson (2021) reported, the number prisoners in England and Wales completing accredited treatment programmes fell by 62% between 2009 and 2019, while the prison population increased, do we have the resources or the will to deliver expensive and long-term treatment on an industrial scale?

Is the cognitive dissonance too great? We live in a society that likes simple answers to complex issues and is intolerant of ambiguity and paradox, where moral absolutes are beguilingly attractive. In the UK, successive governments have stressed their toughness on crime, while politicians and the media have created a discourse that stigmatises those who break the law, creates a false dichotomy between victims and offenders, and presents the criminal justice system as a zero-sum game in which any sympathetic or liberal treatment of offenders is seen as "a slap in the face for victims" (Drake & Henley, 2014; p.147). In such an environment, is it too difficult to consider that a person can be both a perpetrator and a victim of crime?

A Paradigm Shift?

In his seminal work *The Structure of Scientific Revolutions*, Thomas Kuhn (1962) described the history of science as a cyclic process with periods of "normal science" during which there is a broad consensus about how the world works, which problems are worth investigating, and which phenomena are important. The end of a period of normal science is marked by crises – experimental results that do not fit existing theories or internal contradictions that are found in those theories. Eventually there is a "revolution" and scientists adopt a new way of understanding the world. Kuhn termed such revolutions *paradigm shifts*. Paradigm shifts radically change the way that people understand the world. For example, the Copernican revolution in astronomy shattered the belief that the earth is the fixed point around which the rest of the universe revolves and replaced it with a model in which the earth is just one of countless similar planets. In contrast, the Einsteinian revolution in physics did not sweep away Newtonian physics but revealed extra layers of complexity that were just as radical in changing our understanding of the forces governing the universe and which opened up whole new areas of physics and cosmology that had not been imagined in a Newtonian universe.

It could also be argued that forensic psychology is currently due a paradigm shift. For example, 30 years after the principles of effective correctional programming were identified (Andrews, Bonta, & Hoge, 1990), programmes that adhere to those principles appear to have limited impact on reducing reoffending (Lösel et al., 2020; Mews, Di Bella, & Purver, 2017). The deficits-based forensic psychological paradigm has made little progress in explaining some of the most obvious and consistent criminological patterns, such as that crime in general, and violent crime in particular, is overwhelmingly committed by men, or that ethnic minorities are consistently overrepresented at all stages of the criminal justice system.

Is a Trauma-Informed Approach a New Forensic Paradigm?

Forensic psychology may be approaching a paradigm shift, but would an approach that considers the impact of trauma be the way forward? Only time will tell the answer to that question. However, this book aims to illustrate some of the reasons why a trauma-informed approach could be a promising way of framing or re-framing many of the issues that affect criminal justice and forensic mental health services.

Firstly, a trauma-informed approach can offer new perspectives on questions that existing approaches to forensic psychology have not really addressed, such as how the different ways that trauma impacts on men and women can offer insights into why most crime is committed by men (which is discussed in Chapter 2), or why children who grow up in care are much more likely than those who live with their birth families to offend (Chapter 5). A trauma-informed approach can also provide a fresh and compassionate understanding of the particular issues that affect marginalised groups such as people with intellectual disabilities (Chapter 6), Deaf people (Chapter 7), and ethnic minorities (various chapters) when they come into contact with the criminal justice system.

Secondly, adopting a trauma-informed approach brings forensic psychology into line with related fields, particularly mental health. The term *trauma-informed care* was coined by Harris and Fallot (2001) who recognised that most people who come into contact with mental health services have experienced trauma, and that services need to recognise this in order to create a safe therapeutic environment that does not inadvertently retraumatise or invalidate survivors. The idea that trauma and mental health are closely connected is widely accepted (Bentall, 2003; Herman, 1992; van der Kolk, 2014). Moreover, developmental trauma is recognised to have profound and lifelong impacts on many other aspects of life apart from mental health, including educational attainment (Houtepen et al., 2020), employability (Topitzes, Pate, Berman, & Medina-Kirchner, 2016), relationship stability (Umberson, Williams, Thomas, Liu, & Thomeer, 2014), substance misuse (Dube et al., 2003), and chronic physical health conditions (Felitti et al., 1998). Trauma-informed principles have now spread from mental health services to child and adult social care, education, and primary care (Akin, Strolin-Goltzman, & Collins-Camargo, 2017; Hamberger, Barry, & Franco, 2019; Mersky, Topitzes, & Britz, 2019; Walkley & Cox, 2013).

Thirdly, being trauma-informed allows for a richer understanding of the complexities of offending and other human behaviours. A theme that emerges strongly throughout this book is how a trauma-informed approach allows for a fuller approach to formulation, embracing not only the biological aspects of autonomic responses to trauma and threat but also the social aspects of social deprivation and exclusion to make a more fully rounded biopsychosocial formulation.

Fourthly, anyone who has worked clinically in the criminal justice or forensic mental health systems will recognise that trauma is commonplace, not just in the lived experiences of many service users but also of many staff. Traumatic events, in the form of physical violence, threats, and intimidation, as well as self-harm, can also be commonplace in these settings. Moreover, experiences of being restrained, locked in a room, moved suddenly without warning or not being involved in important decisions about one's own care can be common experiences for residents in forensic settings and can be retraumatising when they mirror early experiences. If we are not aware of these parallels, or of their potential impact, they may have profound impact on not only on the people that we care for but also on ourselves and our colleagues. This book therefore not only considers the impact of trauma on service users in criminal justice and forensic mental health settings, it also considers the impact on staff and on organisations.

Another perspective offered by the trauma-informed approach is the importance of listening to what service users have to tell us. The principles of trauma-informed approaches to mental health include collaboration and the empowerment of survivors to determine their own futures, which can be challenging in some forensic settings. A trauma-informed approach also involves a shift from asking "what is wrong with you" to "what happened to you" (Harris & Fallot, 2001), and for this reason we have included accounts from service users in most chapters.

A Note of Caution

We should be cautious about seeing trauma-informed working as a panacea. Trauma is probably not a relevant factor in the case of every offender. Trauma-based formulations may not be helpful for everyone. Some people, for example, argue that seeing somebody through the lens of their abusive experiences is itself stigmatising and losing sight of them as whole people; it can also feel to some people like being labelled or misunderstood. For others, being on the receiving end of a diagnosis has been a useful experience; once they had read the description of the diagnosis, they felt relief, felt understood or recognised. Some people wear their diagnoses as a badge of honour and challenge those who do not have that diagnosis to acknowledge their difference. Others have critiqued from a feminist perspective what they describe as "mother blaming", encouraging us to move away from accounts of trauma that focus on individuals and to focus on abusive systemic processes. There is also a fear that a developmental perspective might lead to a devaluing of medication or biological interventions when most practitioners know that for many people medications can offer a significant piece of the intervention jigsaw. All of these perspectives have a kernel of truth to them that we ignore at our peril.

About This Book

The book is divided into five sections. Section 1 makes the case for placing trauma at the centre of forensic practice. Chapter 1 examines why the link between trauma and crime has been overlooked in the past. It then presents what will be a central and recurring theme throughout the book, that it is not trauma or adversity *per se* that leads to crime but pervasive adversity that leaves survivors with a chronic sense of threat and lack of safety. We propose that it is people's attempts to manage this sense of threat and achieve a sense of safety that leads to a range of survival behaviours that can include offending. Chapter 1 concludes by reviewing the growing body of evidence that links childhood adversity to the central eight criminogenic needs identified by Bonta and Andrews (2016). Chapter 2 examines the issue of gender. Any explanatory framework for offending must account for the very different patterns of offending by men and women. This chapter argues that there are important differences in the types of adversity, and more importantly in the meaning of adversity to individuals and to groups that mean that men and women respond very differently to trauma and adversity. Chapter 3 considers how to approach forensic risk assessment in a trauma-informed way. This is an area where a trauma-informed approach can greatly enrich our understanding of complex processes and interaction. The chapter focuses in particular on the importance to risk assessment of triggering contextual factors and altered states of consciousness that can occur both in response to trauma and in relation to offending behaviour. Chapter 4 looks at the links between trauma, personality disorder, and offending. Despite great progress over the last 20 years in our understanding of people with a diagnosis of "personality disorder", those in forensic services who are given this diagnosis are still often stigmatised and misunderstood. Considering these service users and their behaviour through the lens of trauma can provide a fresh and compassionate approach to their care and treatment.

Section 2 focuses on groups who are particularly vulnerable to trauma. Each chapter is written by a professional expert who works with a particular client group, supported, wherever possible, by personal accounts from experts by experience that illustrate the particular forms of adversity and trauma faced by that group, and the links between adversity and offending. Each chapter also presents practical advice on working with that client group in a trauma-informed way. Chapter 5 explores the reasons why children in the UK who have been in care are 50 times more likely to go to prison than those who have not. Chapter 6 discusses the particular challenges facing those with intellectual disabilities, while Chapter 7 discusses the unique challenges facing Deaf people. Finally, Chapter 8 explores why military veterans are so heavily represented in the criminal justice system.

Section 3 focuses on some of the responses to trauma that are not always recognised as such in forensic settings. Again, service user narratives form an important element of these chapters to illustrate the impact that trauma has had on their lives, and each chapter includes practical guidance from clinicians. Perhaps one of the more obvious responses to trauma, particularly in forensic settings, is self-harm, and Chapter 9 explores the relationship between trauma and non-suicidal self-injury (NSSI) and the service-wide approach to managing NSSI in the UK's National High Secure Healthcare Service for Women. Substance use, both in the community and in institutions, is another widespread response to trauma. Chapter 10 considers the links between trauma and substance use and reviews current approaches to treatment. In recent years, trauma-based models of psychotic experiences have increasingly complemented and in many cases supplanted the medical approach that often regarded these experiences as primarily biologically based. Chapter 11 develops that trauma-informed understanding of psychotic experiences and applies it to violent behaviour. Clinicians have perhaps trodden carefully around the link between trauma and sexual offending, for fear of being seen to "make excuses". There is, however, growing evidence of a multitude of pathways from early trauma and adversity to sexual offending, and these are explored in Chapter 12. Chapter 13 considers how many violent offenders experience trauma symptoms resulting from their own offending. This is another area that clinicians have perhaps avoided from fear of being seen as "minimising" the seriousness of a person's offending, but offence-related trauma can present significant challenges to forensic practitioners, particularly when there is also pre-existing trauma, and the chapter presents a framework for working with offence-related trauma.

Section 4 describes aspects of treatment in different forensic settings. Therapeutic communities originally grew out of the attempts by pioneers such as Wilfred Bion and Thomas Main to treat traumatised soldiers during the Second World War. The need to address trauma is therefore perhaps better integrated into therapeutic communities than into other forensic services. This section begins with chapters from two established therapeutic communities. Chapter 14 described Glebe House, a therapeutic community for young men with histories of harmful sexual behaviours, while Chapter 15 describes HMP Grendon, a prison-based therapeutic community for adult men. In Chapter 16, the challenges of running a trauma service in a Young Offenders' Institution are discussed, while Chapter 17 applies a trauma-informed approach to adult prison environments. Finally in this section, Chapter 18 considers the challenges of working in the community with forensic clients across a variety of agencies.

Section 5 addresses organisational issues. Trauma-informed forensic care is not only about addressing the trauma histories of people in our care. It is also important to acknowledge that forensic settings can often be violent and unpredictable places and that staff who work in them often come with their own trauma histories and have to work in those same dangerous and unpredictable environments as well as dealing with the vicarious trauma of the people in their care. This section addresses the organisational issues involved in delivering trauma-informed care. Chapter 19 explores the issues involved in setting up and delivering a trauma-informed community youth justice service while Chapter 20 explores how implementing a trauma-informed approach in a secure hospital setting can enable healthier and more compassionate ways of working that benefit both staff and patients. Chapter 21 explores in more depth the challenges facing staff in forensic institutions and how a trauma-informed approach can help to address these. Chapter 22 describes how implementing trauma-informed practices in a secure hospital has promoted culture change. Finally in this section, Chapter 23 looks at restorative justice. Trauma-informed forensic care sits uncomfortably in a society and a criminal justice system that values punishment and retribution over rehabilitation and restoration and this chapter describes how a restorative justice approach complements a trauma-informed approach. We round the book off with a discussion of some of the emerging themes from this book, and some suggestions for the future of trauma-informed forensic practice.

Finally, it is important to say at the outset that this book is about material that is traumatic. The content of the chapters in this volume will inevitably be triggering for some of those reading it. Whilst there are no detailed accounts of abusive experience, there are frequent references to different kinds of abuse and adversity as well as service user accounts of the impact of trauma on their lives. The reader is therefore encouraged to think carefully about how they are going to manage the material that they are reading about. All too often in the forensic field attention to our own reactions to this kind of material is ignored. It is critical for those working clinically and academically with this kind of material that the ways in which it can impact on us is considered and measures taken to make sure that our well-being is looked after. We are all human and can all be troubled in complex ways by this kind of material. Part of the message of this book is that we should not ignore trauma, whether it is in society at large, our organisations, our service users, or indeed in ourselves.

Conclusion

Giving evidence to the Parliamentary Select Committee on Public Accounts in 2005, then HM Prison Service Director General Phil Wheatley stated "…if we crowd prison so much that staff cannot care for prisoners and the place begins to feel just like a big sausage machine, that is dangerous" (Wheatley, 2005). Many practitioners who have worked in the criminal justice or forensic mental health systems will have encountered the sausage machine analogy or will be able to identify with it. It speaks not just of the relentless workload and uncomfortable physical conditions but also the way in which organisations can dehumanise those they are supposed to care for and those who are supposed to care, making them less than human objects to be "processed". In organisations that should be focused on caring for some of the most damaged and vulnerable in society that is both a tragedy and a scandal. Our greatest hope in editing this book is that a trauma-informed approach will provide a framework that reintroduces, or perhaps introduces for the first time, a more compassionate approach to forensic practice that sees service users and colleagues as vulnerable, hurt, resilient, but above all, human.

References

Akin, B. A., Strolin-Goltzman, J., & Collins-Camargo, C. (2017). Successes and challenges in developing trauma-informed child welfare systems: A real-world case study of exploration and initial implementation. *Children and Youth Services Review, 82*, 42–52. doi:10.1016/j.childyouth.2017.09.007

Allison, E., & Grierson, J. (2021, May 17). England and Wales prisoners taking fewer rehabilitation courses. *The Guardian*, Retrieved from www.theguardian.com/

Andrews, D. A., Bonta, J., & Hoge, R. D. (1990). Classification for effective rehabilitation: Rediscovering psychology. *Criminal Justice and Behavior, 17*(1), 19–52. doi:10.1177/0093854890017001004

Bentall, R. P. (2003). *Madness explained: Psychosis and human nature.* Penguin.

Bergman, K. (2014). *Swedish crime fiction: The making of Nordic Noir.* Mimesis.

Bonta, J., & Andrews, D. A. (2016). *The psychology of criminal conduct.* Abingdon: Routledge.

Bowlby, J. (1944). Forty-four juvenile thieves: Their characters and home-life. *International Journal of Psychoanalysis, 25*, 19–52.

de Viggiani, N. (2012). Trying to be something you are not: Masculine performances within a prison setting. *Men and Masculinities, 15*(3), 271–291. doi:10.1177/1097184X12448464

Drake, D. H., & Henley, A. J. (2014). 'Victims' versus 'offenders' in British political discourse: The construction of a false dichotomy. *The Howard Journal of Criminal Justice, 53*(2), 141–157. doi:10.1111/hojo.12057

Dube, S. R., Felitti, V. J., Dong, M., Chapman, D. P., Giles, W. H., & Anda, R. F. (2003). Childhood abuse, neglect, and household dysfunction and the risk of illicit drug use: The adverse childhood experiences study. *Pediatrics, 111*(3), 564–572. doi:10.1542/peds.111.3.564

Elliott, D. E., Bjelajac, P., Fallot, R. D., Markoff, L. S., & Reed, B. G. (2005). Trauma-informed or trauma-denied: Principles and implementation of trauma-informed services for women. *Journal of Community Psychology, 33*(4), 461–477. doi:10.1002/jcop.20063

Felitti, V. J., Anda, R. F., Nordenberg, D., Williamson, D. F., Spitz, A. M., Edwards, V., & Marks, J. S. (1998). Relationship of childhood abuse and household dysfunction to many of the leading causes of death in adults: The adverse childhood experiences (ACE) study. *American Journal of Preventive Medicine, 14*(4), 245–258. doi:10.1016/S0749-3797(98)00017-8

Fitton, L., Yu, R., & Fazel, S. (2020). Childhood maltreatment and violent outcomes: A systematic review and meta-analysis of prospective studies. *Trauma, Violence, & Abuse, 21*(4), 754–768. doi:10.1177/1524838018795269

Fontes, L. A., & Plummer, C. (2010). Cultural issues in disclosures of child sexual abuse. *Journal of Child Sexual Abuse, 19*(5), 491–518. doi:10.1080/10538712.2010.512520

Hamberger, L. K., Barry, C., & Franco, Z. (2019). Implementing trauma-informed care in primary medical settings: Evidence-based rationale and approaches. *Journal of Aggression, Maltreatment & Trauma, 28*(4), 425–444. doi:10.1080/10926771.2019.1572399

Harris, M., & Fallot, R. (2001). *Using trauma theory to design service systems. New directions for mental health services,* Jossey-Bass, San Francisco, CA.

Herman, J. L. (1992). *Trauma and recovery: From domestic abuse to political terror.* Pandora.

Hillis, S., Mercy, J., Amobi, A., & Kress, H. (2016). Global prevalence of past-year violence against children: A systematic review and minimum estimates. *Pediatrics, 137*(3), e20154079. doi:10.1542/peds.2015-4079

Houtepen, L. C., Heron, J., Suderman, M. J., Fraser, A., Chittleborough, C. R., & Howe, L. D. (2020). Associations of adverse childhood experiences with educational attainment and adolescent health and the role of family and socioeconomic factors: A prospective cohort study in the UK. *PLoS Medicine, 17*(3), e1003031. doi:10.1371/journal.pmed.1003031

Kuhn, T. S. (1962). *The structure of scientific revolutions.* Chicago: University of Chicago Press.

Lösel, F., Link, E., Schmucker, M., Bender, D., Breuer, M., Carl, L., ... & Lauchs, L. (2020). On the effectiveness of sexual offender treatment in prisons: A comparison of two different evaluation designs in routine practice. *Sexual Abuse, 32*(4), 452–475. doi:10.1177/1079063219871576

Mersky, J. P., Topitzes, J., & Britz, L. (2019). Promoting evidence-based, trauma-informed social work practice. *Journal of Social Work Education, 55*(4), 645–657. doi:10.1080/10437797.2019.1627261

Mews, A., Di Bella, L., & Purver, M. (2017). *Impact evaluation of the prison-based core sex offender treatment programme.* London: Ministry of Justice.

Moskowitz, A., Heinimaa, M., & van der Hart, O. (2019). Defining psychosis, trauma, and dissociation: Historical and contemporary conceptions. In A. Moskowitz, M. J. Dorahy, & I Schäfer (Eds), *Psychosis, trauma and dissociation: Evolving perspectives on severe psychopathology* (pp. 7–29). Wiley. doi:10.1002/9781118585948.ch1

National Institute for Health and Clinical Excellence. (2009). Antisocial personality disorder: Treatment, management and prevention (NICE Clinical Guideline 77). NICE.

National Institute for Health and Clinical Excellence. (2017) A mental health of adults in contact with the criminal justice system (NICE Clinical Guideline 66). NICE.

O'Leary, P. J., & Barber, J. (2008). Gender differences in silencing following childhood sexual abuse. *Journal of Child Sexual Abuse, 17*(2), 133–143. doi:10.1080/10538710801916416

Owen, C., & Statham, J. (2009). *Disproportionality in child welfare: The prevalence of black and minority ethnic children within 'looked after' and 'children in need 'populations and on child protection registers in England.* University of London.

Thornberry, T. P., Ireland, T. O., & Smith, C. A. (2001). The importance of timing: The varying impact of childhood and adolescent maltreatment on multiple problem outcomes. *Development and Psychopathology, 13*(4), 957–979. doi:10.1017/S0954579401004114

Topitzes, J., Pate, D. J., Berman, N. D., & Medina-Kirchner, C. (2016). Adverse childhood experiences, health, and employment: A study of men seeking job services. *Child Abuse & Neglect, 61*, 23–34. doi:10.1016/j.chiabu.2016.09.012

Umberson, D., Williams, K., Thomas, P. A., Liu, H., & Thomeer, M. B. (2014). Race, gender, and chains of disadvantage: Childhood adversity, social relationships, and health. *Journal of Health and Social Behavior, 55*(1), 20–38. doi:10.1177/0022146514521426

van der Kolk, B. (2014). *The body keeps the score: Mind, brain and body in the transformation of trauma.* Penguin.

Walkley, M., & Cox, T. L. (2013). Building trauma-informed schools and communities. *Children & Schools*, *35*(2), 123–126. doi:10.1093/cs/cdt007

Wheatley, P. (2005). Retrieved from https://publications.parliament.uk/pa/cm200506/cmselect/cmpubacc/788/5121905.htm

Widom, C. S. (1989). The cycle of violence. *Science*, *244*(4901), 160–166. doi:10.1126/science.2704995

World Health Organisation. (2020). *Child maltreatment*. Retrieved from www.who.int/news-room/fact-sheets/detail/child-maltreatment

PART I

Trauma and Offending

1

CHILDHOOD MALTREATMENT AND ITS LINKS TO OFFENDING

Phil Willmot

The importance of childhood trauma has been largely overlooked in forensic psychology. Some of the most widely quoted theories of offending based on low self-control (Gottfredson & Hirschi, 1990), moral development (Kohlberg & Hersh, 1977), personality (Hare, 1993), or a combination of factors (Bonta & Andrews, 2016), have little or nothing to say about the impact of childhood adversity. There are perhaps many reasons why the impact of trauma has been overlooked, some of which were discussed in the introduction. For the purposes of this chapter, two reasons stand out. The first is that childhood adversity is an extremely broad term. For example, the term childhood sexual abuse covers experiences as diverse as long-term incestuous abuse by a carer and a single episode of rape by a stranger. While the consequences of these different experiences may both be profound, they are also likely to be very different (Estes & Tidwell, 2002). The nature and impact of each traumatic episode will be unique. However, it is still possible to identify many of the characteristics of childhood adversity that are particularly toxic in terms of links to offending behaviour, and the first section of this chapter discusses those characteristics.

A second important reason why the link between childhood adversity and offending has been overlooked is that the relationship is extremely complex. As with the nature of trauma, the link between trauma and offending will be unique for each individual, but there are some clear patterns. The second part of this chapter briefly summarises these developmental processes and attempts to integrate them with what we already know about key criminogenic factors.

What Patterns of Childhood Adversity Are Associated with Offending?

While rates of adversity among children who go on to offend as adults are generally higher than among those that do not (Thornberry, Ireland, & Smith, 2001; Widom,

DOI: 10.4324/9781003120766-3

1989), maltreatment or adversity of some sort appears to be a widespread feature of childhood (Hillis, Mercy, Amobi, & Kress, 2016), and prospective studies of child abuse survivors show that the majority do not go on to offend (Fitton, Yu, & Fazel, 2020). A history of adversity or maltreatment is therefore insufficient *per se* to predict adult criminal behaviour. However, several different but overlapping patterns of childhood adversity appear to be particularly common among young people and adults involved in the criminal justice system.

Complex Trauma

van der Kolk (2005) defines complex trauma as

> the experience of multiple, chronic and prolonged, developmentally adverse traumatic events, most often of an interpersonal nature (e.g., sexual or physical abuse, war, community violence) and early-life onset. These exposures often occur within the child's caregiving system and include physical, emotional, and educational neglect and child maltreatment beginning in early childhood.
>
> *p. 402*

Brown, Wanamaker, Greiner, Scott, and Skilling (2021) report that 70% of young females and 60% of young males in a Canadian correctional sample had histories of complex trauma, and that a history of complex trauma was associated with high levels of criminogenic needs.

Ford et al. (2012) proposed that complex trauma and delinquency are linked via direct and indirect pathways. The direct pathway involves post-traumatic stress disorder (PTSD) symptoms of diminished arousal reactions coupled with maladaptive hyperarousal which result in episodes of reactive rage and violence. In the indirect pathway, trauma symptoms disrupt the normal development of both secure attachment to caregivers and self-regulatory capacity. These in turn lead to other problems including poor impulse control, substance misuse, impaired information processing, maladaptive thinking, and association with delinquent peers.

Poly-Victimisation

There are various definitions of poly-victimisation, but their common element is exposure to multiple types of traumatic events. Finkelhor, Ormrod, and Turner (2007) suggested various reasons why poly-victimisation is so toxic, including that the debilitating emotional impact of victimisation undermines the ability of children to protect themselves, or that repeated victimisation leads to lower self-esteem or a sense of learned helplessness. Rates of poly-victimisation are significantly higher among justice-involved boys and girls (Ford, Elhai, Connor, & Frueh, 2010; Wood, Foy, Layne, Pynoos, & James, 2002). Among justice-involved young people, poly-victims report more severe PTSD symptoms, emotional and behavioural problems, suicide risk, and substance misuse problems than other trauma survivors (Ford, Grasso, Hawke,

& Chapman, 2013). Ford, Charak, Modrowski, and Kerig (2018) found a direct link between poly-victimisation and substance misuse among justice-involved adolescents, while PTSD symptoms mediated the link between poly-victimisation and increased irritability.

Betrayal Trauma

Betrayal trauma is defined as childhood abuse perpetrated by individuals whom the child cares for, depends on, or trusts (Freyd, 1996). Freyd proposed that abuse of this type is particularly damaging and is processed and remembered differently from other forms of abuse or trauma because the victim is physically and emotionally dependent on their abuser. Freyd proposed that emotional numbing enables victims of betrayal trauma to preserve their relationship with their caregiver and persist in behaviours that elicit caregiving. While this dissociation can be adaptive during childhood, betrayal trauma is associated with a range of severe long-term consequences, including emotional numbing, avoidance and a compromised ability to detect betrayal in relationships that leaves survivors at increased risk of repeated victimisation later in life (Gobin & Freyd, 2009). Kerig, Bennett, Thompson, and Becker (2012) found that justice-involved young people who had experienced betrayal trauma experienced numbing specifically for the emotions of fear and sadness, and that this was associated with callous/unemotional traits.

Experiences of Racism

People from ethnic minorities are overrepresented in the criminal justice system in many countries of the global north (Cunneen & Tauri, 2019; Webster, 2018), and any review of the links between maltreatment and offending ought to consider the link between experiences of racism and offending behaviour. Because much of the literature on childhood maltreatment has focused on abuse and neglect within the home, racism, which usually occurs outside the home, has often been overlooked as a form of developmental trauma. Nevertheless, Kirkinis, Pieterse, Martin, Agiliga, and Brownell (2018) found that experiences of racial discrimination were significantly associated with trauma symptoms.

Much of the focus in the forensic literature has been on the impact of structural or institutional racism on the lives of people from ethnic minorities, with relatively little research into the impact of interpersonal racism or internalised beliefs resulting from chronic exposure to racism (Trent, Dooley, & Dougé, 2019). Most research in this area is based on the experiences of African Americans. Unnever and Gabbidon (2011) have developed a comprehensive model of African American offending which argues that chronic and pervasive experiences of racial discrimination affect the physical and mental health of African Americans in a similar way to other forms of chronic trauma. Among its other elements, their model proposes that racist stereotypes alienate young African Americans and, in particular, African American men from white-dominated institutions like schools and the justice system. This leads to feelings of anger, depression, and hopelessness that African American men feel they have to suppress in order to avoid conforming to those same stereotypes which portray them as aggressive or threatening. This leads to a cycle of emotional avoidance, rumination, and self-medication with drugs or alcohol, all of which increase the risk of offending. While Unnever and Gabbidon's theory is based on African Americans' unique history and experiences of racial trauma and injustice, many of the processes and mechanisms they describe will probably also apply to other minority ethnic groups.

What complex trauma, poly-victimisation, betrayal trauma, and racism all have in common is that they are likely to severely compromise the child's sense of safety. In the case of complex trauma or betrayal trauma, a carer, who ought to be the source of safety and protection, becomes the source of danger. In the case of poly-victimisation and racism, the threat is unpredictable but pervasive. As Maslow (1987) has pointed out, after physiological needs, the need for safety is the most basic of human needs, without which, higher level needs for connection and esteem cannot be consistently met. A chronic and pervasive lack of safety in childhood may therefore be a common feature to many who go on to criminal lifestyles because of the disruptive impact that this lack of safety has on the child's ability to meet other key needs.

Adolescent Maltreatment

There is some evidence that maltreatment that begins or extends into adolescence is particularly associated with adolescent antisocial behaviour (Ireland, Smith, & Thornberry, 2002; Stewart, Livingston, & Dennison, 2008), though not all studies have found this (Mersky, Topitzes, & Reynolds, 2012). Kerig and Becker (2015) suggest several reasons why this might be the case, including: that children are resilient and the impact of maltreatment can be mitigated once the maltreatment is stopped; that the additional changes and stresses of adolescence make older children less resilient to the impact of maltreatment; and that child protection services may be less or effective for older children, particularly if they present with antisocial behaviours that prevent them from being seen as survivors of maltreatment. Support for this final hypothesis was found by Ryan, Herz, Hernandez, and Marshall (2007) who found that young people who entered the juvenile justice system from the child welfare system were sentenced more harshly than their peers. Herz, Ryan, and Bilchik (2010) found that this was particularly true for African American young people.

What Are the Mechanisms That Link Childhood Adversity to Offending?

While we do not know enough about the complex relationships between childhood adversity and offending, several possible mechanisms suggest themselves.

Neuropsychological Impact

Chronic exposure to threat and trauma can have a profound neuropsychological impact. The prefrontal cortex is the site of many higher cognitive functions including executive control over behaviour, emotions and attention, goal-directed behaviour, abstract reasoning, and social connection. Exposure to severe stress markedly impairs the functions of the prefrontal cortex (Arnsten, Raskind, Taylor, & Connor, 2015), and this is consistent with polyvagal theory (Porges, 2011), which proposes that when the sympathetic (flight/flight) or dorsal vagal (freeze) threat response systems are activated the frontal cortex goes "offline" so that physical and mental resources can be dedicated to the immediate goal of ensuring survival. Chronic stress can lead to loss of dendritic connections in the prefrontal cortex and a corresponding increase in connection within the amygdala (Arnsten et al., 2015). This means that a person exposed to chronic and pervasive trauma may end up living with their prefrontal cortex "offline" for long periods. Because of the prefrontal cortex's role in executive cognitive functions, this would make it difficult for them to manage their behaviour or emotions, or to plan, learn, or make complex decisions. As the prefrontal cortex is also involved in social engagement, impairment in its function will also have a negative impact on the person's ability to engage effectively with others.

Disrupted Attachment

Where a carer or attachment figure is a chronic source of threat, this can lead to severely disrupted attachment. The central importance of attachment to the development of the child's interpersonal relationships, self-regulatory and mentalisation abilities, and self-concept means that when the attachment figure is the source of maltreatment, all these systems can be impaired (Cook et al., 2005; Huang et al., 2020).

Cognitive and Attitudinal Impact

Childhood abuse by carers is also likely to result in the development of negative perceptions of self, other, and relationships in general. Patterson (1993) described a "cascade of impairment" through which significant others become frustrated by a child's dysregulated and aggressive behaviour, leading to a cycle in which the child's sense of rejection or defectiveness increases and their behaviour becomes more dysregulated and aggressive. Ford, Chapman, Mack, and Pearson (2006) argued that when a child loses their self-respect and sense of control, especially if it is done deliberately by a trusted person, the child is likely to resort to "survival coping", i.e., presenting a tough façade of defiance and callousness to hide their shame and vulnerability.

Social Learning of Abusive Behaviour

Children who are frequently exposed to abusive behaviour by carers learn that such behaviour can be effective and learn to victimise others (Reckdenwald, Mancini, & Beauregard, 2013), while Olweus (1993) proposed a similar mechanism underlying bullying in schools.

PTSD Symptoms

Childhood maltreatment is related to increased risk of mental health problems, with physical abuse and neglect associated with increased risk for depression and sexual abuse associated with PTSD, low self-esteem, and anxiety (Turner, Finkelhor, & Ormrod, 2006). Rates of PTSD are significantly higher among justice-involved young people than their peers (Wood et al., 2002). PTSD symptoms are correlated with both the frequency and severity of delinquent behaviour among young people (Becker & Kerig, 2011) and are understood to disrupt emotional processing (Rauch & Foa, 2006) and executive function (Olff, Polak, Witteveen, & Denys, 2014). PTSD symptoms such as irritability, impulsiveness, emotional numbing, and hypersensitivity to threat may also increase the risk of antisocial behaviour (Becker & Kerig, 2011; Kerig & Becker, 2012).

Trauma and Criminogenic Needs

A dominant paradigm within forensic psychology over the last 20 years, and one that has had most impact on forensic interventions, has been the Risk Need Responsivity model (RNR: Bonta & Andrews, 2016). An important element of this paradigm is the so-called "need principle", which is based on research that shows that the greatest reductions in re-offending are associated with providing treatment that targets dynamic risk factors. The RNR model identifies the *central eight* criminogenic needs: a history of antisocial behaviour, pro-criminal attitudes, pro-criminal associates, antisocial personality traits, family/marital relationship problems, substance abuse, school/work, and leisure/recreation problems, though Bonta and Andrews make almost no mention of childhood adversity or maltreatment as a precursor to these risk factors. However, there is evidence that links maltreatment to each of these factors through a combination of the above mediating factors.

Problematic Relationships

Childhood abuse has a devastating effect on the victim's sense of self and others, and their understanding of relationships (Herman, 1992). Children maltreated by their carers must rely for comfort and support on someone who is also a source of unpredictable fright. Not surprisingly, such children are at significantly increased risk of developing disorganised attachment styles (Cyr, Euser, Bakermans-Kranenburg, & van IJzendoorn, 2010) that may impair their ability to form stable attachments in late life.

Repeated experiences of maltreatment or rejection in childhood are likely to lead to a sense of self as unloved, inadequate, and incompetent (Hart, Binggeli, & Brassard, 1997). Children who perceive themselves in this way and who expect others to despise and reject them are more likely to blame themselves for negative experiences and have problems eliciting and responding to social support.

Maltreated children are rated as less prosocial and socially competent by their teachers (Kim & Cicchetti, 2003) and are significantly less popular and more likely to be rejected by their peers (Trickett, Negriff, Ji, & Peckins, 2011). In adulthood, survivors of betrayal trauma experience more problems in intimate relationships than others (Owen, Quirk, & Manthos, 2012).

Men and women who have experienced betrayal trauma report being less trusting in general and in intimate relationships (Gobin & Freyd, 2014), and for men, a sense of mistrust mediated the relationship between trauma exposure and the use of intimate partner aggression (LaMotte, Taft, & Weatherill, 2016).

Poor School and Employment Performance

Living in an abusive or neglectful home is associated with a wide range of poor outcomes at school, including academic performance, behaviour and attendance, and aspirations (Kurtz, Gaudin, Wodarski, & Howing, 1993). Self-regulation, which is correlated with secure attachment (Pallini, Chirumbolo, Morelli, Baiocco, Laghi, & Eisenberg, 2018), is strongly associated with both academic performance and positive classroom behaviour (McClelland & Cameron, 2011). It is perhaps not surprising that children, who spend significant periods of time with their polyvagal threat response systems activated and their frontal cortices offline, will find it difficult to reason, plan, or engage in abstract reasoning, all skills that are essential if they are to benefit from education.

Pereira, Li, and Power (2017) found that exposure to childhood abuse or neglect was associated with a range of employment-related outcomes at age 50, including poor qualifications, increased risk of long-term sickness, unemployment, and financial insecurity. Outcomes were primarily mediated by poor educational ability and, to a lesser extent, mental health problems.

Antisocial Attitudes

Bonta and Andrews suggest three groups of antisocial attitudes: *neutralisations* that minimise feelings of guilt or shame by denial or blaming, *identification with criminal others,* and *rejection of convention.*

- **Neutralisations.** Bonta and Andrews draw parallels between neutralisation and the concept of moral disengagement, which Bandura (2002) defined as "cognitive restructuring of inhumane conduct into a benign or worthy one" (p.101). Hyde, Shaw, and Moilanen (2010) found that early parental rejection was associated with reduced empathy in young boys, and significantly predicted adolescent moral disengagement. Wang et al. (2017) found that moral disengagement partially mediated the relationship between childhood maltreatment and adolescent bullying behaviour.
- **Identification with Criminal Others.** Many criminal gangs regard themselves as families (Ruble & Turner, 2000), and DeVito's (2020) study of US gang members found that they frequently reported a lack of consistent secure attachment figures during childhood, as a result of parental death, divorce, parental substance abuse or absence. Gangs provided a surrogate family that provided connection, validation, respect, and safety. Perhaps because they are more likely to experience physical

or sexual abuse within the home, female gang members are more likely to regard gangs as a source of safety (Sutton, 2017).

- **Rejection of Convention.** Bonta and Andrews define rejection of convention as "devalu[ing] the social institutions of work and education, and the institutions of law and order" (p.141). It is perhaps not surprising that people who have struggled to engage successfully with education or employment would be devaluing of these institutions. Mistrust of institutions is linked to devaluing them and people who have experienced betrayal trauma report higher levels of general mistrust of others as well as higher levels of relationship-specific mistrust (Gobin & Freyd, 2014). Unnever and Gabbidon (2011) argue that historical and lived experiences of negative stereotypes, discrimination and racial injustice, in which the police, courts, prisons, state and federal governments have been complicit have led many African Americans to see these agencies as oppressive and lacking legitimacy.

There is further evidence of links between trauma exposure and attitudes towards violence:

- **Violence-Supportive Attitudes.** Baron and Forde (2020) found a direct association between experiences of childhood abuse or neglect and criminogenic schemas that included a hostile view of relationships, a focus on immediate rewards, and a cynical orientation towards conventional norms and rules. These schemas mediated the relationships between childhood maltreatment and violent behaviour and between childhood maltreatment and association with criminal peers. Baron and Forde suggested that experiences of maltreatment promote a hostile and mistrustful view of relationships that undermines empathy for others, that children exposed to manipulation, exploitation, and neglect learn that future rewards promised by delaying gratification are unlikely, and that children exposed to models and rules that promote contempt towards conformist morals are likely to develop a cynical view of conventional norms. Unnever (2014) found that African Americans who "bought into" racist stereotypes were more likely to offend.
- **Violent Fantasies.** Maniglio (2010) suggested that some survivors of childhood maltreatment may develop feelings of helplessness, inferiority, and lack of control with which they cope by withdrawing from the real world and taking refuge in a fantasy world in which they are strong and powerful. Maniglio's review of studies into sexual homicides found that childhood maltreatment, social difficulties, a sense of inadequacy, and sadistic sexual fantasies were common features among sexual murderers. Support for this model came from Daversa and Knight (2007) who found that the relationship between childhood abuse and the use of sexual fantasy for coping by adolescents convicted of sexual offences was mediated by feelings of sexual inadequacy.
- **Violent Scripts.** While much of the research on fantasy and offending has focused on sexual fantasies and their links to sexual offending, it seems likely that similar processes may link violent fantasies and violent offending. There is, however, evidence that exposure to violence during childhood shapes violence scripts, that is, assumptions and expectations about violence. Wilkinson and Carr (2008)

explored the experiences of minority ethnic young men from New York who had recent experience as perpetrators or victims of violent crime. Virtually all participants had experienced exposure to community violence. A common script was the need to respond to insults or disrespect with aggression in order to save face. Wilkinson and Carr also reported that frequent exposure to violence also led to desensitisation and to moral disengagement.

Antisocial Personality Traits

Bonta and Andrews (2016) define antisocial personality traits in terms of the DSM-5 criteria for antisocial personality disorder (American Psychiatric Association, 2013), which include deceitfulness, impulsiveness, irresponsibility, and lack of remorse, all of which can be linked to childhood maltreatment.

- **Deceitfulness and Manipulativeness.** Manipulation is a frequent element of childhood abuse, for example in being groomed into sexual abuse or in being controlled during and after abuse to ensure the child's compliance and silence. It is likely therefore that survivors of grooming and manipulation will learn to use these techniques on others, particularly if they are young or physically vulnerable, making direct confrontation or physical resistance dangerous. Since maltreated children often lack the social competencies to negotiate and persuade others at school (Kim & Cicchetti, 2003), they are thought to be more likely to resort to threats or manipulation.
- **Impulsiveness.** Secure attachment to caregivers in childhood is an important factor in the development of emotional and behavioural self-regulation and inter-personal competence (Bowlby, 1973; Sroufe, 2005), and childhood maltreatment is linked to emotional dysregulation and impulsive behaviour in adulthood (Oshri, Sutton, Clay-Warner, & Miller, 2015). Children's ability to regulate themselves is understood to be shaped by repeated experiences of caregivers' sensitive regulation of their distress, which fosters a sense of security, and this ability is impaired by early experiences of abuse or neglect by caregivers. Children and young people who are unable to regulate the intensity of emotions and impulses may engage in a range of behaviours that can be understood as attempts to self-regulate, including aggression towards the self and others and substance misuse.
- **Irresponsibility.** The development of responsibility overlaps with constructs such as moral development, empathy, and prosocial values and develops in childhood through interactions with family, peers, schools, and communities (Wray-Lake & Syvertsen, 2011). Children growing up with caregivers who model irresponsible behaviour or values through their neglect or abuse, or who fail to form prosocial peer groups or engage with school, or who grow up in high crime communities with little sense of cohesion are less likely to develop responsible attitudes or behaviours.
- **Lack of Remorse.** Maltreated children may learn to cope with distressing emotions through emotional numbing, which can develop into emotional detachment and callousness. Freyd (1996) argued that this is particularly likely in survivors

of betrayal trauma. Kerig, Bennett, Thompson, and Becker (2012) found that the association between trauma exposure and callous-unemotional traits was mediated by emotional numbing.

Criminal Associates

Because of their difficulties in regulating their emotions (Schwartz & Proctor, 2000), maltreated children are more likely to be excluded from conventional peer groups due to their aggressive behaviour (Dishion, Patterson, Stoolmiller, & Skinner, 1991). Because of their disengagement from school, they are therefore more likely to become isolated or to associate with antisocial peers (De Vito, 2020; Sutton, 2017).

Substance Abuse

Substance abuse can function as a coping mechanism that enables abuse survivors to alleviate distress or trauma symptoms (Sturza & Campbell, 2005), but it can also exacerbate other criminogenic needs, including relationship problems (Fairbairn et al., 2018). Adolescents who have experienced childhood maltreatment, particularly poly-victimisation and sexual abuse, are at increased risk of substance abuse (Bergen, Martin, Richardson, Allison, & Roeger, 2004; Ford, Elhai, Connor, & Frueh, 2010; Hamburger, Leeb, & Swahn, 2008). Attachment relationships and substance use both function to regulate emotions and both share similar neurobiological mechanisms (Burkett & Young, 2012). Abuse survivors with an avoidant attachment style appear particularly likely to use substances to cope (Hayre, Goulter, & Moretti, 2019). Hayre et al. suggested that young people with an avoidant attachment style may be less likely to disclose their activities or seek support from their parents, and more likely to rely for support on peers who also engage substance misuse.

Leisure/Recreation

The relationship between childhood adversity and lack of prosocial leisure and recreation activities may be similar to the link with education and employment. Young people who struggle with self-control and who live in "survival mode" with their frontal cortex offline may well struggle to engage in structured recreational activities.

Osgood, Wilson, O'Malley, Bachman, and Johnston (1996) found that young people who engaged in unstructured socialising with peers were more likely than others to engage in antisocial behaviour, drug and alcohol use, and risk-taking behaviours such as dangerous driving. Osgood et al. found support for their hypothesis that three features of unstructured socialising combined to increase risk of delinquency: exposure to antisocial peers, lack of adult supervision, and the greater opportunity to engage in antisocial behaviour provided by the lack of structure. While there is no evidence on the links between childhood adversity and use of leisure time, it could be hypothesised that all three features would be more common in survivors of childhood adversity. Young people from abusive or neglecting families

24

may be more motivated to avoid contact with or supervision by their parents. As well as increasing their likelihood of associating with antisocial peer, their poorer interpersonal skills, mistrust of others, and unpopularity with prosocial peers may mean they are less likely to become involved in structured activities such as sport.

Criminal History

The principle that "past behaviour is the best predictor of future behaviour" is applied widely in psychology, rather than specifically to the field of trauma. However, there are still some reasons why trauma survivors may be more likely to have a criminal record.

Running away from home is both a consequence of maltreatment, a risk factor for further abuse, and a risk factor for delinquency, with homeless young people more likely to engage in crime to support or protect themselves (McCarthy & Hagan, 1991). Studies of women's pathways into offending have highlighted that many women first come into contact with the criminal justice system because of behaviours they engage in to escape or cope with abuse, such as drug use, sex work, and shoplifting while homeless (Brennan, Breitenbach, Dieterich, Salisbury, & Van Voorhis, 2012; Chesney-Lind, 1989), though McCarthy and Hagan reported a similar pattern for some young homeless men.

As a consequence of institutional racism, people of colour are more likely to have a criminal record. In the US, people of colour are arrested at higher rates, charged more severely, are more likely to be convicted and more likely to be imprisoned than their white counterparts, even for crimes that both groups engage in at comparable rates (Barabas, Dinakar, & Doyle, 2019), while similar findings have been found in the UK (Uhrig, 2016).

Protective Factors

Even among young people who have been exposed to severe trauma, offending is not inevitable. For example, Turner, Shattuck, Finkelhor, and Hamby (2016) reported that 68% of young people who identified as poly-victims reported having not engaged in property-related delinquency, and 52% reported having not engaged in violent delinquency. A number of protective factors have been identified that appear to mitigate the impact of trauma.

Individual Protective Factors

Consistent with criminological literature that shows a strong relationship between low self-control and antisocial behaviour (Pratt & Cullen, 2000), high levels of self-control among survivors of childhood maltreatment has been found to protect against future offending (Wright, Turanovic, O'Neal, Morse, & Booth, 2019). Wright et al. also found low depression to be protective. Among African Americans, having a positive sense of racial identity moderates the criminogenic impact of racism (Isom, 2016).

Social Protective Factors

Academic and occupational achievement, reflected by attending and graduating from college and having a sense of job satisfaction, have all been identified as protecting survivors of childhood maltreatment from future violence as protective (Widom, 2017; Wright et al., 2019). Where relationships with primary carers are abusive, there is evidence that caring and supportive relationships with others can be protective. For example, a close relationship with siblings or involvement in team sports have both been found to reduce the risk that physically abused boys would later become involved in violent crime (Kruttschnitt, Ward, & Sheble, 1987).

Summary: The Long-Term Impact of Childhood Maltreatment

The links between maltreatment and offending involve multiple pathways, but a common feature appears to be a chronic and pervasive lack of safety. This lack of safety impacts on the young person's autonomic threat responses, their attachment to carers, and their developing schemas about themselves, others, and the world. Young people are also resilient and resourceful and most find alternative ways to achieve a sense of safety, one of which may be to engage in crime and antisocial behaviour.

While we cannot say that developmental trauma is a precursor to offending in every case, certain types of trauma do appear to increase the risk of offending, and particularly of serious offending (Duke, Pettingell, McMorris, & Borowsky, 2010; Fox, Perez, Cass, Baglivio, & Epps, 2015). There appear to be multiple mechanisms underlying this link (neuropsychological, attachment, cognitive, social learning), which is mediated by the central eight criminogenic needs.

Further Reading

Herman, J. (2015). *Trauma and recovery: The aftermath of violence from domestic abuse to political terror.* Basic Books. For readers wanting an introduction to the trauma literature, Herman's book, originally published in 1992, was an important landmark in the field and is still relevant.

Unnever, J.D. & Gabbidon, S.L. (2011). *A theory of African American offending: Race, racism and crime.* Routledge. A comprehensive but accessible account of how the lived experiences of African American men relates to their overrepresentation in the criminal justice system. Although specific to African Americans, much of it will apply to other groups and countries.

References

American Psychiatric Association. (2013). *Diagnostic and statistical manual of mental disorders (DSM-5®).* Washington DC: American Psychiatric Association.

Arnsten, A. F., Raskind, M. A., Taylor, F. B., & Connor, D. F. (2015). The effects of stress exposure on prefrontal cortex: Translating basic research into successful treatments for post-traumatic stress disorder. *Neurobiology of Stress, 1,* 89–99. doi:10.1016/j.ynstr.2014.10.002

Bandura, A. (2002). Selective moral disengagement in the exercise of moral agency. *Journal of Moral Education, 31*(2), 101–119. doi:10.1080/0305724022014322

Barabas, C., Dinakar, K., & Doyle, C. (2019). Technical flaws of pretrial risk assessments raise grave concerns. Retrieved from https://dam-prod.media.mit.edu/x/2019/07/16/TechnicalFlawsOfPretrial_ML%20site.pdf

Baron, S. W., & Forde, D. R. (2020). Childhood trauma, criminogenic social schemas, and violent crime. *Deviant Behavior, 41*(8), 991–1004. doi:10.1080/01639625.2019.1596534

Becker, S. P., & Kerig, P. K. (2011). Posttraumatic stress symptoms are associated with the frequency and severity of delinquency among detained boys. *Journal of Clinical Child & Adolescent Psychology, 40*(5), 765–771. doi:10.1080/15374416.2011.597091

Bergen, H. A., Martin, G., Richardson, A. S., Allison, S., & Roeger, L. (2004). Sexual abuse, antisocial behaviour and substance use: Gender differences in young community adolescents. *Australian and New Zealand Journal of Psychiatry, 38*(1–2), 34–41. doi:10.1111/j.1440-1614.2004.01295.x

Bonta, J. & Andrews, D. A. (2016). *The psychology of criminal conduct.* Routledge. doi:10.4324/9781315677187

Bowlby, J. (1973). *Attachment and loss. Vol. 2: Separation: Anxiety and anger.* Basic Books.

Brennan, T., Breitenbach, M., Dieterich, W., Salisbury, E., & Van Voorhis, P. (2012). Women's pathways to serious and habitual crime: A person-centered analysis incorporating gender-responsive factors. *Criminal Justice and Behavior, 39,* 1481–1508. doi:10.1177/0093854812456777

Brown, S. L., Wanamaker, K. A., Greiner, L., Scott, T., & Skilling, T. A. (2021). Complex trauma and criminogenic needs in a youth justice sample: A gender-informed latent profile analysis. *Criminal Justice and Behavior, 48,* 175–194. doi:10.1177/0093854820964513

Burkett, J. P., & Young, L. J. (2012). The behavioral, anatomical and pharmacological parallels between social attachment, love and addiction. *Psychopharmacology, 224*(1), 1–26. doi:10.1007/s00213-012-2794-x

Chesney-Lind, M. (1989). Girls' crime and women's place: Toward a feminist model of female delinquency. *Crime & Delinquency, 35*(1), 5–29. doi:10.1177/0011128789035001002

Cook, A., Spinazzola, P., Ford, J., Lanktree, C., Blaustein, M., Cloitre, M., … van der Kolk, B. (2005). Complex trauma in children and adolescents. *Psychiatric Annals, 35,* 390–398. doi:10.3928/00485713-20050501-05

Cunneen, C., & Tauri, J. M. (2019). Indigenous peoples, criminology, and criminal justice. *Annual Review of Criminology, 2,* 359–381. doi:10.1146/annurev-criminol-011518-024630

Cyr, C., Euser, E. M., Bakermans-Kranenburg, M. J., & van IJzendoorn, M. H. (2010). Attachment security and disorganization in maltreating and high-risk families: A series of meta-analyses. *Development and Psychopathology, 22*(1), 87–108. doi:10.1017/S0954579409990289

Daversa, M. T., & Knight, R. A. (2007). A structural examination of the predictors of sexual coercion against children in adolescent sexual offenders. *Criminal Justice and Behavior, 34,* 1313–1333. doi:10.1177/0093854807302411

De Vito, K. (2020). Seeking a secure base: Gangs as attachment figures. *Qualitative Social Work, 19*(4), 754–769. doi:10.1177/1473325019852659

Dishion, T. J., Patterson, G. R., Stoolmiller, M., & Skinner, M. L. (1991). Family, school, and behavioral antecedents to early adolescent involvement with antisocial peers. *Developmental Psychology, 27*(1), 172–180. doi:10.1037/0012-1649.27.1.172

Duke, N. N., Pettingell, S. L., McMorris, B. J., & Borowsky, I. W. (2010). Adolescent violence perpetration: Associations with multiple types of adverse childhood experiences. *Pediatrics, 125*(4), e778–e786. doi:10.1542/peds.2009-0597

Estes, L. S., & Tidwell, R. (2002). Sexually abused children's behaviours: Impact of gender and mother's experience of intra-and extra-familial sexual abuse. *Family practice, 19*(1), 36–44. doi:10.1093/fampra/19.1.36

Fairbairn, C. E., Briley, D. A., Kang, D., Fraley, R. C., Hankin, B. L., & Ariss, T. (2018). A meta-analysis of longitudinal associations between substance use and interpersonal attachment security. *Psychological Bulletin, 144*(5), 532–555. doi:10.1037/bul0000141

Finkelhor, D., Ormrod, R. K., & Turner, H. A. (2007). Poly-victimization: A neglected component in child victimization. *Child Abuse & Neglect, 31*(1), 7–26. doi:10.1016/j.chiabu.2006.06.008

Fitton, L., Yu, R., & Fazel, S. (2020). Childhood maltreatment and violent outcomes: A systematic review and meta-analysis of prospective studies. *Trauma, Violence, & Abuse, 21*(4), 754–768. doi:10.1177/1524838018795269

Ford, J. D., Chapman, J., Connor, D. J., & Cruise, K. R. (2012). Complex trauma and aggression in secure juvenile justice settings. *Criminal Justice & Behavior, 39*, 694–724. doi:10.1177/0093854812436957

Ford, J. D., Chapman, J., Mack, J. M., & Pearson, G. (2006). Pathways from traumatic child victimization to delinquency: Implications for juvenile and permanency court proceedings and decisions. *Juvenile and Family Court Journal, 57*(1), 13–26. doi:10.1111/j.1755-6988.2006.tb00111.x

Ford, J. D., Charak, R., Modrowski, C. A., & Kerig, P. K. (2018). PTSD and dissociation symptoms as mediators of the relationship between polyvictimization and psychosocial and behavioral problems among justice-involved adolescents. *Journal of Trauma & Dissociation, 19*(3), 325–346. doi:10.1016/j.chiabu.2013.01.005

Ford, J. D., Elhai, J. D., Connor, D. F., & Frueh, B. C. (2010). Poly-victimization and risk of posttraumatic, depressive, and substance use disorders and involvement in delinquency in a national sample of adolescents. *Journal of Adolescent Health, 46*(6), 545–552. doi:10.1016/j.jadohealth.2009.11.212

Ford, J. D., Grasso, D. J., Hawke, J., & Chapman, J. F. (2013). Poly-victimization among juvenile justice-involved youths. *Child Abuse & Neglect, 37*(10), 788–800. doi:10.1016/j.chiabu.2013.01.005

Fox, B. H., Perez, N., Cass, E., Baglivio, M. T., & Epps, N. (2015). Trauma changes everything: Examining the relationship between adverse childhood experiences and serious, violent and chronic juvenile offenders. *Child Abuse & Neglect, 46*, 163–173. doi:10.1016/j.chiabu.2015.01.011

Freyd, J. J. (1996). *Betrayal trauma: The logic of forgetting childhood abuse.* Harvard University Press.

Gobin, R. L., & Freyd, J. J. (2009). Betrayal and revictimization: Preliminary findings. *Psychological Trauma: Theory, Research, Practice, and Policy, 1*, 242–257. doi:10.1037/a0017469

Gobin, R. L., & Freyd, J. J. (2014). The impact of betrayal trauma on the tendency to trust. *Psychological Trauma: Theory, Research, Practice, and Policy, 6*(5), 505–511. doi:10.1037/a0032452

Gottfredson, M. R., & Hirschi, T. (1990). *A General Theory of Crime.* Stanford University Press.

Hamburger, M. E., Leeb, R. T., & Swahn, M. H. (2008). Childhood maltreatment and early alcohol use among high-risk adolescents. *Journal of Studies on Alcohol and Drugs, 69*(2), 291–295. doi:10.15288/jsad.2008.69.291

Hare, R. D. (1993). *Without conscience: The disturbing world of the psychopaths among us.* Guilford Press.

Hart, S. N., Binggeli, N. J., & Brassard, M. R. (1997). Evidence for the effects of psychological maltreatment. *Journal of Emotional Abuse, 1*(1), 27–58. doi:10.1300/J135v01n01_03

Hayre, R. S., Goulter, N., & Moretti, M. M. (2019). Maltreatment, attachment, and substance use in adolescence: Direct and indirect pathways. *Addictive Behaviors, 90*, 196–203. doi:10.1016/j.addbeh.2018.10.049

Herman, J. (1992). *Trauma and recovery: The aftermath of violence from domestic abuse to political terror.* Basic Books.

Herz, D. C., Ryan, J. P., & Bilchik, S. (2010). Challenges facing crossover youth: An examination of juvenile-justice decision making and recidivism. *Family Court Review, 48*(2), 305–321. doi:10.1111/j.1744-1617.2010.01312.x

Hillis, S., Mercy, J., Amobi, A., & Kress, H. (2016). Global prevalence of past-year violence against children: A systematic review and minimum estimates. *Pediatrics, 137*(3), e20154079. doi:10.1542/peds.2015-4079

Huang, Y. L., Fonagy, P., Feigenbaum, J., Montague, P. R., Nolte, T., & Mood Disorder Research Consortium. (2020). Multidirectional pathways between attachment, mentalizing, and posttraumatic stress symptomatology in the context of childhood trauma. *Psychopathology, 53*(1), 48–58. doi:10.1159/000506406

Hyde, L. W., Shaw, D. S., & Moilanen, K. L. (2010). Developmental precursors of moral disengagement and the role of moral disengagement in the development of antisocial behavior. *Journal of Abnormal Child Psychology, 38*(2), 197–209. doi:10.1007/s10802-009-9358-5

Ireland, T. O., Smith, C. A., & Thornberry, T. P. (2002). Developmental issues in the impact of child maltreatment on later delinquency and drug use. *Criminology, 40*(2), 359–400. Doi:10.1111/j.1745-9125.2002.tb00960.x

Isom, D. (2016). Microaggressions, injustices, and racial identity: An empirical assessment of the theory of African American offending. *Journal of Contemporary Criminal Justice, 32*(1), 27–59. doi:10.1177/1043986215607253

Kerig, P. K., & Becker, S. P. (2012). Trauma and girls' delinquency. In S. Miller, L. Leve & P. Kerig (Eds), *Delinquent girls: Contexts, relationships, and adaptation* (pp.119–143). Springer. doi:10.1007/978-1-4614-0415-6_8

Kerig, P. K., & Becker, S. P. (2015). Early abuse and neglect as risk factors for the development of criminal and antisocial behavior. In J. Morizot & L. Kazemian (Eds), *The development of criminal and antisocial behavior* (pp.181–199). Springer. doi:10.1007/978-3-319-08720-7

Kerig, P. K., Bennett, D. C., Thompson, M., & Becker, S. P. (2012). "Nothing really matters": Emotional numbing as a link between trauma exposure and callousness in delinquent youth. *Journal of Traumatic Stress, 25*(3), 272–279. doi:10.1002/jts.21700

Kim, J., & Cicchetti, D. (2003). Social self-efficacy and behavior problems in maltreated and nonmaltreated children. *Journal of Clinical Child and Adolescent Psychology, 32*(1), 106–117. doi:10.1207/S15374424JCCP3201_10

Kirkinis, K., Pieterse, A. L., Martin, C., Agiliga, A., & Brownell, A. (2018). Racism, racial discrimination, and trauma: A systematic review of the social science literature. *Ethnicity & Health*, 1–21. doi:10.1080/13557858.2018.1514453

Kohlberg, L. & Hersh, R. (1977). Moral development: A review of the theory. *Theory into Practice, 16* (2), 53–59. doi:10.1080/00405847709542675

Kruttschnitt, C., Ward, D., & Sheble, M. A. (1987). Abuse resistant youth: Some factors that may inhibit violent criminal behavior. *Social Forces, 66*, 501–519. doi:10.2307/2578752

Kurtz, P. D., Gaudin Jr, J. M., Wodarski, J. S., & Howing, P. T. (1993). Maltreatment and the school-aged child: School performance consequences. *Child Abuse & Neglect, 17*(5), 581–589. doi:10.1016/0145-2134(93)90080-O

LaMotte, A. D., Taft, C. T., & Weatherill, R. P. (2016). Mistrust of others as a mediator of the relationship between trauma exposure and use of partner aggression. *Psychological Trauma: Theory, Research, Practice, and Policy, 8*(4), 535–540. doi:10.1037/tra0000157

Maniglio, R. (2010). The role of deviant sexual fantasy in the etiopathogenesis of sexual homicide: A systematic review. *Aggression and Violent Behavior, 15*, 294–302. doi:10.1016/j.avb.2010.02.001

Maslow, A. H. (1987). *Motivation and personality* (3rd Ed.). Harper & Row.

McCarthy, B., & Hagan, J. (1991). Homelessness: A criminogenic situation? *The British Journal of Criminology, 31*(4), 393–410. doi:10.1093/oxfordjournals.bjc.a048137

McClelland, M. M., & Cameron, C. E. (2011). Self-regulation and academic achievement in elementary school children. *New Directions for Child and Adolescent Development, 133*, 29–44. doi:10.1002/cd.302

Mersky, J. P., Topitzes, J., & Reynolds, A. J. (2012). Unsafe at any age: Linking childhood and adolescent maltreatment to delinquency and crime. *Journal of Research in Crime and Delinquency, 49*(2), 295–318. doi:10.1177/0022427811415284

Olff, M., Polak, A. R., Witteveen, A. B., & Denys, D. (2014). Executive function in posttraumatic stress disorder (PTSD) and the influence of comorbid depression. *Neurobiology of Learning and Memory, 112*, 114–121. doi:10.1016/j.nlm.2014.01.003

Olweus, D. (1993). *Bullying at school: What we know and what we can do.* Blackwell Publishers.

Osgood, D. W., Wilson, J. K., O'Malley, P. M., Bachman, J. G., & Johnston, L. D. (1996). Routine activities and individual deviant behavior. *American Sociological Review, 61*(4), 635–655. doi:10.2307/2096397

Oshri, A., Sutton, T. E., Clay-Warner, J., & Miller, J. D. (2015). Child maltreatment types and risk behaviors: Associations with attachment style and emotion regulation dimensions. *Personality and Individual Differences, 73*, 127–133.

Owen, J., Quirk, K., & Manthos, M. (2012). I get no respect: The relationship between betrayal trauma and romantic relationship functioning. *Journal of Trauma & Dissociation, 13*(2), 175–189. doi:10.1080/15299732.2018.1440479

Pallini, S., Chirumbolo, A., Morelli, M., Baiocco, R., Laghi, F., & Eisenberg, N. (2018). The relation of attachment security status to effortful self-regulation: A meta-analysis. *Psychological Bulletin, 144*(5), 501–531. doi:10.1037/bul0000134

Patterson, G. R. (1993). Orderly change in a stable world: The antisocial trait as a chimera. *Journal of Consulting and Clinical Psychology, 61*(6), 911–919. doi:/10.1037/0022-006X.61.6.911

Pereira, S. M. P., Li, L., & Power, C. (2017). Child maltreatment and adult living standards at 50 years. *Pediatrics, 139*(1), e20161595. doi: 10.1542/peds.2016-1595

Porges, S. W. (2011). *The polyvagal theory: Neurophysiological foundations of emotions, attachment, communication, and self-regulation.* W. W. Norton & Company.

Pratt, T. C., & Cullen, F. T. (2000). The empirical status of Gottfredson and Hirschi's general theory of crime: A meta-analysis. *Criminology, 38*, 931–964. doi:10.1111/j.1745-9125.2000.tb00911.x

Rauch, S., & Foa, E. (2006). Emotional processing theory (EPT) and exposure therapy for PTSD. *Journal of Contemporary Psychotherapy, 36*(2), 61–65. doi:10.1007/s10879-006-9008-y

Reckdenwald, A., Mancini, C., & Beauregard, E. (2013). The cycle of violence: Examining the impact of maltreatment early in life on adult offending. *Violence and Victims, 28*(3), 466–482. doi:10.1891/0886-6708.VV-D-12-00054

Ruble, N. M., & Turner, W. L. (2000). A systemic analysis of the dynamics and organization of urban street gangs. *The American Journal of Family Therapy, 28*(2), 117–132. doi:10.1080/019261800261707

Ryan, J. P., Herz, D., Hernandez, P. M., & Marshall, J. M. (2007). Maltreatment and delinquency: Investigating child welfare bias in juvenile justice processing. *Children and Youth Services Review, 29*(8), 1035–1050. doi:10.1016/j.childyouth.2007.04.002

Schwartz, D., & Proctor, L. J. (2000). Community violence exposure and children's social adjustment in the school peer group: The mediating roles of emotion regulation and social cognition. *Journal of Consulting & Clinical Psychology, 68*(4), 670–684. doi:10.1037//0022-006X.68.4.670

Sroufe, L. A. (2005). Attachment and development: A prospective, longitudinal study from birth to adulthood. *Attachment & Human Development, 7*(4), 349–367. doi:10.1080/14616730500365928

Stewart, A., Livingston, M., & Dennison, S. (2008). Transitions and turning points: Examining the links between child maltreatment and juvenile offending. *Child Abuse and Neglect, 32*, 51–66. doi:10.1016/j.chiabu.2007.04.011

Sturza, M. L., & Campbell, R. (2005). An exploratory study of rape survivors' prescription drug use as a means of coping with sexual assault. *Psychology of Women Quarterly, 29*(4), 353–363. doi:10.1111/j.1471-6402.2005.00235.x

Sutton, T. E. (2017). The lives of female gang members: A review of the literature. *Aggression and Violent Behavior, 37*, 142–152. doi:10.1016/j.avb.2017.10.001

Thornberry, T. P., Ireland, T. O., & Smith, C. A. (2001). The importance of timing: The varying impact of childhood and adolescent maltreatment on multiple problem outcomes. *Development and Psychopathology, 13*(4), 957–979. doi:10.1017/S0954579401004114

Trent, M., Dooley, D. G., & Dougé, J. (2019). The impact of racism on child and adolescent health. *Pediatrics, 144*(2), e20191765. doi:10.1542/peds.2019-1765

Trickett, P. K., Negriff, S., Ji, J., & Peckins, M. (2011). Child maltreatment and adolescent development. *Journal of Research on Adolescence, 21*(1), 3–20. doi:10.1111/j.1532-7795.2010.00711.x

Turner, H. A., Finkelhor, D., & Ormrod, R. (2006). The effect of lifetime victimization on the mental health of children and adolescents. *Social Science & Medicine, 62*, 13–27. doi:10.1016/j.socscimed.2005.05.030

Turner, H. A., Shattuck, A., Finkelhor, D., & Hamby, S. (2016). Polyvictimization and youth violence exposure across contexts. *Journal of Adolescent Health, 58*(2), 208–214. doi:10.1016/j.jadohealth.2015.09.021

Uhrig, N. (2016). *Black, Asian and minority ethnic disproportionality in the criminal justice system in England and Wales.* London: Ministry of Justice.

Unnever, J. D. (2014). A theory of African American offending: A test of core propositions. *Race and Justice, 4*(2), 98–123. doi:10.1177/2153368714531296

Unnever, J.D. & Gabbidon, S.L. (2011). *A theory of African American offending: Race, racism and crime.* Routledge.

van der Kolk, B. A. (2005). Developmental trauma disorder: Toward a rational diagnosis for children with complex trauma histories. *Psychiatric Annals, 35*(5), 401–408. doi:10.3928/00485713-20050501-06

Wang, X., Yang, L., Gao, L., Yang, J., Lei, L., & Wang, C. (2017). Childhood maltreatment and Chinese adolescents' bullying and defending: The mediating role of moral disengagement. *Child Abuse & Neglect, 69*, 134–144. doi:10.1016/j.chiabu.2017.04.016

Webster, C. (2018). 'Race', ethnicity, social class and juvenile justice in Europe. In B. Goldson (Ed.), *Juvenile justice in Europe* (pp.148–161). Routledge. doi:10.4324/9781315194493

Widom, C. S. (1989). The cycle of violence. *Science, 244*(4901), 160–166. doi:10.1126/science.2704995

Widom, C. S. (2017). Long-term impact of childhood abuse and neglect on crime and violence. *Clinical Psychology: Science and Practice, 24*(2), 186–202. doi:10.1111/cpsp.12194

Wilkinson, D. L., & Carr, P. J. (2008). Violent youths' responses to high levels of exposure to community violence: What violent events reveal about youth violence. *Journal of Community Psychology, 36*(8), 1026–1051. doi:10.1002/jcop.20278

Wood, J., Foy, D. W., Layne, C., Pynoos, R., & James, C. B. (2002). An examination of the relationships between violence exposure, posttraumatic stress symptomatology, and delinquent activity: An "ecopathological" model of delinquent behavior among incarcerated adolescents. *Journal of Aggression, Maltreatment & Trauma, 6*(1), 127–147. doi:10.1300/J146v06n01_07

Wray-Lake, L., & Syvertsen, A. (2011). The developmental roots of social responsibility in childhood and adolescence. *New Directions for Child and Adolescent Development, 134*, 11–25. doi: 10.1002/cd

Wright, K. A., Turanovic, J. J., O'Neal, E. N., Morse, S. J., & Booth, E. T. (2019). The cycle of violence revisited: Childhood victimization, resilience, and future violence. *Journal of Interpersonal Violence, 34*(6), 1261–1286. doi:10.1177/0886260516651090

2

TRAUMA, VIOLENCE, AND GENDER

Phil Willmot and Yasmin Siddall

Introduction

Patterns of offending by men and women are different. Official recorded crime and self-reported delinquency by women are less serious, begin later in adolescence, and are less persistent than male criminality and delinquency (Cernkovich & Giordano, 1987; Lanctôt & LeBlanc, 2002). Above all, offending by men is much more common; in 2019, men accounted for 73% of all convictions, and 95% of the prison population in the UK (Ministry of Justice, 2020). However, many of the most widely used explanatory models of offending have little to say about these differences (Bonta & Andrews, 2016; Gottfredson & Hirschi, 1990; Kohlberg, 1976).

In this chapter we draw on the Power Threat Meaning Framework (Johnstone and Boyle et al., 2018) to examine the differences between men and women, or boys and girls, in how they experience maltreatment and adversity, what it means to them, and how they respond to it. Although the primary focus of this chapter is on gender differences, we acknowledge that it is also important to consider the intersectionality of other characteristics and identities such as race, socioeconomic status, sexual orientation, age, language, spirituality, religion, education, and physical/mental ability. These often overlap and operate together, creating different forms or types of discrimination and privilege.

Space does not allow for anything like a comprehensive analysis of the relationship between gender and offending, let alone of these intersectionalities. Instead, we aim to illustrate how the Power Threat Meaning Framework can help clinicians to incorporate the often overlooked issue of gender into their formulations.

The Power Threat Meaning Framework

The Power Threat Meaning Framework was developed primarily as an alternative to predominantly medical and biological models of mental health, though it can also be

DOI: 10.4324/9781003120766-4

applied to understanding the needs of people who offend or behave in other challenging ways. The assumptions underpinning the framework are:

- many mental health and behavioural problems can be understood as consequences of the negative operation of power;
- the threat and meaning posed by the negative operation of power leads to distress and prevents people from meeting their core emotional needs; and
- many psychiatric symptoms or behavioural problems can be understood as responses that the person has learned to protect themselves or to meet core emotional needs in other ways.

The framework's focus on the negative operation of power as a basis for understanding behaviour and its emphasis on the uniqueness of each individual's experiences and the meanings they ascribe to them, makes it a promising framework for starting to examine the link between adversity and offending, and how different patterns emerge in men and women.

Power: What Happens to People?

The framework describes power as operating in various forms including biological/embodied power, coercive power, economic power, social and cultural capital, and interpersonal power, most of which privilege white, male, heterosexual, wealthy, educated, and mentally healthy people (Boyle and Johnstone, 2020). Here we only have space to briefly consider the first two of these.

Embodied Power

The peak age for aggression in both boys and girls is around two, with girls being only slightly less aggressive (Tremblay et al., 1999). With the development of language and interpersonal skills, physical aggression becomes less frequent, though the reduction is faster among girls. Levels of verbal and indirect aggression in boys and girls remain similar into adolescence (Card, Stucky, Sawalani, & Little, 2008). Several factors have been suggested as inhibiting physically aggressive behaviour in women. Firstly, women across different cultures have been found to experience fear more intensely than men, both in general (Brebner, 2003) and specifically fear of retaliation (Eagly & Steffen, 1986), though these differences appear to reflect differential socialisation rather than biological differences. Secondly, level of empathy and guilt, both of which can inhibit aggressive behaviour, are generally higher among women than men (Baron-Cohen & Wheelwright, 2004), but are inhibited in women by the administration of testosterone (van Honk et al., 2011), suggesting a biological component.

Coercive Interpersonal Power

Overall, men are more likely than women to have experienced potentially traumatic events (though a focus on discrete events arguably excludes the impact of systemic misogyny and other forms of discrimination), and more likely to have experienced non-sexual assault, accidents, combat, fire or disasters, or serious illness, though women are twice as likely to experience PTSD (Tolin & Foa, 2006). Men, and those from ethnic minorities, are also more likely to have witnessed others being killed or injured (Cronholm et al., 2015; Tolin & Foa). Women are more likely to have experienced sexual assault, both in childhood and as an adult (Komarovskaya, Booker Loper, Warren, & Jackson, 2011; Tolin & Foa). Sexual abuse of young girls is more likely to be perpetrated by caregivers or family members (Wamser-Nanney & Cherry, 2018). Adolescent girls are more likely to be sexually abused by adult acquaintances or adolescent partners, whereas boys are more likely to be abused by juvenile family members, juvenile acquaintances, or juvenile strangers (Gewirtz-Meydan & Finkelhor, 2020). There is some evidence that sexual abuse of boys is more likely to occur before puberty, whereas girls are more likely to be abused after puberty (Chaplo et al., 2017; Gewirtz-Meydan & Finkelhor). Sexual abuse of girls tends to be more severe and chronic than sexual abuse of boys (Ullman & Filipas, 2005).

Studies of justice-involved individuals show higher rates of childhood abuse, particularly sexual abuse within the home among incarcerated women than men (Baglivio et al., 2014), while men were more likely to have experienced or witnessed violence outside the home (Wood et al., 2002). Among female prisoners, physical and sexual assault as adults are the most commonly reported traumatic experiences (Karatzias et al., 2018), while for male prisoners, the most common experiences are witnessing someone else being killed or seriously injured, being assaulted themselves, and childhood sexual abuse (Maschi, Gibson, Zgoba, & Morgen, 2011; Weeks & Widom, 1998).

Finally, the gender differences described in this section may need to be treated with an element of caution. Most of the studies described here involve self-report measures of trauma which are likely to be influenced to some degree by culturally determined biases about what constitutes abuse and about the forms of trauma that are "acceptable" for men and women to experience.

Threat: How Does This Affect People?

Threat refers to the risks that the negative influence of power may prevent an individual from meeting their core needs. Threat here refers not just to physical threats but also the threat to health, emotional well-being, and quality of life caused by neglect, poor health, disability, or deprivation. Within forensic practice, the Good Lives model (GLM: Ward, 2002) is widely used to frame offending behaviour as resulting from needs that are unmet, or in ways that are ineffective or harmful. While different patterns of adversity are likely to present different threats, experiences of chronic or repeated adversity or maltreatment, particularly by carers who should be providing a secure base, are likely to severely compromise the child's sense of safety. As Maslow (1987) has pointed out, after basic needs for food and shelter, the need for safety is the most basic of human needs, without which, higher level needs for connection and esteem cannot be consistently met.

There is a lack of research on the differential impact of intrafamilial and extra-familial maltreatment. However, maltreatment in the home is likely to cause relational harm, including disrupted attachments, feelings of abandonment, betrayal, shame, hostility, lack of protection, or entrapment. It may also be associated with strong feelings of shame and pressure to keep the maltreatment secret (Herman, 1992). In contrast, maltreatment outside is more likely to be committed by peers or strangers and the harm may be more social, for example, feelings of isolation or exclusion, loss of status or identity, a sense of injustice or social defeat. For young people experiencing multiple forms of adversity both inside the home and outside, the sense of danger and disconnection from others is likely to be more pervasive, unrelenting, and harmful.

Rose and Rudolph (2006) present evidence that, as a result of gendered socialisation, goals of interpersonal connection and intimacy in relationships are more important to girls, whereas goals of agency and status are more important to boys. As a result, maltreatment that threatens the sense of connection to others may be particularly distressing for girls, while for boys, maltreatment that threatens their sense of agency or status may be more distressing.

Meaning: What Sense Do People Make of This?

Gender can have a powerful impact on the meaning of adverse events, particularly for individuals or communities that hold traditional ideals of masculinity that reflect toughness, independence, and agency, and of femininity as reflecting sensitivity, subordination, and passivity. For example, sexual abuse is likely to be particularly shameful for girls in communities where sex is linked to notions of honour and shame (Gill & Harrison, 2019), but also for boys who hold traditional views of masculinity (Easton, Saltzman, & Willis, 2014). Alternatively, men may avoid identifying themselves as victims by reframing physical abuse as "character building" disciplinary punishment and/or by saying their abuse was justified by their behaviour (Gueta & Chen, 2016).

The role of patriarchal and sexist world views, in which masculinity is defined in terms of domination and control of women is well established in the areas of male-perpetrated sexual and domestic violence (Flood & Pease, 2009). However, there is a growing awareness of the links between masculinity and crime more generally, and in the relationship between masculinity and incarceration (Maguire, 2020). Connell (1995) developed the concept of *protest masculinity*; in societies where male superiority and privilege are assumed, socially and economically marginalised men who do not benefit from what Connell (2000) describes as the "patriarchal dividend" will tend to act in overly masculine ways such as through aggression and crime, in order feel superior.

Threat Responses: What Do People Do to Survive?

The Power Threat Meaning Framework reframes many mental health symptoms and problematic behaviours as threat responses that enable the person to survive and to meet their needs in response to overwhelming power and threat and offending behaviour can also be understood in this way. There is a lack of direct research into gender differences in the links between needs and offending. However, there are various pieces of evidence that suggest that men and women may commit crime in general, and violence in particular to achieve different goals, or to achieve similar goals in different ways.

For example, many women first come into contact with the criminal justice system through behaviours they engage in to achieve safety by escaping abusive homes – for example drug use, sex work, or shoplifting – whereas this pattern appears less common among men (Chesney-Lind, 1989; Daly, 1994). Gueta and Chen (2016) observed that male prisoners often reported becoming involved in crime in order to fulfil the role of "breadwinner" and to support their families, whereas female prisoners reported being motivated by power and status.

When it comes to violent crime, gender differences appear to be influenced by widespread cultural assumptions that regard violence by men as acceptable or even admirable in certain circumstances, while violence by women is often seen as shameful or deviant. It has been argued that status or respect as a motivation for violence is predominantly found in men (McDermott, 2015), particularly in criminal and other subcultures that hold a view of masculinity that values dominance strength and independence (Copes & Hochstetler, 2003). Leadbeater, Kuperminc, Blatt, and Hertzog (1999) found that adolescent boys were more likely to express distress through aggressive and delinquent behaviour, whereas adolescent girls were more likely to respond with inward-focused responses such as depression, suicidal ideation, and eating disorders. Leadbeater et al. suggested that these responses reflect the greater societal emphasis on aggression and self-assertion in boys and on socialising, self-regulation, and emotional sensitivity in girls. Sutton (2017) reported that male gang members were more likely to report joining a gang to earn money and reported greater neighbourhood disadvantage than female members, while female gang members were more likely to describe their gang as a surrogate family that provided a sense of belonging. Female gang members reported coming from high crime neighbourhoods and feeling unsafe in multiple environments.

One of the few types of violent crime where gender differences have been studied is intimate partner violence. Among heterosexual couples, men report being more likely to initiate violence and to use violence to exert power or dominance, whereas women are more likely to report using violence in self-defence or retaliation (Hamberger & Guse, 2002).

Personal Narratives: Vea and Paul

Vea and Paul are patients in the National High Secure Healthcare Service for Women and the Men's Personality Disorder Service respectively at Rampton Hospital. Their names and personal details have been changed to protect their identities. Their personal narratives demonstrate the multi-factorial contextual Power Threat Meaning approach, incorporating social, psychological, and biological factors.

A collaborative discussion, based on the Power Threat Meaning Framework: Guided Discussion document (Johnstone and Boyle et al., 2018), provided a way for Vea and Paul to reflect and consider the framework in relation to their own life experiences.

Vea and Paul were guided to discuss and reflect on the following questions:

- What has happened to you? (i.e., How is power operating in your life?)
- How did it affect you? (i.e., What kind of threats does this pose?)
- What sense did you make of it? (i.e., What is the meaning of these situations and experiences to you?)
- What did you have to do to survive? (i.e., What kinds of threat responses are you using?)
- What are your strengths? (i.e., What access to power resources do you have?)
- What is your story? (i.e., Pulling of these reflections together)

Vea's Story

Some of Vea's experiences have been modified to protect her identity. The name **Vea** means **seen**. This name seemed fitting given Vea believes she was never truly **seen** by anyone.

What Happened to Me?

My biological mother abused alcohol and drugs and I was born prematurely. My biological father was incarcerated for a serious offence. I never knew him. I was adopted as a baby. I have no memory of my biological parents.

My adoptive parents cared for lots of other children. The household was always busy and noisy, and to some degree it did not feel stable. I often sensed unfairness between the children within the household. I felt I wasn't noticed, listened to, or understood.

I am mixed heritage. I looked and felt different to my adopted family and amongst my peers at school. I am always aware of my difference and I never felt I fitted in anywhere. I was sexually abused in my early teens. When I disclosed this abuse, I was not believed. I displayed challenging behaviour at school and home. I often felt I was disciplined more harshly than others. I felt I was misunderstood, unloved, and unfairly treated.

I was placed back into care as a teenager. I felt completely rejected by my adopted family. I moved frequently between placements across the country. I had no control or say about when or where. I was completely powerless and helpless. I felt totally at the mercy of the social services.

Financially, I had extremely limited funds. This limited my options and opportunities. When living on my own, I did whatever I could to make money. This involved prostitution and sometimes putting myself in extremely vulnerable and terrifying situations.

As a woman, I felt quite empowered when using my body and my looks to get certain needs met (financial, safety, security, connection). This felt good at times; however, some of the situations I put myself in ended up being dangerous, unhealthy and were traumatising. The memories still haunt me.

I feel incredibly ashamed of myself and angry at everyone who has ever let me down. I envy those who are more privileged or fortunate than myself. I used drugs to numb these difficult feelings, but they continued to fester underneath. My illegal drug use has also exposed me to some extremely difficult and traumatic situations.

How Did This Affect Me?

Relationally I have always struggled interpersonally throughout my life. I never felt I 'fitted in' anywhere. I struggled to trust, feel safe and connect with people. I always expect my relationships to end. I often end up pushing people away by being too intense with them, so they eventually end up rejecting or abandoning me.

Emotionally I sometimes find it difficult to feel anything; to connect with my emotions. When I do connect with my emotions (negative or positive), I struggle to regulate them. They are far too intense and all consuming. I sometimes lose control. It has catastrophic when I have lost control. I have severely hurt other people, as well as myself.

Socially/in the community I feel vulnerable in social situations, I struggle to fit in and to feel as though I 'belong' with others. My anxiety usually worsens in these situations and I sometimes act in unnatural ways e.g. by being too loud or showing off. I often feel ashamed about my behaviour afterwards.

Economically/materially I am poor. I have never had much money, and when out of the care of inpatient services, I struggled to meet my basic needs. I did whatever I could to make money. I feel both angry and ashamed about this.

Environmentally I lived in some places which were unsafe. Often quite deprived areas where there was a lot of crime and access to drugs. It was difficult to relax and to feel safe in these places. I had to be hypervigilant.

Bodily My body was regularly invaded. I struggled to know what was appropriate and what wasn't. People didn't always respect my personal space or boundaries. I have struggled physically. I have areas of chronic pain and have caused significant debilitating injuries to parts of my own body. I have cycled through periods of binging, purging, and starving.

Identity I have no clear sense of identity. I had little support to be able to develop my own beliefs, values, and identity. I often feel ashamed about myself.

Some circumstances made the threats I was exposed to harder to survive. I experienced a range of adverse experiences from even before my birth, onwards. I did not feel protected or loved by my parents or carers. I felt betrayed and let down, even by the organisations which were meant to protect me. I did not have anyone I could confide in about the threats, and when I did, I wasn't believed. Over the years, I faced several threats from several different perpetrators. Some of these were deliberate acts of harm towards me from other people. Some were repeated and ongoing. I felt I had little control over them and was unable to escape. Some of the threats were physically invasive and multi-layered.

What Sense Did I Make of What Happened to Me?

What I believe, feel and experience:

- Unsafe, afraid, and attacked – *"I always have to be on guard. No one can be trusted"*
- Different, alienated, isolated, and lonely – *"I have never felt as though I belonged or fitted in. I have always felt different, excluded and alone"*
- Bad, unworthy – *"I'm not good. I'm a monster"*
- Shamed, humiliated – *"I am unlovable. There is something wrong with me. Everyone sees it"*
- Abandoned and rejected – *"People always leave me. They don't like me"*
- Betrayed – *"My family and professionals have betrayed me. I feel angry at everyone who has ever let me down"*
- Emotionally overwhelmed – *"I can't manage my feelings. Sometimes I feel too deeply"*
- Emotionally empty – *"Sometimes I feel nothing at all"*
- Sense of injustice and unfairness – *"Why me? Why was I treated so differently? I hate them!"*
- Hopeless – *"It will never change"*

What Did I Have to Do to Survive?

I have survived in different ways. My threat responses have different functions and differ depending on the context or situation I am in.

I am hypervigilant and at times, paranoid and suspicious. I struggle to sleep and relax. I am always on 'guard', watching and waiting for the next threat. I know it is coming eventually! I 'read' into things 'too much', overthinking. I am just trying to protect myself.

I disconnect or numb difficult feelings through dissociation, disconnection, fragmentation, and substance misuse. I learnt how to effectively dissociate early on in life. This helped protect me from intense, painful feelings and situations. Unfortunately, I have in the past, had little control over this and struggled to manage myself in dissociated states. I can be dangerous to other people and myself and have caused significant harm to people when in this state.

I give in and submit. Sometimes, when I lack confidence, I give up easily. I don't even try to help myself. I self-sabotage. I try to appease people as it feels easier than opposing them.

I fight and overcompensate. I argue. I have been physically violent, or I act out and show off. I feel intense anger and rage. I am usually much more violent and punitive towards myself than to others.

I avoid. I hide and flee. I am not always open about how I feel with people.

I struggle to remember. I either don't process events at the time, or I struggle to recall them as it feels too painful and shameful to think about what I have done.

I use drugs and alcohol to moderate my feelings. To soothe, detach, or to stimulate.

Sometimes I feel hopeless and wish to die. Other times, I need support and I struggle to ask for help, verbally, in a healthy way.

I hurt myself to regulate my feelings. My tolerance for pain is extremely high. Sometimes I don't feel any physical pain at all.

What Are My Strengths?

In my early life, I had few strengths, other than my physical fitness, sporting and singing ability, I felt I had little else to draw on as a resource, other than my looks.

During my adult life, whilst in services, I developed more resources and strengths. These have helped me significantly. I draw on these resources and feel less of a need to resort to my previous unhealthy threat responses to survive.

I have experienced caring, secure relationships. I still test these from time to time, but deep down, I know I can trust more now.

I have supportive friends. I don't have many, but the few I have is more than I've ever had in my whole life. I feel less uncomfortable about being different now, and realise that, everyone is in fact unique, and that's okay.

I have experienced a sense of community, belonging and social support.

I have had access to information, knowledge, and alternative views, widening my understanding of myself and the world around me. This has helped me to have a more mature outlook on things.

I have developed more skills and abilities. I use these to cope and I am less likely to hurt myself and others now.

I listen to my body and my mind more. I realise now, that when something feels 'off', my body is usually trying to warn me.

I have experienced compassion from others, and I have become much more compassionate towards others. Sometimes it is hard to be compassionate towards myself, but I do try.

I have felt much more connected and appreciative of the world, particularly of nature.

I have learned better ways to manage my emotions and to healthily express my thoughts and feelings.

I have been able to begin to process and heal some of my earlier trauma and pain. I know this will take time but being able to start this has been life changing.

I have learned how to express myself more. I now write, talk and am much more creative.

My confidence and self-esteem have grown. I still have some way to go, but it's a start.

Paul's Story

What Happened to Me?

I was sexually abused at a very early age. My so-called mother was a drunk. She had several different partners coming and going. I was like a football for them.

When my mother was married to my stepfather it felt like I got a kicking every day, I'd get locked in cupboards. My PE lessons were hit and miss, more miss because I was "very clumsy" apparently and I was always taking notes to school saying how clumsy I was, and I couldn't play PE because I was badly bruised.

If I did show any emotion I'd just get beaten and beaten and beaten and abused in one way or form or another. If it wasn't name calling, it's being beaten, if it's not being beaten, I'm having my head held under the water in the bath.

I was the oldest in my family. From about eleven years old I hardly went to school because I had to look after my siblings, cooking, cleaning, wiping their backsides, taking them round the parks, you name it. My mother was too interested in pills and booze and going out trying to find fellas.

We were like a magnet for people who abused people. My younger sister ended up being abused by several different people. She also ended up on porn films when she was about 13. We attracted those types of people because we were that vulnerable and helpless.

I was 15 when I finally got away. I would run away regularly, and the police would pick me up, and I would tell them my mother was violent and they would just take me back home anyway and say that she loves you. I told the social services and nothing happened. The school, social services, everybody was trying to convince me to go home. In the end I just gave up. I'd go home, and as soon as I got outside the door my anxiety went right up through the roof. The last time they brought me back, my mother was waiting for me. She had my clothes in bin bags and she said "there's your clothes, I don't want you anymore". I sat in that car and I cried my eyes out, one because of the rejection and two because I was so damn relieved to be out of that.

After that I went to a care home, but I didn't really fit in. I was there for about a month and then they put me in a foster home with a lovely lady called Sue. I was there for about 5 or 6 months and it was brilliant. I stopped wetting the bed, I had a life, I had friends for a little while. That was the first time I had some stability in my life.

41

After that I got my own flat. I ended up being a prisoner in my own home because when I came out of my house I would just freak out around people and had these urges to attack them and the voices in my head were saying hit them, hit them, hit them. I went to the doctor and they referred me to this unit. On a good day I'd turn up and try to explain what I was going through, but I could barely talk back then or even think straight, even on a good day. There were times that I said to them that I needed help otherwise one day I was going to hurt someone really bad. I'd keep these appointments up for a little while until things got really bad and I really feared going out because of hurting other people, and I would end up not getting another appointment. I was in fear of getting attacked, hurt or rejected by other people. It was just easier to be alone, away from everybody, so I isolated myself as a prisoner in my own house.

When I was locked up I got my social work file and it said that I was at risk from being born basically, so they knew. The school would report me for not turning up, or the hospital reported me for having broken fingers; they'd turn up and then they'd go away again. They knew.

How Did This Affect Me?

Lack of safety. It was one of those things where I couldn't do right for doing wrong, every single thing was wrong. Even when I followed their every instruction it was wrong. I developed a skill very early on of not showing any emotion. It was survival.

Because of my appearance I got bullied at school, so I was constantly fighting outside, trying to survive and I was constantly fighting at home, trying to survive, but in a different way. At home I had to fight to keep my emotions in check and try my damnedest to try to please them even though everything was wrong, or at least stay out of their way.

Lack of connection. It's indescribable, the feeling of not being wanted, there wasn't many days go by where I didn't have the thought of ending my own life, because of all them problems. I just wanted to crawl into a hole and die, I just wanted it all to end.

Inability to express emotions. It got beat in to me so it was a natural thing for me, I didn't just shut other people out I shut myself out, I shut my own emotions out, I wasn't even allowed to feel and when I did I was too afraid of losing it.

What Did This Mean to Me?

I saw everybody as a threat. And I mean everybody, even though they said that they were trying to help me, it drove me bloody crazy, people were bringing me stuff that I didn't want, and I saw it as a threat.

One of the worst things is defectiveness, I continued all the abuse, but in my head. I saw everything everybody ever said to me and I just kept it repeating to myself. I felt like everybody around me was normal and I was abnormal, I felt like a non-human, like an alien, like I wasn't from this planet. I felt like the whole world didn't understand or wasn't even interested.

What Did I Do to Survive?

I became numb, I became shut off from everything. When I spoke, I spoke in a flat tone, I had virtually no facial expressions, my body language was non-existent; I was really difficult to read. It was like a massive wall that's very difficult to penetrate or get over.

I was a magnet for bullies... I was passive; I was so frightened I couldn't say no, and when I did say no they'd take no notice anyway and would just continue.

So, I'd stay away from everybody, to stay away from harm and harming others. I wanted to live on a desert island on my own so there was no one else around, no people around, no problems. But when I was alone, I wasn't away from all the torment and the flashbacks and the memories, so it stuck with me anyway.

I hated drinking, I can't stand the taste or the smell of it. But with the nightmares and the flashbacks, all that intense feeling, it took the edge off. So for a short time, it was nice. But then it was followed by other problems. I used to smoke cannabis too; all the tension from my body would go. I'd go into this dreamland where there was nothing, no pain, no bad memories, no abuse, no flashbacks, no torment, just pure escape; it was ecstasy. But I couldn't afford to go out and buy it all the time.

But then people would push me so far and I'd lose it. I was regularly fighting in and out of school at a very early age. I got in to such an uncontrollable rage I just couldn't control myself, it wasn't just me hitting them and going away, I'd be hitting them, knocking them to the ground, then jumping on top of them, trying to smash their head open and I had to be dragged away because I was screaming with rage and I couldn't stop myself. All my emotions would come out, every single thing, so even after I finished, I was bawling, I was throwing up, I was crying my eyes out. I would be totally, mentally and emotionally wiped out and not for a day or two, but a week or more. I'd feel so guilty about my uncontrollable rage.

I would try and keep my emotions to myself and keep that rage in because of how far it could go, I didn't know when it would stop. I couldn't stop it, so I ended up being a target, and people would push me and push me and then when I got into that rage where I couldn't stop and was dragged off they would be the ones crying.

I became prickly and hostile towards others to prevent them from hurting me, I didn't know I was being prickly towards them, I would just be sarcastic all the time. I got the point where I couldn't cope with being around people, I would just keep myself to myself. It's hard to look back and see how standoffish and unfriendly I was, just staring at everyone because I was so fearful of them attacking me. I wouldn't take my eyes of them just in case they would creep up on me when I wasn't looking, I became the aggressor.

I wanted to have relationships and have a normal life like everybody else, and I did have a few but most wouldn't last. All the abandonment and rejection I'd had as a kid played out later on in life by pushing other people away before they rejected me; any sign of any relationship breakup I would just stay away. I ended up with abusive partners. For some strange reason when I saw someone that I really liked I was really passive and I didn't go near them, but the people that came to me I would partner up with and would live that life of abuse again.

What Is Life Like Now?

I came here and I started building relationships with the psychologists. It took me 6 months to build my first relationship. Just to get talking and when that psychologist moved on and I moved on to another psychologist it took me maybe 5 months. The psychologist that I am working with now, it took me weeks to open up. By this point I had done a lot of DBT-based work, speech and language therapy. I started working with this psychologist around 2 years ago and she introduced me to a number of books which helped me understand myself in a more trauma-based way, to unlock what I am feeling and thinking and why, and link the trauma to the feeling. I read a lot of self-help books and this has helped me because people say things to you and you don't quite believe, but when you read the exact same thing in a book you think it must be true, so it helps me build trust. Even now I find it very difficult to trust after 9 years of therapy.

I've been here for 9 years now and I've learned a lot of new skills. It doesn't stop the trauma or the PTSD or the nightmares, it doesn't help me concentrate but it helps me get through the day. For the first time I am actually building relationships, not with just one or two people but with everybody and I am able to maintain and repair and I'm learning how to speak to people, even how to elaborate myself. For the first time in my life I have got a life. For me it's coming out of the darkness into the light.

Conclusions

Although what Vea and Paul experienced was very different, their descriptions of the impact are strikingly similar. Neither felt safe or connected to others, even as adults. Both were let down, not just by their families, but by professional agencies that should have protected them, leaving them with a chronic sense of mistrust and injustice that frustrated their desire to feel connected to others. Both felt overwhelmed by unmanageable emotions that sometimes led them to behave extremely destructively.

Vea and Paul also describe many similar strategies for survival: being hypervigilant to threat, dissociating from overwhelming emotions or using drugs and alcohol to numb them; and being trapped in an endless cycle of wanting connection to others but being hurt or hurting others when they found it, leading to a sense of frustration and despair.

These narratives also point to some of the gendered patterns described in the first part of the chapter. Paul described being sexually abused from an early age, though the impact on his later sexual development in his narrative is unclear. Vea describes being sexually abused in her early teens and, we might speculate that that experience influenced her decision to engage in sex work, like many justice-involved women (Chesney-Lind, 1989), to establish some sense of agency and control in her life. Vea also refers to managing her distress through self-harm, a pattern that is much more common among women than men (see Chapter 9), as well as creating a sense of control over her body through binging, purging, and starving. These observations perhaps suggest a more general pattern – that there is a broader range of "socially acceptable" responses to trauma for women, whereas the range of "acceptable" or "normal" outlets for men in some communities may be limited to stoical detachment, heavy drinking and violence.

Like most forensic practitioners, both authors of this chapter work exclusively with patients of one gender and so we rarely consider our patients' behaviour through the lens of gender. Collaborating on this chapter has revealed the similarities and differences in pathways from adversity to violence in men and women. It also shows that we have much more to understand about the different experiences of adversity faced by men and women, how they and society regard those experiences, and how they adapt to survive. The Power Threat Meaning Framework, with its core, compassionate assumption that emotional distress and troubled behaviour are understandable responses to life circumstances, provides a promising framework for this exploration.

Further Reading

Maguire, D. (2020). *Male, failed, jailed: Masculinities and revolving-door imprisonment in the UK*. Springer International. An accessible and compassionate examination of how different forms of masculinity, in the context of social deprivation and exclusion, contribute to male offending.

Motz, A., Dennis, M., & Aiyegbusi, A. (2020). *Invisible trauma: Women, difference and the criminal justice system*. Routledge. A psychoanalytically informed account of the development of violence and other offending, identifying pathways for change to address trauma within the lives of women and their children. It highlights the role of emotional, social, and cultural forces in traumatising women who come into contact with the criminal justice system.

References

Baglivio, M. T., Epps, N., Swartz, K., Huq, M. S., Sheer, A., & Hardt, N. S. (2014). The prevalence of adverse childhood experiences (ACE) in the lives of juvenile offenders. *Journal of Juvenile Justice, 3*(2).

Baron-Cohen, S., & Wheelwright, S. (2004). The empathy quotient: An investigation of adults with Asperger syndrome or high functioning autism, and normal sex differences. *Journal of Autism and Developmental Disorders, 34*(2), 163–175. doi:10.1023/B:JADD.0000022607.19833.00

Bonta, J., & Andrews, D.A. (2016). *The psychology of criminal conduct*. Routledge. doi:10.4324/9781315677187

Brebner, J. (2003). Gender and emotions. *Personality and Individual Differences, 34*(3), 387–394. doi:10.1016/S0191-8869(02)00059-4

Boyle, M., & Johnstone, L., (2020). *A Straight Talking Introduction to the Power Threat Meaning Framework*. PCCS Books.

Card, N. A., Stucky, B. D., Sawalani, G. M., & Little, T. D. (2008). Direct and indirect aggression during childhood and adolescence: A meta-analytic review of gender differences, intercorrelations, and relations to maladjustment. *Child Development, 79*(5), 1185–1229. doi:10.1111/j.1467-8624.2008.01184.x

Cernkovich, S., & Giordano, P. C. (1987). Family relationships and delinquency. *Criminology, 25*(2), 295–319. doi:10.1111/j.1745-9125.1987.tb00799.x

Chaplo, S. D., Kerig, P. K., Modrowski, C. A., & Bennett, D. C. (2017). Gender differences in the sequelae of childhood sexual abuse: An examination of borderline features, dissociation, emotion dysregulation, and delinquent behaviors among detained adolescents. *Journal of Child and Adolescent Trauma, 10*(1). doi:10.1007/s40653-016-0122-z

Chesney-Lind, M. (1989). Girls' crime and women's place: Toward a feminist model of female delinquency. *Crime & Delinquency, 35*(1), 5–29. doi:10.1177/0011128789035001002

Connell, R. (1995). *Masculinities*. Polity.

Connell, R. (2000). *The men and the boys*. Polity.

Copes, H., & Hochstetler, A. (2003). Situational construction of masculinity among male street thieves. *Journal of Contemporary Ethnography, 32*(3), 279–304. doi:10.1177/0891241603032003002

Cronholm, P. F., Forke, C. M., Wade, R., Bair-Merritt, M. H., Davis, M., Harkins-Schwarz, M., … & Fein, J. A. (2015). Adverse childhood experiences: Expanding the concept of adversity. *American Journal of Preventive Medicine, 49*(3), 354–361. doi:10.1016/j.amepre.2015.02.001

Daly, K. (1994). *Gender, crime, and punishment*. New Haven, CT: Yale University Press.

Eagly, A. H., & Steffen, V. J. (1986). Gender and aggressive behavior: A meta-analytic review of the social psychological literature. *Psychological Bulletin, 100*(3), 309–330. doi:10.1037/0033-2909.100.3.309

Easton, S. D., Saltzman, L. Y., & Willis, D. G. (2014). "Would you tell under circumstances like that?": Barriers to disclosure of child sexual abuse for men. *Psychology of Men & Masculinity, 15*(4), 460–469. doi:10.1037/a0034223

Flood, M., & Pease, B. (2009). Factors influencing attitudes to violence against women. *Trauma, Violence, & Abuse, 10*(2), 125–142. doi:10.1177/1524838009334131

Gewirtz-Meydan, A., & Finkelhor, D. (2020). Sexual abuse and assault in a large national sample of children and adolescents. *Child Maltreatment, 25*(2), 203–214. doi:10.1177/1077559519873975

Gill, A. K., & Harrison, K. (2019). 'I am talking about it because I want to stop it': child sexual abuse and sexual violence against women in British South Asian communities. *British Journal of Criminology, 59*(3), 511–529. doi:10.1093/bjc/azy059

Gottfredson, M. R., & Hirschi, T. (1990). *A general theory of crime*. Stanford, CA: Stanford University Press.

Gueta, K., & Chen, G. (2016). Men and women inmates' accounts of their pathways to crime: A gender analysis. *Deviant Behavior, 37*(12), 1459–1472. doi:10.1080/01639625.2016.1189753

Hamberger, L. K., & Guse, C. E. (2002). Men's and women's use of intimate partner violence in clinical samples. *Violence Against Women, 8*(11), 1301–1331. doi:10.1177/107780102237406

Herman, J. (1992). *Trauma and recovery: The aftermath of violence from domestic abuse to political terror*. Basic Books.

Johnstone, L. & Boyle, M. with Cromby, J., Dillon, J., Harper, D., Kinderman, P., Longden, E., Pilgrim, D. & Read, J. (2018). *The power threat meaning framework: Towards the identification of patterns in emotional distress, unusual experiences and troubled or troubling behaviour, as an alternative to functional psychiatric diagnosis*. Leicester: British Psychological Society.

Karatzias, T., Power, K., Woolston, C., Apurva, P., Begley, A., Mirza, K., … & Purdie, A. (2018). Multiple traumatic experiences, post-traumatic stress disorder and offending behaviour in female prisoners. *Criminal Behaviour and Mental Health, 28*(1), 72–84. doi:10.1002/cbm.2043

Kohlberg, L, (1976). Moral stages and moralization: The cognitive-developmental approach. In T. Lickona (Ed.), *Moral development and behavior-theory, research and social issues* (pp.31–53). New York: Holt, Rinehart and Winston.

Komarovskaya, I. A., Booker Loper, A., Warren, J., & Jackson, S. (2011). Exploring gender differences in trauma exposure and the emergence of symptoms of PTSD among incarcerated men and women. *Journal of Forensic Psychiatry & Psychology, 22*(3), 395–410. doi:10.1080/14789949.2011.572989

Lanctôt, N., & LeBlanc, M. (2002). Explaining adolescent females' involvement in deviance. *Crime and Justice, 29*, 113–202. doi:10.1086/652220

Leadbeater, B. J., Kuperminc, G. P., Blatt, S. J., & Hertzog, C. (1999). A multivariate model of gender differences in adolescents' internalizing and externalizing problems. *Developmental Psychology, 35*(5), 1268–1282. doi:10.1037/0012-1649.35.5.1268

Maguire, D. (2020). *Male, failed, jailed: Masculinities and revolving-door imprisonment in the UK.* Springer International.

Maschi, T., Gibson, S., Zgoba, K. M., & Morgen, K. (2011). Trauma and life event stressors among young and older adult prisoners. *Journal of Correctional Health Care, 17*(2), 160–172. doi:10.1177/1078345810396682

Maslow, A. H. (1987). *Motivation and personality* (3rd Ed.). New York: Harper & Row.

McDermott, R. (2015). Sex and death: Gender differences in aggression and motivations for violence. *International Organization, 69*, 752–775. doi:10.1017/S0020818315000065

Ministry of Justice. (2020). *Statistics on women and the criminal justice system 2019.* Ministry of Justice.

Rose, A. J., & Rudolph, K. D. (2006). A review of sex differences in peer relationship processes: Potential trade-offs for the emotional and behavioral development of girls and boys. *Psychological Bulletin, 132*(1), 98–131. doi:10.1037/0033-2909.132.1.98

Sutton, T. E. (2017). The lives of female gang members: A review of the literature. *Aggression and Violent Behavior, 37*, 142–152. doi:10.1016/j.avb.2017.10.001

Tolin, D. F., & Foa, E. B. (2006). Sex differences in trauma and posttraumatic stress disorder: A quantitative review of 25 years of research. *Psychological Bulletin, 132*(6), 959–992. doi:10.1037/0033-2909.132.6.959

Tremblay, R. E., Japel, C., Pérusse, D., McDuff, P., Boivin, M., Zoccolillo, M., & Montplaisir, J. (1999). The search for the age of "onset" of physical aggression: Rousseau and Bandura revisited. *Criminal Behavior and Mental Health, 9*(1), 8–23. doi:10.1002/cbm.288

Ullman, S. E., & Filipas, H. H. (2005). Gender differences in social reactions to abuse disclosures, post-abuse coping, and PTSD of child sexual abuse survivors. *Child Abuse & Neglect, 29*(7), 767–782. doi:10.1016/j.chiabu.2005.01.005

van Honk, J., Schutter, D. J., Bos, P. A., Kruijt, A. W., Lentjes, E. G., & Baron-Cohen, S. (2011). Testosterone administration impairs cognitive empathy in women depending on second-to-fourth digit ratio. *Proceedings of the National Academy of Sciences, 108*(8), 3448–3452. doi:10.1073/pnas.1011891108

Wamser-Nanney, R., & Cherry, K. E. (2018). Children's trauma-related symptoms following complex trauma exposure: Evidence of gender differences. *Child Abuse & Neglect, 77*, 188–197. doi:10.1016/j.chiabu.2018.01.009

Ward, T. (2002). Good lives and the rehabilitation of offenders: Promises and problems. *Aggression and Violent Behavior, 7*(5), 513–528. doi:10.1016/S1359-1789(01)00076-3

Weeks, R., & Widom, C. S. (1998). *Early childhood victimization among incarcerated adult male felons.* US Department of Justice, Office of Justice Programs, National Institute of Justice, Washington DC.

Wood, J., Foy, D. W., Layne, C., Pynoos, R., & James, C. B. (2002). An examination of the relationships between violence exposure, posttraumatic stress symptomatology, and delinquent activity: An "ecopathological" model of delinquent behavior among incarcerated adolescents. *Journal of Aggression, Maltreatment & Trauma, 6*(1), 127–147. doi:10.1300/J146v06n01_07

3

TRAUMA-INFORMED RISK ASSESSMENT AND INTERVENTION

Understanding the Role of Triggering Contexts and Offence-Related Altered States of Consciousness (ORASC)

Lawrence Jones

Exhortations to "open the black box" of dynamic risk factors (Ward, 2021 and, in a different way, Case, 2021; Woldgabreal, Day, & Tamatea, 2020; Mayson, 2019) invite us as practitioners to begin to develop a more elaborated view of the psychological, biological, and socio-cultural processes underpinning dynamic risk. This chapter aims to offer one strand of exploration in response to this: the nature of psychological processes underpinning the link between trauma and dynamic risk. The risk assessment and intervention literature has not typically looked at the ways in which trauma influences dynamic risk processes. More specifically, two neglected areas for consideration in conducting trauma-informed risk assessments and interventions will be highlighted: *triggering contextual factors* and *triggered altered states of consciousness* and shifts in the capacity for agency.

An integrative resource loss- and gain-based framework, based on the work of Layne and Hobfoll (2020) and Layne, Briggs, and Courtois (2014), for conceptualising the link between trauma and dynamic risk processes will be offered. The central argument is that trauma responses impact in complex ways on resource acquisition and resource conservation processes, and these responses require something to activate or trigger them. Activating processes are *endogenous* and *exogenous* (Baskin-Sommer et al., 2021). Exogenous or contextual risk-exacerbating and/or protective scaffolding processes therefore need to be worked with, when assessing and intervening with dynamic risk, alongside endogenous shifts in thinking and feeling linked with traumagenic offence-related altered states of consciousness (ORASC) and associated changes in capacity for agency.

DOI: 10.4324/9781003120766-5

The conservation of resources model (COR: Layne & Hobfoll, 2020), developed to understand post-traumatic adjustment trajectories, offers a useful model for understanding return-to-offending processes. Characterising the potential impact of trauma as involving a depletion of resources, broadly defined, this offers a framework for an integrative understanding of the complex role of trauma in offence processes (Jones, 2020a; 2020b).

The model describes the useful idea of *resource caravans* (Layne & Hobfoll 2020), defined as "clusters of resources (e.g., self-esteem, mastery, coping skills, social support, physical health, wealth, personal relationships) that collect together, accumulate, accrue in their beneficial effects, and 'travel' with their host over time" (Hobfoll, 2012a; p.91). It contrasts these with **risk factor caravans** defined by Layne and Hobfoll (2020) as a

> constellation of co-occurring risk factors that accumulate in number, 'travel' with their host over time, increase the host's risk for subsequent exposure to and vulnerability to the harmful effects of additional risk factors, and accrue and 'cascade forward' in their harmful effects across development.
>
> *p.91*

The model proposes that resource loss caravans linked with trauma and adversity are more rapid and consequently need to be targeted first in intervention before going on to work on resource gain cycles.

This approach offers a language to describe the complex "domino effects" of developmental responses to traumatic experiences, past and ongoing (Stein, Wilmot, & Soloman, 2016). This same domino effect language is useful for thinking about the development of offending.

In understanding offending, the idea of malignant "resource *gain* cycles" is also relevant. This is the idea that some kinds of resource seeking and acquisition can be harmful to self and others, as well as forming a means for escaping different kinds of harm, privation, and adversity. Ward's *approach goal* offending (Ward & Siegert, 2002) is an example of this. Offending that is *approach explicit* is about meeting core needs but doing this in a harmful manner, which can also take on a compulsive accelerating quality (see also Hodge's notion of *addiction to crime*, e.g., Hodge, McMurran, & Hollin, 1997, but also Katehakis, 2016 on sexual compulsivity and Lovern & Rock, 2021, on substance misuse, all linked with trauma histories).

Resource-focused functional analysis – identifying the function of behaviour in attaining and conserving resources – fits with the COR theory of trauma impact (e.g., Layne & Hobfoll, 2020), and both Cloitre, Cohen, Ortigo, Jackson, and Koenen's (2020) clinical model of trauma, and evolutionary systems models (Arnhart, 1998; Gilbert, 2020; Jones, 2016; Leedom; 2014; Liotti, 2017; Panksepp, 1998). Typically, trauma has been seen as only involving the fear and the attachment systems. However, evolutionary models linking trauma and offending propose that all evolved systems can be adversely impacted by different kinds of adversity (Jones, 2016). This suggests a broader set of domains: dominance, play, sexual, caring, in addition to fear and attachment, which are conceptualised as "wired into" the brain, and are motivated towards establishing a set of key evolutionarily important resources (experienced as needs, each with its own internal working model; Leedom, 2014). These resources were identified by Ward (2002) as underpinning the *goods* in the good lives model; based in part on Arnhart's (1998) evolutionary theory linking evolved motivational needs with the Aristotelean notion of a *good life*.

Offending is, then, a way of attaining resources – often in adverse (e.g., violent, impoverished, racist, sexist, homophobic, or resource depleted) or traumatising contexts, or environments that remind the individual of experiences of these in the past – that theoretically can be obtained in more prosocial ways. If trauma and adversity can precipitate negative resource cycles that can result in a cascade of downstream adverse consequences, then offending, looked at through this lens, is a resource gain strategy, and can be triggered by resource loss cycles/processes linked with trauma responses to either reminders/triggers or current traumagenic contexts.

Evolutionary approaches highlight different resource acquisition and maintenance strategies adapted for different environments. The safer and more predictable versus dangerous and unpredictable distinction, highlighted in Durrant's (2017) work on *life history,* is useful for classifying environments where resource loss cycles are more likely, but also where "fast" or "slow" patterns of adaptation are more appropriate (Del Giudice, 2020). Trauma responses are adaptations to a dangerous or unpredictable context using "fast" strategies rather than "slow" strategies. Fast strategies involve often rapid, unthinking heuristically driven (system 1 processes, Kahneman, 2011), immediate resource acquisition-oriented behaviours aimed at survival in contexts of social and material resource scarcity. Slow strategies involve deliberative, planful, socially focused and invested behaviours aimed at maximising resources in a safe predictable environment.

The idea that for a good lives plan to be developed, the individual needs to address a range of needs in different domains can be extended if we think about the way that certain needs develop a motivational monopoly, and that the reason for this is that, for any particular individual, one or more of the evolved systems has been impacted by experiences (of deprivation or excess primarily, but not exclusively, in early life) that result in that system becoming foregrounded in ways that may have been functionally adaptive at some stage. For example, as a consequence of developmental experiences: the fear system can be linked with perceptions of, and reactions to, lack of safety; the sexual system can become fixated on an age group or sexual activity following experiences of abuse and develop an all-encompassing compulsive quality; the dominance system can result in an overarching need for power and control; the attachment system can be shaped in such a way that the individual becomes vulnerable to rejection, abandonment, or loss (real or imagined). See Table 3.1.

The question is: how we can work with and understand different resource loss and resource gain processes in an individual's life? Both the pathway to offending and the pathway to mental health difficulties are driven by *current* (often traumatic and not just historical) adversity that is compounded and fed by early accumulated trauma and oppressive experiences mediated by resource losses of different kinds.

In summary then, trauma, adversity, and oppression/lack of power are all processes linked with depletion of resources. Trauma responses are, in part, evolved adaptations

Table 3.1 Resource loss in relation to evolved systems, trauma, and contextual triggers

Evolutionary systems (Gilbert, Liotti, Panksepp)	"Goods" (Ward)	Goods as resource requirements (evolutionary function)	Trauma impact on resource acquisition processes	Past and current environmental Precipitator	Protective environmental factors	Offending to obtain resources
Play	Play Happiness Creativity	Adaptation resources Social connection and status	Inhibited play Rigid thinking Poor problem solving	Social prohibition, Cultures that don't value play	Support for recreation Valuing creativity and playfulness	Substance misuse Recreational violence "creative" offending e.g., fraud Rigidly controlling behaviour
Threat	Life Knowledge (in relation to predictability) Inner peace Happiness	Existential resources, survival	Fear for life Unpredictability Inner turmoil Unhappiness	Unpredictability High threat situations Abuse Poverty Racism, sexism, homophobia	Predictable environments and relationships Absence of threat Economic resources Non-racist, non-sexist, non-homophobic social scaffolding	Pre-emptive violence Substance misuse Defensive violence Offending to manage negative emotions
Achievement, dominance, status, power	Knowledge (as in achievement) Work Agency Creativity	Inclusive fitness Social safety	Low status Defectiveness Lack of felt agency Repressed creativity Oppression	Powerlessness Lack of opportunities Lack of responses for overbearing domineering behaviour	Opportunities for achievement, status, work, education, cultural engagement offering status.	Status-oriented violence, Shame-based offending, Controlling, bullying behaviour

			Preoccupation with dominance and control; Self-regulation difficulties	Dismissive, controlling, oppressive, or stigmatising cultures	Validating, supportive, non-controlling, non-stigmatising, trauma-informed culture	Theft to get material resources to establish status
Attachment	Relatedness	Existential resources; Survival	Rejection; Abandonment; Grief	Loss of attachment figures or threat thereof; Neglect; Abuse; Lack of opportunity to form attachment	Secure attachment opportunities; Supportive consistent long-lasting relationships	Relational violence, stalking, sexual offending; Offending to meet safety needs not achieved through attachment
Social connection	Connection	Resources associated with collaboration	Social alienation; Moral injury	Ostracising othering cultures; Refugee contexts; Loss	Opportunities for cultural engagement and belonging	Violence and anti-social orientation linked with feeling like an "outsider"
Care	Connection; Relatedness; Happiness	Progeny survival	Fear of harm to offspring	Loss or threat of loss of progeny	Support for parental role	Over protection, violence linked with protecting children from real or imagined threats
Sexual	Connection; Relatedness; Happiness	Reproduction	Vandalised "love maps"; Sexual compulsivity	Cultures of sexual prohibition or valorising sexual abuse e.g., as a way of "doing masculinity"; Neglect leading to exposure to abuse or premature sexual experience	Opportunities for meaningful relationships; Modelling of culturally informed non-abusive ways of "doing masculinity" available	Sexual offending

to unpredictable, unsafe, resource-depleted environments; and offending linked with trauma is one response aimed at restoring or attaining resources. The ways in which both the context and the individual's state of consciousness impact on and shape resource dynamics will be a the theme of the chapter. In the next section triggering processes will be explored.

Triggering and Precipitating Processes for Resource Needs

Trauma experiences, whether acute or chronic, have an impact on the whole person and their social contexts. This impact has been identified as taking a number of different forms, termed here *trauma process* (TP). The concept of a "trigger" is used to describe a current experience that reminds the individual of a past intense experience (e.g., trauma or substance misuse, experience; Lovern & Rock, 2021) that, as a consequence of the intensity, sets in train a sequence of psychological reactions that result in the individual transitioning through a number of discrete shifts in state of consciousness (Putnam, 2016) and resulting in a state in which the individual is at increased risk of acting in a manner that is consonant with the TP goals deriving from the original experience(s) (see Table 3.2).

Jones (2015, 2016) argued that a key task is to identify ways of linking the *risk mechanisms* deriving from developmental factors that allow clinicians to understand triggering processes for dynamic risk factors. Trauma-derived dispositions such as strengths, vulnerability, or fragility need to be triggered in order to enter into a *realisation process* and to be played out. Table 3.3 illustrates how this kind of process operates.

Trauma processes are different in the context of different personality configurations and developmental or neuropsychological presentations. Trauma processes, for instance, play out very differently in the context of autistic spectrum disorders or externalising personality traits. The kinds of states of consciousness, psychological

Table 3.2 Manifestation and precipitation processes

Manifestation/precipitation of trauma processes	*Examples*
Triggering reminders and ongoing trauma	People who remind them of abusers, smells, activities, TV programmes… .
Ruminative self-incitement	Revenge thoughts, fantasies, planning aimed at offsetting/resolving trauma experiences
Social contagion vulnerability	Rejection trauma resulting in a need to please peers – which becomes problematic when peers are engaging in offending behaviour
Exposure to availability of offending routes to meeting resource needs	Exposure to drugs, availability of weapons, pro-offending cultures
Pervasive mood states ("positive" – "manic" – or "negative" e.g., depression numbness or anxiety) derived from trauma experiences	Accumulating sense of anticipation or frustration resulting in increased probability of offending of different kinds

Table 3.3 Trauma-triggering process

Trauma experience	Trauma process (TP)	Precipitating process/triggers (PP)	Initiating transition	Transitioning states	Offence-related altered states of consciousness (ORASC)	Trauma process Conclusion completion
e.g., Witnessing violence	Intrusive bodily experience of fear and hypervigilance. Dissociative structural and processual mechanisms. Diathesis or installation of vulnerability to PPs	Reminders. Or chain reminders (Briere 2019) e.g., being made to feel ashamed by being teased, this then reminding the person of feeling shame at the time of witnessing violence for not having protected the victim	Shock, trauma-related orienting reactions. Paralleling the reactions at the time of the original trauma	Rapid or gradual emergence of myopia, cognitive abeyance. Emotional escalation associated with bodily transitions, increasing felt irresistibility of action urges, loss of metacognitive stances – less mentalisation. Increased salience of triggered system reinforcers (establishing operations). Increased "feeling of knowing" in relation to beliefs/schema associated with trauma consonant actions	e.g., myopia, automatisation of behaviour/loss of felt agency, witnessing self-acting (passenger states) rather than willing self to act, or mind-blindness. Intense sense of blinkered agency in the context of mind-blindness	Process of shifting from ORASC and TRASC (Trauma Related Altered State of Consciousness) to NWC (Normal Waking Consciousness) Frewen & Lanius (2015)

processes played out at the time of an offence are critical to making sense both of the offending and the trauma-related contribution to offending. Equally important, however, is that each of these states is *culturally embedded and interpreted* and played out according to the culturally derived interpretational "rules" in which they occur. It is to this area we turn now.

Situational Approach to Safety and Risk Assessment

Looking at risk through the trauma and diversity lens highlights the importance of understanding triggering contexts in the development of offending behaviour. This invites us to move from a position of doing risk assessments that focus on the individual to one in which we also assess the context into which individuals are placed. Baskin-Sommers et al. (2021) highlight complex interactions between endogenous and exogenous processes in the development of offending behaviour.

Cloitre et al. (2020) propose the resource loss model of trauma, arguing that trauma represents either loss of psychological or material resources in the context of resource-deprived environments. They argue that "the traumatised state is not static. If resource regeneration does not occur, the result is not stasis, but rather *continued resource loss and degeneration*" (p.6, my emphasis). Hobfoll (2012b) describes the way in which the socio-environmental context can either "support, foster, enrich, and protect the resources of individuals families and organisations… or they can detract, undermine, obstruct, or impoverish peoples resource reservoirs" (p.229).

Contexts can also be characterised by the extent to which trauma exposure or threat is an *ongoing feature* (see Table 3.1), ongoing traumatic stress as opposed to post-traumatic stress. Stein, Wilmot, and Soloman (2016) argue that many contexts are characterised by ongoing threat and that in these contexts traumatic symptoms represent a rational fear. Intrusive thoughts about the past are supplemented by intrusive thoughts about *the future*. Traumatised behaviour is based on concrete threats, not imagined ones and is therefore still *adaptive*.

Ongoing trauma (including e.g., being embedded in oppressive cultures or being relationally alienated) or trauma reminders present a destabilising context for the individual. Offending is a compensatory resource acquisition process. Violence, for example, can be about acquiring safety or status resources. The individual uses offending as a way of reinstating or acquiring resources in situations of scarcity, privation, adversity, or reminders of trauma. In *good lives* terms this is attaining goods, often in the context of resource loss or scarcity.

Hobfoll et al.'s (2009) idea that individuals who lack resources are more vulnerable to resource loss and at greater risk of being exposed to additional and ongoing resources loss processes, is critical to this understanding. Contextual assessment, therefore, should include an analysis of the extent to which the current context is presenting the individual with ongoing traumatic experiences or threats and the extent to which the context provides or deprives resources for the individual.

Adverse aspects of the current context that are likely to be triggering are likely to be those that most resemble the contexts of earlier trauma. It is common therefore that both reminders and current trauma are overlapping domains in terms of their potential for precipitating reactions aimed at conserving or establishing resources.

Dynamic risk assessment then needs to look at the context an individual is moving into as well as their own capacities to cope. This can be seen as a specific kind of scenario planning that focuses on the traumagenic resource scarcity profile of the post-release environment, e.g., how impoverished, exposed to crime, punitive, trauma-uninformed, neglectful, and unstimulating and exposed to drugs is it? This is not about the individual; it is about lack of adequate provision post-release. At worst it is about the extent to which people are set up to fail.

Aspects of the context that are going to contribute to negative resource cycles will both make meeting needs through offending more salient and make trauma responses more easily triggered. These processes interact and are consequently difficult to disentangle.

Whilst releases from custody is often an eagerly sought-after outcome, it is also potentially very stressful. Relationships with people in prison are lost abruptly and the individual has to enter a changed world, often being accommodated in settings where they know few if any other people. In addition, they have to start to look after themselves and engage in new activities like job seeking and forming relationships. Inevitably, if there is a trauma history this experience of rapid resource loss will run the risk of being triggering for the individual.

Exogenous and Endogenous Processes

Exposure to Endogenous Trauma-Maintaining or Triggering Social Contexts That Feel Unsafe in Different Ways

Table 3.1 highlights the way that trauma and adverse experiences can impact in a range of different ways through different evolved systems and in the context of different cultures. Neglect is a unique kind of contextual trauma that often gets missed. Exposure to people around the individual not respecting their boundaries, or who are engaging in offence-related behaviour that trigger offence approach goals for the individual, is a kind of neglect. Also, the extent to which offending generally results in non-conviction, or lack of a constructive response, will create the neglectful context for neglected states of mind where the individual is reminded of neglected experiences as a child where they could "get away with murder" and engage in offending with impunity.

Other contextual triggers include exposure to substance misuse subcultures and toxic versions of masculinity, associated with cultural disparaging of vulnerability that results in wanting to conceal vulnerability that parallels the contexts that were around in childhood or/and those that were in place at the time of the offence.

Exposure to external and internalised racism (contextually triggered and scaffolded) that are offence-context paralleling for the individual are also harming. Similarly, exposure to sexism, ableism, ageism, classism, homophobia in ways that reinforce external and internalised self-condemnatory narratives needs to be identified and assessed. In addition to exposure to racism, absence of exposure to a culture that one belongs to is traumatic. This state of privation can be cumulatively troubling.

Risk factors will not be realised if the context does not support or trigger them. Oppressive, traumagenic, and trauma-triggering contexts are likely to release processes that realise the negative resource cycles linked with mental health deterioration and offending behaviour. Table 3.4 illustrates different kinds of contextual factors.

Table 3.4 Illustrative checklist of contextual-triggering processes requiring assessment

Contextual features	Trauma process
Level of poverty in area moving to on release	Risk of ongoing trauma Range of poverty-related experiences reminding individual of past states of poverty linked with trauma and triggering reactions
Distance from previous trauma-triggering contexts	To what extent is the person being reminded of the trauma, to what extent are they vulnerable to re-traumatisation linked e.g., with social networks
Availability of support from family	Loss, rejection, abandonment, loneliness
Evidence of crises in family or close friends	Others' trauma as stressful and also triggering
Availability of cultural resources and opportunities to feel as if you belong	Cultural alienation
Availability of secure attachment opportunities	Loneliness, lack of attachment-derived self-regulation experiences
Absence of connection and belonging – availability of community	Experiences of social and cultural alienation associated with stigma if culture is not "main stream"
Personal economic resources	Poverty-linked loss/lack of status, hunger, lack of enjoyment
Level of crime in area moving to	Increased chances of being victim and also being reminded of being a victim in the past
Availability of work or meaningful education	Social alienation, loss of status
Trauma and diversity awareness of accommodation and probation services	Insensitivity resulting in lack of appropriate scaffolding and support
Absence of racism, sexism, homophobia, ableism	If these are present, then microaggressions will continue to accumulate and compound trauma linked with stigma and prejudice
Availability of meaningful crisis support	Resource loss spiral develops momentum quickly in initial stages
Absence of strong containing relationships	Feeling alone and boundaryless

In evolutionary terms, contexts can be classified as being dangerous and unpredictable, requiring a *fast* life history strategy or predictable requiring a *slow* one. Trauma responses and offending are often responses to unpredictable and dangerous contexts (Durrant, 2017). In unpredictable dangerous contexts, responses need to be quick. In the next section we turn to the psychological processes triggered by traumagenic contexts focusing specifically on shifts in agency and consciousness.

Endogenous Trauma-Linked Mechanisms: Offence-Related Altered States of Consciousness (ORASC)
Endogenous State Processes

Schmidt and Vermetten (2017) highlight the significance of altered states of consciousness in understanding the ways in which trauma operates. They conceptualise the impact of trauma on consciousness as involving *changes in the maintenance of consciousness*; on a "spectrum from feeling briefly disconnected from reality to losing consciousness, amnesic spells/gaps in memory" along with associated changes in behaviour on a "spectrum reaching from brief periods of absentmindedness to seizure like attacks (spectrum from intrusions to Psychogenic Non-Epileptic Seizures)" (p.80) driven by various brain networks, i.e., "networks mediating emotion regulation, awareness, executive/cognitive control, attention, self-referential processing, and motor functions". They highlight the "corticolimbic pathway as critical for these processes" (p.80) and problematic regulation of emotion resulting in either emotional numbing or unstable mood played out behaviourally through loss of interest or emotional instability.

The following quotes illustrate the significance of states of consciousness in the commission of offences.

> Both rapists said they felt badly about what they had done…They said that in their normal state of mind they could not comprehend how they could brutalise another human being. But they knew they would do it again if they were in the same emotional state of frustration and anger that preceded the rapes.
>
> *p.204*

> One of the rapists said that consideration of punishment would have made no difference because when he was in the state that led him to rape, nothing could stop him. He pointed out that after the rape he wept and despised himself for having brutalised another human being but, before the rape, concern for the victim and even his own welfare never occurred to him.
>
> *p.241; Epstein, 1982, cited in Gilbert (2013, 1989)*

These quotes capture a critical aspect of working with risk and safety with people who have experienced trauma and who have offended, that challenges one of the central assumptions behind interventions with this group in the past: the assumption of consistent agency. That is, the assumption that an individual's sense of, and capacity for, agency is consistent over time. Many therapies aim to work towards an individual admitting to themselves that they are/were an agent at the time of the offence and thereby acknowledging that they can choose not to behave in certain ways in the future. Whilst this is a desirable state of affairs in terms of trying to bring about change, what happens if the reality is different from this?

The mind operates in a heterogeneous array of states, not all of which are characterised by the same kinds of capacity for agency. The history of therapy is replete with accounts of trauma victims being told that their narratives are distorted in some way and people being told that they are lying, manipulative, or have been suggestible when they give accounts of trauma. The lesson from this history is, surely, that we need to take survivors' accounts more seriously, and accounts of loss of, or changes in conscious agency, as exemplified in these quotes, remind us of this imperative. We need to take accounts of different ways of thinking, feeling, seeing, and experiencing in different states of consciousness seriously. "It just happened" might mean that the person experienced this behaviour as not coming from the same source as their usual sense of agency. This doesnt, of course, mean that sometimes some people might not be telling the truth.

Katehakis (2016), in discussing compulsive sexual behaviour, cites the service user phrase "being in the bubble" as reflecting the way in which the mind is "hijacked" by dissociative fantasy states during episodes of compulsive sexual arousal. The phrase "being in a bubble" is commonly encountered when working with people who have offended also. It is useful to try and understand what is meant by this for each individual case. Katehakis characterises "being in the bubble" in relation to sexual compulsivity (frequently linked with early experiences of sexual abuse) as being linked with activation of evolved systems – the wanting, incentive or craving system, driven by dopamine, and the sexual arousal system. Associated with this is a state of anticipatory euphoria and a reduced ability to think and engage in executive activities – frontal lobe functions associated with thinking, planning, changing set, and perspective taking – as well as reduced ability to regulate or inhibit affective states. Fantasy, Katehakis argues, activates shifts in the state of consciousness linked with anticipatory craving (and euphoric recall) and reduced self-control.

Offence-related altered states of consciousness (ORASC) – contrasted with *normal waking consciousness* and *trauma-related altered states of consciousness* (NWC and TRASC: Frewen & Lanius, 2015) – are aimed at avoiding resource loss particularly, but not exclusively, in unpredictable dangerous contexts or contexts that remind the individual of past experiences of these, where frontal lobe functions involved with predicting future behaviour is less adaptive, by entering into a state of cognitive abeyance and social disconnection (see Jones, 2020c, on cognitive abeyance). In an ORASC, other people can become less important; feelings may no longer have the same pull on the individual (or certain emotions take on a motivational monopoly); the loss of resources linked with maintaining social contract with others is avoided as they are no longer emotionally significant to the individual.

In Chapter 13, the evidence for people being traumatised by their own offending is presented. The likelihood is that these experiences are a combination of current traumatic experience and past trauma experiences that are triggered prior to and during the offending process. In other words, TRASC and ORASC can actually be the same thing. TRASC and ORASC are states associated with evolved systems and reflect the underlying psychological processes whereby these systems impact on behaviour. When a context triggers a resource loss crisis or significant resource acquisition opportunity, different evolved systems are triggered and, once activated, impact on behaviour through system 1 processes (intuitive, automatic, unconscious, and effortless thinking, Kahneman, 2011; Toates, Smid, & van den Berg, 2017: see Table 3.5).

These shifts in state of consciousness are often linked with risk of offending (Moskowitz, 2004; Chapter 11). Jones (2016, 2020a, 2020c) argues that offending behaviour is often linked with ORASC. Corr and Morsella (2015) describe the central role that consciousness has in self-regulation, offering a unified perspective and facilitating agency. Changes in consciousness can involve different kinds of change in capacity to self-regulate in an agentic manner. These changes can also be linked with fragmentation in the experience of self and an associated range of different responses reflecting different parts of the self, linked with dissociative states. In behavioural terms these states can be conceptualised as establishing operations.

Table 3.5 Intrusive and agentic/deliberative processes

Intrusive automatic non-intentional system 1 processes reflecting adaptation to unpredictable dangerous "fast" contexts, or reminders of these	*Deliberative system 2 processes reflecting adaptation to predictable "slow" contexts*
Does not require working memory	Remembering in active manner (requires working memory)
Forgetting (thoughts, perceptions, feelings [interoception] and states)	Choosing
Amnesia	Willing, planning, generating options
Intrusive thoughts, rumination	Suppressing
Intrusive emotions, arousal, sexual arousal	Imagining, fantasising, "mentalising", empathising
Intrusive memories, flashbacks, reliving	Frontal lobe activation
Intrusive emotions	
Fear, anger, joy, disgust, shame, guilt	

⟵⟶ Shading into each other and interacting.

Fragmented autobiography	Flexible/showing plasticity
Overly general memory	Metacognition
Urges, cravings, impulses	Self-regulation
Anticipation	Mindfulness
Myopia	Attentional agility and capacity to shift set
Altered states of consciousness, including inhibition of system 2 processes, dissociation, attentional diffusion, or hyper focus	Being aware of self and others (and respective needs, minds, feelings, states)
Hypervigilance, fight, flight or freeze, numbing	
Frontal lobe decommissioned	
Sexual arousal (e.g., in context of being sexually abused) stereotypical/lacking plasticity	

The trauma literature highlights the way that trauma-linked shifts in state are linked with parasympathetic activation that is

> mediated by anaesthetic and dissociative neurochemicals, namely, endogenous opioids and endocannabinoids that reduce the perception of physical pain as well as emotional pain. Moreover, the release of these anaes- thetic neurochemicals results in a lowering of consciousness and interferes with the integration of information, for example, information processing. The organism is concerned with survival and minimizing the use of energy, and reflects the core of the dissociative experience.
>
> *Lanius, 2014; p.21*

It is no coincidence that substance misuse, with its associated altered states of con- sciousness (Lovern & Rock, 2021), is also linked both with managing distress linked with trauma but also "disinhibition" and an altered risk of offending.

Lanius (2014) writes

> In previously traumatized individuals, re-accessing reminders of traumatic events results in opioid activation... This opioid activation, if sufficiently strong, may not only result in a perceived lack of fear but it is also likely to produce amnesia, thus conferring a further barrier toward mounting active defensive responses such as fight or flight. That is, if there is no access to the memory of being traumatized, the likelihood of intentional defensive behavior will be much reduced.
>
> *p.96*

Durrant (2017) highlights lack of plasticity or responsiveness to the environment as a factor in the development of risk processes. Trauma and resourcelessness, past and present, activates processes that privilege system 1 (designed for "fast" evolu- tionary environments) based activity (Kahneman, 2011), accompanied by ORASC and deactivates system 2 ways of coping, all diminishing plasticity.

A systematic review by Couette, Mouchabac, Bourla, Nuss, and Ferreri (2020) concluded that that social cognition is comprehensively disturbed in individuals with a PTSD diagnosis. People with this diagnosis experience a reduced ability to mentalise what others think, feel, or believe; they can also be massively altered in their perception of basic emotional expressions in others and their capacity for affective empathy – all adaptations for survival in "fast" environments that are inevitably risk- inciting and counterproductive for safety planning. It is not clear however the extent to which the "deficits" they identify are state dependent.

Kyte, Jerram, and DiBiase (2020) describe the brain opioid theory of social attachment (BOTSA) and the way that ruptures in attachment can result in an increase in risk taking behaviour and difficulties in regulating behaviour. Trauma his- tories are identified as being associated with endogenous opiate systems exhibiting release patterns linked with surviving abusive contexts. LeRoy, Knee, Derrick, and Fagundes (2019) also highlight the patterns of behaviour linked with the trauma of loss. Leaving prison is, in some ways, a recapitulation of past loss experiences and will trigger this response, characterised by disorganisation followed by seeking behaviour (partially mediated by absence of endogenous opioids).

In the next section we turn to the significant ways in which people make sense of these experiences.

Evolved Systems and Attributing Meaning to the Disruption of Agency in Triggered States

From an evolutionary perspective, trauma reactions are responses deriving from evolved motivational systems aimed at survival and reproduction requiring social and material resources linked with significant shifts in states of consciousness. From a personal meaning perspective what is difficult about this is that the individual does not understand their reactions as being *evolved systems* and, what is more, often interprets the mechanisms whereby evolved systems have their impact, such as intrusive shifts in state, in an idiosyncratic and culturally flavoured way. "Why am I having intrusive thoughts about being sexually abused?" can be answered in a number of ways. In the absence of an evolutionary perspective the answer could be "because I want to" and then an explanation addressing the question "why do I want to?" is called for. Answers to this might be or include "because I enjoyed it" followed by questions about "why did I enjoy it?", often accompanied by feelings of self-disgust and shame.

The point here is that a significant component of the impact of trauma comes out of the way in which the individual, based on culture, makes sense of what are essentially unchosen reactions and emotions intruding on and changing their consciousness. A common attribution is that the thoughts have been chosen and that the unchosen reactions are attributable to the current situation. Kube, Berg, Kleim, and Herzog (2020) write "… based on an intense emotional reaction, the brain infers … that there must be a source of threat that explains the interoceptive state (i.e., 'I'm scared, therefore there must be something threatening')" (p.451).

There are two pathways when thinking about the impact of trauma: the conscious agentic deliberative pathway (e.g., "I am going to make sure that nobody does that to me again" or "I'm going to get revenge" or "why should I have to suffer and be abused when others aren't?") and an intrusive less conscious pathway that then has to be processed and made sense of. A bodily reaction that the individual might not attribute to being a memory, they simply have feelings e.g., of panic if it is the fear system, or sexual arousal if it is the sexual system. Figure 3.1 and Table 3.6 illustrate the kinds of meanings attributed to intrusive experiences.

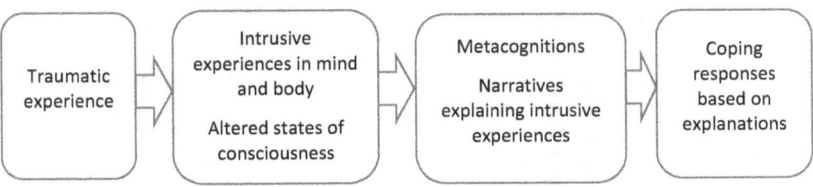

Figure 3.1 Process of interpreting intrusive trauma-related experiences

Table 3.6 Illustration of culturally driven interpretations of trauma-related intrusive experiences and shifts in state

Evolved system intrusive mechanism	Personal, culturally informed explanation for intrusion: answering the question "why is this happening to me?", "I'm having these thoughts and feelings because"	Personal, culturally informed, resolution belief	How this can be played out in behaviour
Intrusive thoughts, emotions, behaviours, states following sexual abuse	"there's something wrong with me"	"I need medical help" "I'm deeply flawed and defective"	Seeking medical solutions. Abdicating responsibility for self-regulation to medical people
	"I must want to think about it"	"I hate myself for wanting to think about it so much""I have to do something to myself to stop/punish this"	Self-harm, self-sabotage, internalised enactment of abusive behaviour, punishing others perceived as victims who "wanted" to be abused
	Body experiences sexual feelings and states of dissociation deriving from the traumatic experience	"I want it and other people also want this because it was "enjoyable"" "Everybody secretly is behaving like this" "Pleasure is 'good' or 'right' pain is 'bad'"	Offending based on the belief or self-deception that the victim will "enjoy" it and won't be harmed by it
	"I want to get revenge"	"I won't feel better until I have had revenge"	Vengeful attacks
Intrusive thoughts, emotions, behaviours, states following violent abuse	"I need to remind myself never to let it happen again"	"I'm going to make up for 'letting it happen' by never 'letting it happen' again" "if I attack first then I can stop these thoughts/feelings from coming/continuing" "people who don't fight are weak and deserve to be attacked"	Hypervigilance and being easily triggered, pattern of pre-emptive assaults, seeking positions of dominance as a way of protecting self/ feeling safe, using sexual "dominance" as a way of securing self-perception as indomitable

Category	Cognitions / emotions / states	Beliefs	Behaviours / risks
Intrusive thoughts, emotions, behaviours, states following emotional abuse	"I need to remind myself about how bad I am in case I forget" / "If I am tough with others I will" / "It's happening again"	"I deserved to be punished and I don't deserve to have a life because I am so bad" / "attack or flee"	Self-harm / Self-destructive behaviour including substance misuse and offending / Attack / Take control to feel safe / Act this out in sexual contexts
	"Everyone hates me" / "Nobody loves me" / "I am unlovable"	"I have to make everyone like me" / "The only way I can have relationships is to force or trap people so they have no choice"	Over compliance and fawning leading to offending when done with perpetrators / Sexual and domestic violence and abuse
Intrusive thoughts, emotions, behaviours, states following exposure to drink, drugs, pornography	"I enjoy thinking about using, so it must be good" / "People who want to stop me are scared and jealous of my fun" / Anticipatory arousal and craving states	"I must use drugs/pornography to feel better" / "Other people should use drugs too – in order to feel good"	Drug use / Pornography use / Dealing and offering others drugs and illegal pornography
Intrusive thoughts, emotions, behaviours, states following loss, rejection and abandonment	"This person 'made me' feel bad" / "They did it on purpose because: / I'm bad, worthless / They hate me / They're bad	"If I'm bad I may as well act bad" / "Hurt, neglect, reject myself" / "Make sure the next relationship doesn't end the same way"	Impulsive futurelessness / Assaults on rejecting figures (real or imagined)

Different cultures have more or less nuanced ways of understanding and/or working with these kinds of experience. From an interventions perspective there is much that could be achieved by stepping away from a Eurocentric approach to consciousness and by learning from other cultures about how to make sense of these experiences and cope with them.

Lived Experience of Trauma- and Offence-Related Altered States of Consciousness (ORASC)

From a trauma responsive risk management/safety planning perspective it is important to recognise trauma symptoms/reactions as early warning signs for the peri–offending platform, i.e., an interpersonal and intrapersonal context in which the ingredients of an offending response can develop. Shifts in mental state characteristic of the individual's offence process need to be identified and worked with.

In Barry's account an actual account from a service user (see Table 3.7) he talks about the "red mist"; this describes two processes: a dissociative process where he

Table 3.7 Case material analysis "Barry" illustrating trauma- and offence-related altered states of consciousness (ORASC)

Narrative (from an actual account)	Comments on shift in state	Possible associated neuropsychological processes
Just after unlocking, like I've got into a red mist... you've become that angry person, you're in a red mist, you can't see your options; you know how a horse can't see outside it's blinkers when it's trotting down the road, basically can't see its options, can't see or think clearly and up ...and end up in seclusion.	The antecedents to this were experiences of rejection and being humiliated by a "peer" that triggered trauma memories of rejection and humiliation. These triggered the attachment system and fear systems as well as a sense of shame and need for status reparation. He describes a shift into an altered state of consciousness he calls the "red mist" and describes it in terms of "not seeing" options, "not seeing" outside, and not seeing or thinking clearly. The account also reflects his ability to step back and become aware of his myopia retrospectively.	Activation of evolved systems linked with attachment, safety, and status. Trauma memories activated as bodily and state shifting processes. Altered states of consciousness are linked with mu opioid (and possibly endocannabinoids) and noradrenaline activity; corticolimbic dynamics and ventral vagal, dorsal vagal, and parasympathetic functioning also shift. Alongside this, the shift in state reflects an inaccessibility of thinking capacities associated with frontal lobe executive functioning.

Table 3.7 Cont.

Narrative (from an actual account)	Comments on shift in state	Possible associated neuropsychological processes
I become so impulsive, it's like I had fallout with a peer, all of a sudden red mist hit me, I punched the wall, I punched the window of the office, hit me, until I realised it because how I, how I'm changing I've met some big challenges and made some big changes.	He describes the suddenness of onset of a shift from not being "impulsive" to a state where he is hitting the wall and the window. The emotion of anger is disinhibited and, initially, he doesn't "realise it" i.e., he isn't conscious of himself in the process.	Limbic system is dysregulated in the absence of executive emotional-regulation.
I do try and pause and rationalise and look at options.	Beginning to shift back into a more deliberative state where thinking is more possible.	Executive functioning beginning to be re-instated.
Sometimes it's overwhelming; that's when I look for other people and get peer support. I've come a long way with peer support… peer support, they try and talk me down with 'just think of the changes you've made, if you do this you'll undo the progress that you've made, all that hard work' they give you thinking time in a way; it's distracting you from that red mist, so you are forgetting about the red mist; I've got a better understanding. I have made big changes with psychology and others.	Description of using social contact and interaction as a way of self-regulating and overcoming his feeling of being overwhelmed.	Triggering social attachment systems as a way of managing the fear system. This then helping to reinforce activation of executive functioning.
red mist is like you run out of options and other relapse prevention skills as well.	An account of loss of agency and sense of choice.	Executive functioning loss described.
I have that little pause button, I break um I stop it before I've exploded".	The pause button is his ability to emotionally self-regulate.	Frontal lobe functioning linked with inhibiting emotional arousal.

loses contact with reality – in the mist you cannot see what is around you – that he specifies as being blinkered, not being able to think of options, and a dysregulated anger process. This is a state then where the problem-solving capacity – frontal lobe functioning – is decommissioned and he is simply left with his anger. This is a kind of behavioural *establishing operation* or schema mode, an unthinking state characterised by impulsive behaviour. In this state the individual experiences themselves as being optionless and futureless (Kerig & Becker, 2010). Emotionless or numb states linked with high frontal inhibition of limbic activity, or emotional "dysregulation" linked with frontal hypoactivity, are critical states to monitor.

Dynamic risk processes require dynamic shifts in state. In neuropsychological terms this means *shifts in function over time*, not simply structural deficits which would be more continuous in nature. Dynamic shifts may therefore be associated with neuro-chemical changes in time as opposed to longer term neuronal changes; however, neurochemical changes can have a longer term impact on structure.

Assessment and Intervention

Layne, Steinberg, and Steinberg (2014) offer a simple heuristic diagram for thinking about the ways in which we can intervene (see Figure 3.2).

The strength of this causal modelling approach is that it highlights a range of different sites of intervention in the causal sequence. When thinking about trauma-derived factors leading into possible offending, the risk factors are the "exogenous" processes and altered states are one kind of mediating mechanism, discussed in this chapter.

Intervention and assessment should, based on this analysis, focus on:

• Assessing and intervening with the context, e.g., how abusive, impoverished, exposed to violence, culturally insensitive, racist, sexist, homophobic, unsafe, emotionally abusive, socially isolating, or lacking opportunities for social contact they are.

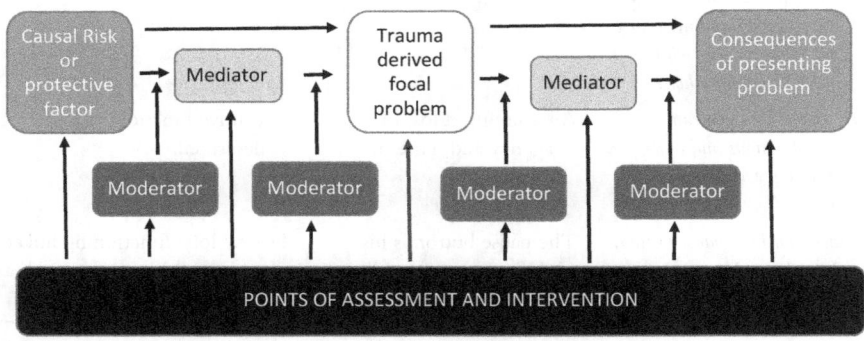

Figure 3.2 Causal model diagram of targets of assessment, intervention, and pathways of influence adapted from Layne, Steinberg, and Steinberg (2014)

- Offering social support and connection opportunities to protect the individual from the impact of trauma-triggering processes.
- Assessing the availability of resources of all kinds in the post-release context – particularly just after release which can be seen as a potentially significant precipitating/triggering experience requiring intensive input to prevent rapid deterioration.
- Assessing for offence-related trauma triggers and associated state repertoire.
- Assessing endogenous resources for managing triggers, dissociation, skills in re-establishing executive functioning or offsetting cognitive abeyance.
- Assessing use of artificially induced altered states, used to cope, that might facilitate offending processes.
- Assessing and intervening with people whilst they are in an offence paralleling altered state, to enable understanding of the dynamics of the state and facilitate state dependent learning.

Recent thinking about the ways in which trauma and adversity impact on memory, shaped through narrative, points to a rethinking of ways in which people have agency. Complex trauma is associated with a variety of memory changes. There is a loss of experienced agency in relation to intrusive thoughts, flashbacks, fight or flight reactions: people enter into, more or less conscious, passive or passenger states, where other sources of action, less driven by agency, "take over".

Psychological processes that have evolved to ensure survival in dangerous, unpredictable, "fast" situations, where there is little time to think, intrude on normal waking consciousness. It is this challenge to the conceptualisation of the self as having agency that is both difficult for traditional models of psychotherapy and offers the chance of innovative ways of working that do not focus on talking alone.

Other ways in which trauma challenges traditional concepts of agency include a recognition of the fundamentally social aspect of the capacity to think and choose. Thinking is something that happens in states of relationship rather than alone; thinking alone is significantly shaped by internalised working models of others (Leedom, 2014). The capacity to think and problem solve is enhanced when it is exercised in the context of relationship. So, one way of conceptualising the impacts of trauma and adversity is to see it as being about the disruption of social scaffolding internal and external to the capacity to create reflective spaces where thinking, generating possibilities, conceptualising other people's reactions and one's own reactions become less possible.

The critical difference linked with this way of conceptualising problems is that *self as agent* becomes *self as passive passenger* or indeed *self as absent*, whilst a way of behaving that has been shaped over millions of years and is often very similar to those of other mammals, takes precedent.

Clinically then, it is imperative for the individual to develop awareness and skills and capacities that can be used *in the context of different states* of mind. The task has to be one in which the problem of both acquisition of skills and executive functioning for directing the delivery of those skills become important issues. When an individual does not work in these ways with these alternative aspects of themselves it is possible that they find themselves reacting in unthinking and prototypically driven patterns of behaviour that are congruent with whatever system has been triggered.

Another aspect of an individual that is foregrounded by this perspective is the possibilities of an individual not being cohesive and just "one person"; it is possible to think of an individual as having a multiplicity of selves, often contradictory, that are linked with different states and different patterns of interacting and relating. Each one of these states and ways of interacting needs to be worked with. Each part becomes a relevant contributor to the overall task of developing improved capacity for self-management and choice. We end up working with different parts or sub personalities, trying to work out a way in which each one of these parts can be understood and incorporated into an overall solution to the individuals' problems (Di Fulvio, 2019; Schwartz, 2016).

The process whereby an evolved system takes hold of an individual's activity needs to be one in which normal experiences of everyday waking consciousness and agency are displaced by more automatic or unchosen states, feelings, thoughts, and behaviours that are congruent with the evolve system. People often describe these processes in a way that captures the passive aspect: "it felt as if I was in the back seat", "it just happened", "I just watched myself doing it", "I forgot what happened" and "I just found myself in the situation afterwards, it just happened". These are kinds of accounts that reflect the individual's attempts to make sense of the experience of evolved systems taking hold of consciousness. They are used in accounts of trauma **and** in accounts of offending; both contexts where dissociation can occur – due to current events or due to triggered past reminders.

The capacity to self-regulate is often construed as intentionally relinquished because this avoids a narrative which is based on a radical shift in mental state and "not being myself". Often the eruption of an evolve system into an individual's behaviour is linked with a way of being social. The fear system for example can shift the individual either into a state of unheeding self-interest or highly dependent seeking for another person to take the role of decider or chooser – safe base in attachment terms – on their behalf. So, it is clear that each evolved system has definite social contextual implications; assessment and intervention of dynamic risk needs to take both of these domains seriously and focus on the nuanced social constructions each individual has of these states derived from the cultures in which they are developed.

Conclusion

Hopefully this chapter has challenged the reader to think about risk through a trauma-informed lens. The importance of assessing and intervening with resources loss and resource privation processes inside the individual and outside the individual has been highlighted. The historical neglect of the contextual powerlessness (lack of resources) of people in understanding offending has led to a neglect of the social responsibility to address this in terms of prevention and change. This social responsibility for preventing offending won't be acknowledged unless it is articulated and assessed. As psychologists we therefore need to be identifying exactly what kinds of resources will be needed when people are released. The requirements from contexts into which people are placed need to be taken seriously and identified. Placing somebody in a bedsit or in a hostel with a negligible income, without the prospect of getting work easily, with no support, with well-intentioned staff who do not have a trauma-informed or diversity-informed perspective, where there is no specialist support for people triggered by current experiences of adversity, and possibly punitive interpretations of ORASC – e.g., thinking they are reacting because they are "evil" or "bloody minded" or "mad" or "inhuman"– is unfair on the person being released and on those providing care for them.

In the future it is hoped that a more nuanced understanding of the kinds of altered states people experience in the context of trauma-related offending can be articulated and researched, along with a more culturally literate, anti-racist, and non-biased approach to understanding and working with the ways that different people make sense of these states in different cultures.

Further Reading

Jones, L. F. (2020a). Violence risk formation: The move towards collaboratively produced, strengths-based safety planning. In Wormith, S., Hogue, T. & Craig, L. (Eds), *The Wiley handbook of what works in violence risk* (pp.99–118).

Putnam, F. W. (2016). *The way we are: How states of mind influence our identities, personality and potential for change*. International psychoanalytic books.

Wiley.Layne, C. M., & Hobfoll, S. (2020). Understanding post-traumatic adjustment trajectories in school-age youth: Supporting stress resistance, resilient recovery, and growth. In E., Rossen (Ed.), *Supporting and educating traumatized students: A guide for school-based professionals* (pp.75–97). Oxford University Press.

References

Arnhart, L. (1998). *Darwinian natural right: The biological ethics of human nature*. State University of New York Press.

Baskin-Sommers, A., Chang, S. A., Estrada, S., & Chan, L. (2021). Toward targeted interventions: Examining the science behind interventions for youth who offend. *Annual Review of Criminology*. Retrieved from www.annualreviews.org/doi/abs/10.1146/annurev-criminol-030620-023027 on August 2021.

Briere, J. (2019). *Treating risky and compulsive behavior in trauma survivors*. Guilford.

Case, S. (2021). Challenging the reductionism of "evidence-based" youth justice. *Sustainability, 13*, 1735. doi:10.3390/su13041735

Cloitre, M., Cohen, L. R., Ortigo, K. M., Jackson, C., & Koenen, K. C. (2020). *Treating survivors of childhood abuse and interpersonal trauma: STAIR narrative therapy*. Guilford Publications.

Corr, P. J., & Morsella, E. (2015). The conscious control of behavior: Revisiting Gray's comparator model. In P. J., Corr, M., Fajkowska, M. W., Eysenck & A., Wytykowska (Eds), *Personality and control*, vol. 4 (pp.15–42).

Couette M., Mouchabac S., Bourla A., Nuss P., & Ferreri F. (2020). Social cognition in post-traumatic stress disorder: A systematic review. *British Journal of Clinical Psychology, 59*, 117–138. doi:10.1111/bjc.12238

Del Giudice, M. (2020). Rethinking the fast-slow continuum of individual differences. *Evolution and Human Behavior, 41*(6), 536–549. doi:10.1016/j.evolhumbehav.2020.05.004

Di Fulvio, E. (2019). *Alternative paradigms in correctional treatment: Internal family systems and the risk –need–responsivity model* (unpublished masters thesis). Pacifica Graduate Institute.

Durrant, R. (2017). Why do protective factors protect? An evolutionary developmental perspective. *Aggression and Violent Behavior, 32*, 4–10. doi:10.1016/j.avb.2016.12.002

Epstein, S. (1982). The unconscious, the preconscious and the self-concept. In J. Suls and A.G. Greenberg (Eds) *Psychological perspectives on the self.* Lawrence Erlbaum Associates.

Frewen, P. A., & Lanius, R. A. (2015). *Healing the traumatized self: Consciousness, neuroscience, and treatment.* W.W. Norton.

Gilbert, P. (1989). *Human nature and suffering.* Lawrence Erlbaum Associates Ltd.

Gilbert, P. (2013). An evolutionary and compassion-focused approach to dissociation. In Kennedy, F., Kennerley, H. & Pearson, D. (Eds), *Cognitive behavioural approaches to the understanding and treatment of dissociation* (190–205). Routledge.

Gilbert, P. (2020). Evolutionary functional analysis: The study of social mentalities, social rank and caring-compassion. In Kirby, J. N. & Gilbert, P. (Eds), *Making an impact on mental health.* (pp.4–42). Routledge.

Hobfoll, S. E. (2012a). Conservation of resources theory: Its implication for stress, health, and resilience. In S., Folkman (Ed.), *The Oxford handbook of stress, health, and coping* (pp.127–147). Oxford University Press.

Hobfoll, S. E. (2012b). Conservation of resources and disaster in cultural context: The caravans and passageways for resources. *Psychiatry: Interpersonal and Biological Processes, 75*(3), 226–231. doi:10.1521/psyc.2012.75.3.227

Hobfoll, S. E., Horsey, K. J., & Lamoureux, B. E. (2009). Resiliency and resource loss in times of terrorism and disaster: Lessons learned for children and families and those left untaught. In D., Brom, R., Pat- Horenczyk & J. D., Ford (Eds), *Treating traumatized children: Risk, resilience and recovery* (pp.150–163). Routledge/Taylor & Francis.

Hodge, J. E., McMurran, M., & Hollin, C. R. (1997). *Addicted to crime?* Wiley.

Jones, L. F. (2015). The Peaks unit: from a pilot for 'untreatable' psychopaths to trauma-informed milieu therapy. *Prison Service Journal, 218*, 17–23.

Jones, L. F. (2016). *Conceptualising trauma informed care in forensic settings.* British Psychological Society Division of Clinical Psychology and Division of Forensic Psychology, joint meeting. Winchester.

Jones, L. F. (2020a). Violence risk formation: The move towards collaboratively produced, strengths-based safety planning. In Wormith, S., Hogue, T. & Craig, L. (Eds), *The Wiley handbook of what works in violence risk* (pp.99–118). Wiley. doi:10.1002/9781119315933.ch5

Jones, L. F. (2020b). Treatment approaches to trauma for those convicted of sexual crime: Interventions globally. In H., Swaby, B., Winder, R., Lievesley, K., Hocken, N., Blagden & P., Banyard (Eds), *Sexual crime and trauma* (pp.1–32). Palgrave.

Jones, L. F. (2020c). Trauma, adverse experiences, and offence-paralleling behaviour in the assessment and management of sexual interest. In G., Akerman, D., Perkins & R. M., Bartels (Eds), *Assessing and managing problematic sexual interests: A practitioner's guide* (pp.251–274). Routledge. doi:10.4324/9780429287695

Kahneman, D. (2011). *Thinking fast and slow.* Farrar, Straus and Giroux.

Katehakis, A. (2016). *Sex addiction as affect dysregulation: A neurobiologically informed Holistic Treatment.* Norton.

Kerig, P. K., & Becker, S. P. (2010). From internalizing to externalizing: Theoretical models of the processes linking PTSD to juvenile delinquency. In S. J., Egan (Ed.), *Posttraumatic stress disorder (PTSD): Causes, symptoms and treatment* (pp.33–78). Nova Science Publishers.

Kube, T., Berg, M., Kleim, B., & Herzog, P. (2020). Rethinking post-traumatic stress disorder – A predictive processing perspective. *Neuroscience & Biobehavioral Reviews, 113*, 448–460. doi:10.1016/j.neubiorev.2020.04.014

Kyte, D., Jerram, M., & DiBiase, R. (2020). Brain opioid theory of social attachment: A review of evidence for approach motivation to harm. *Motivation Science, 6*, 12–20.

Lanius, U. F. (2014). Dissociation and endogenous opioids: A foundational role. In U. F., Lanius, S. L., Paulsen & F. M., Corrigan (Eds), *Neurobiology and treatment of traumatic dissociation: Toward an embodied self* (pp.81–104). Springer Publishing Company.

Layne, C. M., Briggs, E. C., & Courtois, C. A. (2014). Introduction to the special section: Using the trauma history profile to unpack risk factor caravans and their consequences. *Psychological Trauma: Theory, Research, Practice, and Policy, 6*(Supplement 1), S1–S8. doi:10.1037/a0037768

Layne, C. M., & Hobfoll, S. (2020). Understanding post-traumatic adjustment trajectories in school-age youth: Supporting stress resistance, resilient recovery, and growth. In E., Rossen (Ed.), *Supporting and educating traumatized students: A guide for school-based professionals* (pp.75–97). Oxford University Press.

Layne, C. M., Steinberg, J. R., & Steinberg, A. M. (2014). Causal reasoning skills training for mental health practitioners: Promoting sound clinical judgment in evidence-based practice. *Training and Education in Professional Psychology, 8*, 292–302. doi:10.1037/tep0000037

Leedom, L. J. (2014). Human social behavioral systems: Ethological framework for a unified theory. *Human Ethology Bulletin, 29*, 39–65.

LeRoy, A. S., Knee, C. R., Derrick, J. L., & Fagundes, C. P. (2019). Implications for reward processing in differential responses to loss: Impacts on attachment hierarchy reorganization. *Personality and Social Psychology Review, 23*, 391–405. doi:10.1177/1088868319853895

Liotti, G. (2017). Conflicts between motivational systems related to attachment trauma: Key to understanding the intra-family relationship between abused children and their abusers. *Journal of Trauma & Dissociation, 18*(3), 304–318. doi:10.1080/15299732.2017.1295392

Lovern, J., & Rock, S. (2021). Beyond craving: Cue-induced dissociative state switches in substance use disorders. *Journal of Psychoactive Drugs, 53*(1), 35–39. doi:10.1080/02791072.2020.1800873

Mayson, S. G. (2019). Bias in, bias out. *Yale Law Journal, 128*, 2218.

Moskowitz, A. (2004). Dissociation and violence: A review of the literature. *Trauma, Violence, and Abuse, 5*, 21–46. doi:10.1177/1524838003259321

Panksepp, J. (1998). *Affective neuroscience: The foundations of human and animal emotions.* Oxford University Press.

Putnam, F. W. (2016). *The way we are: How states of mind influence our identities, personality and potential for change.* International psychoanalytic books.

Schmidt, U., & Vermetten, E. (2017). Integrating NIMH research domain criteria (RDoC) into PTSD research. In M. A., Geyer, B. A., Ellenbroek, C. A., Marsden, T. R. E., Barnes & S. L., Andersen (Eds), *Current topics in behavioral neurosciences* (pp.1–23). Springer.

Schwartz, R. C. (2016). Perpetrator parts. In M., Sweezy & E. L., Ziskind (Eds), *Innovations and elaborations in internal family systems therapy.* Routledge.

Stein, J. Y., Wilmot, D. V., & Solomon, Z. (2016). Does one size fit all? Nosological, clinical, and scientific implications of variations in PTSD Criterion A. *Journal of Anxiety Disorders, 43*, 106–117. doi:10.1016/j.janxdis.2016.07.001

Toates, F., Smid, W., & van den Berg, J. W. (2017). A framework for understanding sexual violence: Incentive-motivation and hierarchical control. *Aggression & Violent Behavior, 34*, 238–253. doi: 10.1016/j.avb.2017.01.001

Ward, T. (2002). Good lives and the rehabilitation of offenders: Promises and problems. *Aggression and Violent Behavior, 7*, 513–528. doi:10.1016/S1359-1789(01)00076-3

Ward, T. (2021). Why theoretical literacy is essential for forensic research and practice. *Criminal Behaviour and Mental Health. 31*, 1–4. doi:10.1002/cbm.2170

Ward, T. & Siegert, R. J. (2002). Toward a comprehensive theory of child sexual abuse: A theory knitting perspective. *Psychology, Crime and Law, 8*(4), 319–351. doi:10.1080/10683160208401823

Woldgabreal, Y., Day, A., & Tamatea, A. (2020). Do risk assessments play a role in the enduring 'color line'? *Advancing Corrections, 10*, 18–28.

4

TRAUMA, PERSONALITY DISORDER, AND OFFENDING

Louise Sainsbury

When working with adults who have offended and been given a diagnosis of personality disorder (PD), it quickly becomes apparent that the majority have experienced multiple traumas. First experiences of traumas are frequently perpetrated by their primary attachment figures, often in the context of significant adversity e.g., domestic violence, substance misuse, poverty, social and economic inequality, discrimination, homelessness, criminality, and the care system. What these words do not describe is the overwhelming experience of terror, rejection, betrayal, loss, helplessness, shame, rage, and insecurity of what is home. Across the reported histories of many individuals is the frequent reporting of general behavioural difficulties in childhood, including difficult temperament, "temper tantrums", running away, aggression, violence, stealing, and substance misuse. Frequently they are labelled as "difficult to manage" children and given diagnoses of oppositional disorder, conduct disorder, Attention Deficit Hyperactivity Disorder (ADHD), and emerging personality disorder that are apparently independent of what has happened to them.

Many individuals were placed in the care of the local authority, increasing the insecurity in their lives, and their "difficult behaviours" often resulted in frequent changes of children's homes and foster family placements. One of the many tragic descriptions I read was of a patient who after six weeks with a foster family was removed because his behaviour had not changed quickly enough; he was eight years old and had already suffered multiple adverse attachments and abuses. Patients have talked about being taken into care and their behaviour "returning to normal" because they were safe, and then being placed back with the family member who had abused them. Most frequently, patients have spoken about how they were not asked "what happened to you?"

This chapter first explores the relationships between childhood trauma, the diagnosis of personality disorder (PD), and offending. Next, a service user's narrative understanding of his pathways from childhood traumas to offending is presented.

DOI: 10.4324/9781003120766-6

Finally, psychological approaches to treatment and requirements of services are discussed. First a note on the diagnosis of PD. UK forensic mental health services are structured around psychiatric diagnoses and a diagnosis or significant traits of PD is frequently the only way individuals gain access to services. The diagnosis of PD has been criticised in terms of its validity and reliability (Livesley, 1998; Ramon, Castillo, & Morant, 2001) and the negative judgements that are frequently held about individuals who are given this diagnosis (Lam, Poplavskaya, Salkovskis, Hogg, & Panting, 2016). A consensus statement for people with complex mental health problems stated that

> If used wholly appropriately, the term personality disorder has some merit in providing a shorthand expression for people who suffer a long-standing pattern of emotional and cognitive difficulties, which interferes with many parts of their everyday life including their relationships, work and social functioning
>
> *Lamb, Sibbald, & Stirzaker, 2018, p.2*

In this chapter I will use the term "given a diagnosis of personality disorder" as it is neutral as to the value or legitimacy of the label and reflects the fact that a psychiatric diagnosis was *given* by others, but not necessarily accepted by the person. I take a position of understanding personality and PD as including neurobiological, somatic, emotional, attentional, cognitive, and behavioural patterns and impacting on sense of self and others and patterns of relating that have varying degrees of fluidity and adaptability, depending on what happened to individuals, their families, and communities.

Studies have reported that individuals given a diagnosis of PD typically report significantly higher rates of childhood traumas compared to community populations and individuals diagnosed with other psychiatric conditions (Battle et al., 2004). The majority of studies have focused on individuals given a diagnosis of borderline PD (BPD: Afifi et al., 2011), reporting rates of childhood trauma as high as 90%, and antisocial PD (ASPD: DeLisi, Drury, & Elbert, 2019). There have been a few studies of other PD diagnoses, including paranoid, avoidant, dependent, and obsessive-compulsive, that have reported higher rates of childhood traumas than that general population (e.g., Tyrka, Wyche, Kelly, Price, & Carpenter, 2009). These studies are limited by the problems with the diagnosis of PD and the overlap of symptom criteria across the subtypes of PD (Tyrer, 2005).

Childhood traumas, adverse attachments, and adversity have been shown to affect the development of all systems that come under the rubric of *personality* (Briere, Hodges, & Godbout, 2010), so it is unsurprising that high rates of trauma are reported by individuals who have been given a diagnosis of PD (Battle et al., 2004). Conversely, having one trusted adult always available has been found to be significant feature of resilience in the face of increasing adversity, particularly for emotional well-being (Bellis et al., 2017).

Whilst high rates of childhood traumas and adversities have been consistently found, a proportion of individuals who had been given a diagnosis of PD did not report childhood traumas. Studies have examined the role of genetics to the aetiology of PD diagnoses, predominantly BPD and to a lesser extent ASPD, with heritability estimates ranging between 40% and 50% for BPD (Luyten, Campbell, & Fonagy, 2020). Much of this research has been carried out using self- or third-party report questionnaires to assess PD traits and temperament, which limits the capacity to disentangle what is temperament and what is the impact of trauma. Later studies have reported that genetics accounts for a declining amount of the variance with increased exposure to traumatic life events (Luyten et al., 2020). Reviews have noted limitations in this area including categorical assessment of PDs and limited reference to problems with PD diagnoses. Boyle and Johnstone (2020) have detailed other forms of adversity, e.g., negative forms of power including gender, race, economic, and ideological, which they argue can provide part of the reason why people who have not suffered obvious trauma experience significant emotional distress. There is evidence that repeated "small T" experiences – being in the out-group, micro aggressions that communicate negative messages, e.g., you are stupid, unwanted, bad – lead to the same physical, emotional, and social consequences as "big T" trauma (Perry, podcast communication in Brown, 2021).

Childhood Traumas and Offending

Individuals who have offended have been found to have far higher rates of childhood traumas, adverse attachments, and adversity than the general population. Studies have consistently found rates of between 50–70% for diagnoses of PD in forensic populations (Fazel & Danesh, 2002). Studies have found that accumulating traumas and adverse childhood experiences contribute to the most serious, violent, and chronic offending (Craig, Piquero, Farrington, & Ttofi, 2017). As noted in Chapter 1, there has been increasing focus on the multiple ways in which childhood traumas can be causal factors for offending. Howard and McMurran (2012) have argued that examining *PD traits* has greater potential for conceptualising the relationships between PD and offending, including impulsiveness, dysregulation of emotions, attitudes to violence, and problem-solving abilities. There is significant consistency across (1) areas of functioning that are affected by childhood trauma and adversity, (2) PD diagnostic traits, and (3) dynamic risk factors (DRFs), e.g., impulsivity, cognitive and emotional regulation, difficulties relating to self and others, and with stress and coping. This is consistent with recent critique of DRFs that these factors are broad concepts that represent a multitude of inter- and intra-personal systems (Ward, 2016).

No specific associations between types of childhood trauma, diagnoses of PD, and types of offending have been found (Altintas & Bilici, 2018). It appears that other factors (e.g., age of victim, chronicity, relationship to perpetrator, available support, protective factors) and the meaning of childhood traumas and adversities specific to the individual are more significant in understanding the pathways to offending behaviours. As summarised in Chapter 1, there are numerous potential relationships between childhood trauma and DRFs, and the identification of specific pathways at an individual level is required to understand the relationships between childhood traumas and adverse attachments, the resulting survival strategies that are subsequently given a diagnosis of PD, and offending.

There are obvious links between the impact of childhood trauma and adversity on the development of self and PD diagnostic traits such as beliefs that others will harm, not protect or nurture, and of themselves as bad, weak, unlovable, and the patterns of coping, that can be formulated as contributing to an individual attempting to gain primary good/basic needs through offending. For example, the experience that the majority of people during childhood harmed you and the feelings of being weak and helpless, can result in learning to gain safety and feelings of strength and powerfulness through violence to fend off would be attackers and avoid feeling or showing vulnerability. This may represent changes in the initial survival adaptations to childhood trauma, e.g., emotional numbing and dissociation may subsequently come to support the suppression of vulnerability and disconnection from emotions that is a factor in later offending. The unique and changing responses of the individual are recognised as arising from interactions between the nature and duration of adverse attachments, trauma, and adversity, the age ranges in which these were experienced, the meaning to the individual, and presence of exacerbating or attenuating factors and that neurobiological response patterns appear to change with age (Perry, Pollard, Blakley, Baker, & Vigilante, 1995).

There has been a focus on understanding the motivations for offending using theories of human motivation e.g., the Good Lives Model (GLM: Ward & Stewart, 2003). The GLM proposes that individuals seek to meet their needs for primary goods (safety, freedom from emotional distress, belonging, autonomy, competence, etc.) and formulates DRFs as aspects of persons and their environments which indicate a higher probability that these goal-directed actions will involve crime (Heffernan, Wegerhoff, & Ward, 2019). This highlights the need to use theories of personality development and functioning, including the impact of childhood trauma.

Impact of Childhood Traumas on Personality Development

Childhood traumas, adverse attachments, and adversity have been found to negatively impact on the development of individuals' neurobiological, affect regulation, somatic, attentional, impulse control, cognitive, relational, self/identity, and behavioural systems (e.g., Anda et al., 2006; D'Andrea, Ford, Stolbach, Spinazzola, & van der Kolk, 2012; Streeck-Fischer & van der Kolk, 2000). These difficulties frequently result in attention deficits, hyperactivity, hypervigilance to threat, impaired mentalisation ability, somatisation, and aggression against self and others (e.g., Streeck-Fischer & van der Kolk, 2000; van der Kolk, 2014). There is a strong consistency between these areas and the diagnostic criteria for PDs, including difficulties with attention, impulse control, emotions, beliefs and thoughts, behaviours, sense of self and others, and patterns of relating to self and others. The symptoms of PD can be understood to have developed as survival mechanisms to minimise threat and regulate emotional distress. This is consistent with the Power Threat Meaning Framework (Boyle & Johnstone, 2020) for understanding a diagnosis of PD as survival adaptations that have become unhelpful and damaging.

Threat, Safety, and Attachment Theory

Attachment theory is an empirically based theory of how normal emotional, psychological, and behavioural development occurs through interactions with the infant's attachment figures (Ainsworth, Blehar, Waters, & Wall, 1978; Bowlby, 1969/1982). Attachment theory has evidenced that children, beginning in infancy, attempt to survive adverse attachments though adapting to their attachment figures to meet their basic needs (primary goods), primarily safety and emotional regulation. In childhood, these resilient survival strategies are internalised as stable representations of self and others that drive patterns of reacting and relating. The nature of childhood traumas and adversity means that there is a lack of emotional and psychological understanding (attunement) that is the necessary relational means by which children internalise secure (healthy) emotional and cognitive understanding (mentalisation) that are central to healthy development.

Attachment theory proposes that through the repeated experiences of attunement and repair of misattunements from (secure) attachment figures, infants' experience being accepted, understood and their basic needs met, and people as safe and predictable. This forms the basis of emotional regulation, in which all emotions are acceptable and tolerable (Bowlby, 1988). These repeated experiences are initially encoded in procedural memory as felt experience. As language develops a parallel system of verbal understanding of self and others develops (Lyons-Ruth, 1999). Insecure, frightening, abusive, and neglecting attachment figures do not provide the safety necessary for healthy development, and infants adapt to maintain proximity to the attachment figure to gain some degree of safety by excluding aspects of themselves which are not acceptable. Three insecure attachment styles have been identified: *avoidant/dismissive* in which emotions and need for others are excluded and independence valued; *ambivalent/preoccupied* in which independence and exploration is excluded and emotions and needs are expressed to maintain the attachment relationship; and *disorganised* characterised by a seemingly chaotic mix of approach and avoidance behaviours, such as walking towards the attachment figure whilst looking away (Hesse & Main, 2000) and high levels of dissociation that represents the unresolvable dilemma of seeking safety from the source of anxiety. Insecure attachment styles are associated with adverse parenting and the disorganised attachment style is more strongly associated with childhood trauma and neglect by attachment figures. High rates of insecure attachment style have been reported for individuals who report a trauma history, those who have offended or been given a diagnosis of PD (Bakermans-Kranenburg & van IJzendoorn, 2009; Hudson & Ward, 1997). In adolescence and adulthood these same strategies often result in being given a PD diagnosis and offending (Fonagy, 2003). For example, aggression and violence as a defended means of relating to others, expression of unprocessed emotion, and re-enactment of trauma.

The Body's Defence System: Fight, Flight, Freeze, and Collapse

The stress response system is in the lower parts of the brain and when its survival strategies of flight, fight, freeze, and collapse are triggered, the higher-level functions including impulse control, reflection, and problem solving are effectively taken "off line" and behaviour is driven autonomically. Studies have shown that childhood trauma and adversity hypersensitises the stress response system to perceiving threat, which effects multiple areas of functioning, including attention, impulsivity, and aggressive and avoidant behaviours (Perry, 2008). PD traits and offending can be formulated as driven by a hypersensitised stress response system. For example, substance misuse can be seen as a flight response to numb emotional pain that disinhibits a hypersensitised attention for threat and increases the likelihood of a fight response of violence. Perry et al. (1995) have described how, as the lower parts of the brain do not hold a concept of time, the stress response system reacts as if the past traumas are occurring now. This can explain why individuals' reactions can appear either out of proportion or "come out of nowhere", and why some individuals who have good insight and knowledge of skills continue to offend.

A consistent narrative from individuals who have offended has been to perceive threat, from either their victim or others and displaced on to their victim. Thus, some offending is a fight response to eliminate perceived or actual threat, often reinforced by beliefs that others will harm and that to feel weak is intolerable. Schore (2003) argued that violence can be understood as the fight response dysregulated by childhood trauma.

Flight responses of suppression of emotion, not seeking support from others, numbing through substances, and avoidance of expected conflict through compliance can lead to increasing emotions and a violent fight response to the next stress or. In some sexual offences, compulsive sexual behaviours are flight responses to numb feelings of inadequacy and gain feelings of acceptance that can contribute directly to offending, for example, through sex with children who are seen as less likely to be rejecting.

The collapse response, in particular dissociation, which functions to protect the individual from unescapable fear or pain, can become highly sensitised responses at times of extreme emotion or a chronic pattern of depersonalisation that can drive violence (Moskowitz, 2004). As Streeck-Fischer & van der Kolk (2000) described, "under stress they pass the dehumanisation that they themselves have experienced onto others" (p.911).

These stress responses are frequently seen across forensic services. Individuals' rejection of services and denial of offending can be understood as flight responses to expected harm and rejection from services. Individuals' complaining about staff and services, often classed as having narcissistic and antisocial PD traits, can be considered fight responses. Both of these can represent distorted means of meeting primary needs, e.g., safety, autonomy. For an individual with a trauma history, people are the threat, and the threat increases with increased proximity. Programmes and therapy can be highly threatening because of the expectations to disclose aspects of themselves. Flight responses of refusing to attend, deflecting or saying very little, fight responses such as dismissing the value of the service or making unrealistic demands, freeze responses of disconnection, and collapse e.g., silent, dissociated, confused, are common in treatment. These reactions are frequently misunderstood as superficially engaging, lack of motivation, or not ready for treatment. Furthermore, as beliefs and values are stored in the higher parts of the brain and implicit biases are stored in the lower parts of the brain, this can explain how someone holds for example anti-violence beliefs and values and still having implicit biases that result in violent behaviour (Perry, 2006). This can guide formulation and intervention with individuals, who emphasise that they do not have pro-offending beliefs and yet continue to react with violence.

Individuals' stress responses patterns can change through repeated predictable experiences of moderate stress and co-regulation with another (Perry, 2006). This requires staff to have the capacity to provide effective containment of the individual through physiological and psychological calmness, attuning to the behaviours as survival strategies and focusing on developing a sense of safety in the moment, thus beginning to relearn the autonomic threat system (Perry, 2008). Focusing on increasing understanding of flight and flight reactions and how to sooth the stress response system before responding can increase resilience (e.g., Dana, 2018). To quote a patient, "breathing, rather than reacting, gives me that five second gap to then be able to think about what I am doing and remember that my aggressive urges are going to make things worse".

Emotional Regulation

Difficulties with emotional regulation, including seeking support from others, is a consistent impact of childhood traumas and is reflected in PD symptoms and DRFs. For example, emotional numbing has been found to be associated with youth aggression, and a mediator between trauma and callous-unemotional traits (Allwood, Bell, & Horan, 2011; Kerig, Bennett, Thompson, & Becker, 2012). Attachment theory suggests that if our emotions are responded to with neglect or punishment, we feel the unacceptability and badness of our emotions and suppress our emotional experience and expression to survive. Inconsistent and unpredictable care in response to our expression of emotions is internalised, as only heightened expressions of emotions are responded to (Fonagy, Steele, Steele, Moran, & Higgitt, 1991). When abuse is by an attachment figure, emotions have to be excluded so as to maintain sufficient proximity to the abusive attachment figure to survive, hence the high rates of dissociation and apparently "odd" behaviours that function to exclude anxiety. These resilient adaptations are internalised and form stable patterns of emotional regulation, underpinned by negative beliefs about others that in adulthood perpetuate emotional difficulties in part by excluding corrective emotional experiences with others.

Capacity to Play

Related to safety and emotional regulation, the capacity to play in childhood is necessary for development. It is through play that a range of responses can be tried and competence developed, including creativity, problem solving, coping, and emotional expression. Streeck-Fischer and van der Kolk (2000) described how during chronic trauma, children are preoccupied with survival, which prevents the capacity to play-fully and curiously try out a variety of ways to engage with the world and exploring self and others is threatening. Play in children who have experienced trauma has been found to be rigid and constricted, with no modification over time (Terr, 1981). There is similar restrictiveness in adults given a diagnosis of PD, and in some DRFs, that perpetuates survival strategies, in which neglect, rejection, violence, and the belief that nothing can change are dominant, and offending is seen as the only option. Lack of self-exploration is often seen in individuals within forensic services, who are too anxious, hopeless, or mistrustful to explore themselves and others or "play" with new ways of being. Role play and experiential techniques have a similar quality to play and can be experienced as threatening or something they have to "get right" to avoid punishment. For some individuals, the spontaneity and fun of play is a reminder of ridicule and punishment, which they respond to with survival strategies, re-enacting abusive or humiliating responses, perpetuating aggression or detachment as responses to change techniques.

Re-enactments

Ardino (2012) reported that a characteristic of trauma is the compulsion to re-enact the trauma and considered that antisocial acting out of unresolved childhood trauma may be a consistent feature in the behaviour of those who offend. Some of the symptoms for BPD (e.g., intense and unstable relationships) and other PDs (e.g., callous unconcern for the feelings of others in antisocial PD; the tendency to misconstrue the actions of others as hostile in paranoid PD; excessive preoccupation with being criticised or rejected in social situations in avoidant PD) may represent manifestations of re-enactments of previous traumas. Part of the compulsion to re-enact is considered to be the need for consistency and predictability with primary experiences, even when these are traumatic, as unpredictability is threatening (Perry, 2008). Ardino (2012) considered that re-enactments may be crucial in understanding how past trauma may be involved in maintaining risk of reoffending. Streeck-Fischer & van der Kolk (2000) highlight that unless caregivers understand re-enactments, they are liable to label the child as oppositional, rebellious, unmotivated, and antisocial. Within adult forensic services re-enactments are often labelled as "manipulative", "antisocial", "therapy-interfering", and "narcissistic" or "settled", "quiet", "loner", "odd", rather than as state-dependent response patterns.

Service User Narrative

The impact of adverse attachments and trauma on development of an individual and pathways to offending are described below by Tom. Tom has been in prison and forensic mental health services, and given several psychiatric diagnoses including PD and paranoid schizophrenia. Tom described his pathway from childhood traumas to the difficulties he had and offending and what was central to his being able to reconnect with himself and others and to be able to think about his offending.

> Because of my dissociation that developed in response to my mum and mainly my dad's difficulties and the bullying I suffered at school, I was not able to learn life's lessons, as you have to be able to remember things; and because of the dissociation, it totally blanked out things that I needed to know and learn to be able to look after and take care of myself. This contributed to my trying to kill myself when I was a teenager. All of life's lessons I've have been taught have been harsh ones, the sexual abuse I've been through, the bullying by the kids on the estate and dad's bullying of mum. These lead to the schemas I developed, it's like the schemas came about through mum and dad. I sometimes couldn't trust the people who were supposed to take care of me because of their problems, Dad's problems. I learnt that people were not safe, my mistrust schema. It's like the people who love me put mistrust in me and all the schemas that came with that. The bullying at school compounded my mistrust, and the sexual abuse compounded it further. I couldn't compute, I couldn't do anything with it, I couldn't understand it, I was like a 'rabbit in head lights' all my life my mind was switched off with overwhelming anxiety. Due to the dissociation, I couldn't work it out. It came out in my relationships and in the pub when I was drunk. I was angry and confused all the time and I was not able to sort it out. I drank until I blacked out to keep the shutters down. When I was stoned, I now know, that this was similar to how I felt when I was zoned out as a kid; the dissociation was a way of keeping the shutters down. Drinking didn't actually keep the shutters down; I was reacting with violence.
>
> After my index offence I went to prison for the first time, which is a frightening, fear provoking, stressful and paranoid place, and I was coming off drugs. This was when I first started hearing voices and seeing things. My mistrust and paranoia increased. I started to believe that my soul had been taken. Through the work I have done I realised that this is dissociation.

Tom described changes he has made and what contributed to him making these. "Being locked up and getting the proper help I needed. I can now think before I act and I know that drugs and alcohol are not the solution". When asked what had contributed to his dissociation and mistrust having reduced, he said his therapist who had worked with him for many years, "Pushing my boundaries but not too quickly". He recalled several years ago that he had been strongly encouraged by a member of his clinical team to attend an occupational therapy group session and his verbally angry refusal, as he felt pushed, albeit positively, too far for where he was at that time. He described that back then that he would not talk to anyone and that his therapist had had to get him talking. He described, "I had become too inward on myself (shrunken boundaries), I was keeping everything inside and I was keeping the shutters down". He described his therapist's persistent and paced pushing and encouragement as central to him being able to change. He described

I only ever experienced coldness during my childhood and this had contributed significantly to my disconnection from myself and my feelings and it feels good to be able to now feel emotions of love and warmth towards myself for achieving something.

Psychological Approaches to a Diagnosis of Personality Disorder and Offending

Psychological therapies have proposed relationships between aspects of personality and violence, e.g., CBT (Beck & Deffenbacher, 2000), attachment theory (Fonagy, 2003), GLM (Ward & Stewart, 2003), and schema therapy (Bernstein, Arntz, & Vos, 2007). CBT is the predominant approach in UK prison and forensic mental health services. The focus on the attitudes, thoughts, emotions, motivations, and behaviours that contributed to offences presupposes that individuals can identify and describe these. Individuals who experienced childhood traumas and adverse attachments and who are given a diagnosis of PD are highly likely to have difficulties in identifying and disclosing their thoughts, emotions, and beliefs about themselves and their offending, and to find this triggering their stress response system, shutting down their cognitive abilities. Childhood traumas impact most at a physiological and emotional level and this is increasingly being recognised across therapies that are incorporating a focus on emotions, the stress-response system, and body focused work (van der Kolk, 2014). Schema therapy is based on and incorporates much of the aspects identified above, and has been extended for use in forensic services; thus, this model is explored in further detail.

Schema Therapy

Schema therapy (ST: Young, Klosko, & Weishaar, 2003) was developed in response to the ineffectiveness of standard CBT with patients given a diagnosis of PD. ST is based on attachment theory, specifically that when basic human needs that are not met in childhood, due to adverse attachments and trauma, children adapt to their attachment figures and traumas, in combination with temperament, in order to survive. Through the internalisation of these experiences, schemas about self, others, and the world develop and the then adaptive survival responses are primarily emotionally encoded. These adaptive survival strategies subsequently become maladaptive coping modes or self-states in non-adverse environments.

The maladaptive modes are loosely linked to the fight, flight, fawn, and collapse/comply stress-response system, e.g., detached avoidant protector mode as flight, bully attack mode as fight and fawn, and compliant surrenderer mode as the fawn response. The pain, fear, loss, and anger of childhood trauma and adversity and resultant schemas are conceptualised as held in the child modes (vulnerable, impulsive, and angry child modes). Critic modes (punitive, demanding) are conceptualised as either the internalisation of the adverse attachment figure or abuser, or a coping mode in which the critic is attempting to meet childhood needs through criticising/punishing their behaviour. Healthy adult mode represents the capacity to reflect, manage responses – including impulses, expressions of need, vulnerability, and anger – effectively and engage effectively in relationships. Schemas and modes are considered to provide an explanatory model for the development and functioning of clusters of traits that are given a diagnoses of personality disorder. The therapeutic relationship is considered central in providing corrective emotional experiences and there is an emphasis on emotion-focused experiential techniques and sensory experiences, to heal and develop resilience (Briedis & Startup, 2020).

Bernstein et al. (2007) proposed that offending often represents maladaptive attempts to meet basic needs. Theorised offending modes include predator, conning manipulator, paranoid over-controller, and self-aggrandiser. These are theorised to be active at the time of an offence and function to stop the individual from feeling "weaker" modes, e.g., vulnerable child mode. Keulen-de Vos et al. (2016) examined the offending of patients given cluster B PD diagnoses and reported more child, paranoid ovecontroller, and detached self-soother modes leading up to, and more, over-compensatory (bully attack and predator) modes during their crimes. They concluded that it appeared that vulnerable feelings, such as shame and abandonment, often played a role in crimes, consistent with studies on reactive aggression. Similar patterns have been consistently seen across patients in forensic settings.

A recent RCT with patients in high security forensic hospitals in the Netherlands and given a diagnosis of predominantly antisocial, other cluster B and paranoid PDs, found that both treatment with individual schema therapy and treatment with other individual therapies (CBT, integrative/eclectic, systemic) showed moderate to large improvements on outcomes of rehabilitation (gaining leave) and PD symptoms after three years, and that ST had superior outcomes (Bernstein et al., 2021). Bernstein et al. found that the ST condition was quicker to lower vulnerabilities and promote strengths and had modest advantages over other treatments in improving traits such as self-control and self-regulation. Further, the ST condition showed rapid improvements in the first two years, which was considered in part due to ST's focus on creating the therapeutic bond. ST does not require individuals to be motivated or "ready for treatment" (Bernstein et al., 2012). Lack of motivation and difficulties in engaging in treatment are considered coping mode responses to schemas, typically mistrust, defectiveness, abandonment, and emotional deprivation triggered by the treatment process (re-enactments).

Schema therapy's focus on conceptualising individuals' maladaptive modes as arising from childhood traumas and adverse attachment and working on these as these occur in response to therapy and services, is central to providing forensic services with a useable and effective model to work with individuals whose survival strategies are often seen as "not treatment ready", "unmotivated", or "just wanting to cause trouble". ST (and similar models) provides a means of developing an integrated understanding of individuals' lives, rather than excluding offending or being only seen as offenders. Service users have reported the helpfulness of ST in understanding themselves and their offending, the emotion focused techniques, and the importance of the safety of the therapeutic relationship (Tan, 2015; Walji, 2015).

ST's developmental frame provides a means of working with individuals' offences that holds these in the context of what has happened to them, formulates their cognitive defences, such as minimising or blaming others, as coping strategies and focuses on meeting underlying needs for safety that enables individuals to explore themselves, their development, and their offending, as demonstrated in Tom's narrative. Developing safety in the therapeutic relationship involves working *in vivo* with maladaptive coping modes including detached protector, paranoid over-controller, and bully attack mode reactions within sessions. Focusing on containing and co-regulating their avoidant (flight) and overcompensation (fight) responses through body-focused work and naming the likely underlying needs and related fears provides emotional experiences of another attempting to understand, contain and support them. This can initially trigger further maladaptive mode responses arising from mistrust and uncertainty of a different response from another to their implicit map of self, others, and world. However, at the same time this experience is still being felt. Alongside this, there is the focus on the emotional links between present triggers for maladaptive mode coping and past attachment adversity and trauma. Working on these links is thus working on reducing survival strategies that are represented in DRFs e.g., offending beliefs and urges, interpersonal aggression, emotional control, difficulties with supervision. For example, using imagery rescripting to reduce bully attack mode to a staff member, whose specific behaviour was a reminder of an adult male perpetrator of childhood physical abuse and humiliation, using present day safe relationships to create safety in the past image, and then using this safety to strengthen healthy adult mode in imagery rescripting of his present-day interactions with the member of staff.

Strengthening healthy adult mode functioning and reducing use of offending modes increases experience of personal strengths and support from others and reduces the strength of mistrust abuse and other schemas. This provides the basis for working on offending using a combination of maladaptive mode mapping of the offence cycle and experiential techniques (e.g., imagery rescripting and gestalt chair work) to strengthen individuals' health adult capacity to contain maladaptive modes and change offending patterns. Applying this to a generalised case example, John had undertaken thinking skills programmes in which DRFs of sexual preoccupation, poor relationships, and poor problem solving (sex with sex workers or one-night stands etc.) were identified driving his sexual violence and outstanding treatment targets. John was described as presenting with a superficial understanding of these DRFs and how to manage these in the future. ST formulated that his experience of avoidant attachment figures resulted in defectiveness and emotional deprivation schemas that contributed to his seeking acceptance and intimacy through detached avoidant protector mode, including sex with sex workers or one night stands as this reduced the risk of rejection. However, this reminded him of his defectiveness and increased his shame and perpetuated his cycle. The build-up of shame, combined with rejection when attempting to develop a meaningful relationship, was formulated to escalate his hypersensitivity to rejection, and when perceiving humiliation from a sex worker or one-night stand, he shifted into bully attack mode, discharging unprocessed emotions through violence against his victims.

In ST the focus was on developing safe emotional connection with his therapist and keyworkers, providing repeated experiences of being understood, accepted, and encouraged to develop. Chair work with his child and maladaptive modes focused on giving voice to these parts of himself and their functions, and strengthening his healthy adult mode to be able to effectively meet his primary needs for acceptance and belonging. Imagery rescripting was used to work with his pain and loss of the emotionally depriving relationship with his parents and subsequent abuses, and the development of his preoccupation with sex. The last part was imagery rescripting on his mode shifts in his offending cycle and developing the basis for his relapse prevention plan including effective means of meeting his basic needs. Outcome goals/measures, in addition to reassessment of DRFs, were directly related to the schema and mode formulation, e.g., increased emotional connection across a range of relationships including with staff, supervisors, and other pro-social peers that provided feelings of acceptance and belonging, as well as increased feelings of competence in relationships and in occupation.

Whether the approach is ST or another trauma-focused model, forensic services would benefit from a model that formulates the impact of adverse attachments and childhood traumas on an individuals' personality and related DRFs, to be able to effectively respond to offending behaviours. The challenge arising from this understanding is the need for services in the face of financial and political demand for "high volume, low touch" therapies (Perry, podcast communication, in Brown, 2021), to deliver intensive long-term treatments by highly trained and experienced staff that provides consistent and predictable relational safety and moderate and predictable stress that builds resilience, which in the longer term can be more cost-effective (Bamelis, Arntz, Wetzelaer, Verdoorn, & Evers, 2015; Ward, 2016).

Further Reading

Perry, B.D., Pollard, R.A., Blakley, T.L., Baker, W.L., & Vigilante, D. (1995). Childhood trauma, the neurobiology of adaptation, and "use-dependent" development of the brain: How "states" become "traits". *Infant Mental Health Journal, 16*(4), 271–291.

Streeck-Fischer, A., & van der Kolk, B.A. (2000). Down will come baby, cradle and all: Diagnostic and therapeutic implications of chronic trauma on child development. *Australian and New Zealand Journal of Psychiatry, 34*(6), 903–918.

Van der Kolk, B.A. (2015). *The body keeps the score: Brain, mind, and body in the healing of trauma.* Penguin Books.

Wallin, D.J. (2007). *Attachment in psychotherapy.* Guilford Press.

References

Afifi, T.O., Mather, A., Boman, J., Fleisher, W., Enns, M.W., MacMillan, H., & Sareen, J. (2011). Childhood adversity and personality disorders: Results from a nationally representative population-based study. *Journal of Psychiatric Research, 45*(6), 814–822. doi:10.1016/j.jpsychires.2010.11.008

Ainsworth, M.D.S., Blehar, M.C., Waters, E., & Wall, S. (1978). *Patterns of attachment: A psychological study of the strange situation.* Hillsdale, NJ: Erlbaum.

Allwood, M.A., Bell, D.J., & Horan, J. (2011). Posttrauma numbing of fear, detachment, and arousal predict delinquent behaviors in early adolescence. *Journal of Clinical Child & Adolescent Psychology, 40*(5), 659–667. doi:10.1080/15374416.2011.597081

Altintas, M., & Bilici, M. (2018). Evaluation of childhood trauma with respect to crim-inal behavior, dissociative experiences, adverse family experiences and psychiatric backgrounds among prison inmates. *Comprehensive Psychiatry, 82,* 100–107. doi:10.1016/ j.comppsych.2017.12.006

Anda, R.F., Felitti, V.J., Bremner, J.D., Walker, J.D., Whitfield, C.H., Perry, B.D., … & Giles, W.H. (2006). The enduring effects of abuse and related adverse experiences in childhood. *European Archives of Psychiatry & Clinical Neuroscience, 256*(3), 174–186.

Ardino, V. (2012). Offending behaviour: The role of trauma and PTSD. *European Journal of Psychotraumatology, 3,* 1–4. doi:10.3402/ejpt.v3i0.18968

Bakermans-Kranenburg, M.J., & van IJzendoorn, M.H. (2009). The first 10,000 adult attachment interviews: Distributions of adult attachment representations in clinical and non-clinical groups. *Attachment & Human Development, 11*(3), 223–263. doi:10.1080/ 14616730902814762

Bamelis, L.L., Arntz, A., Wetzelaer, P., Verdoorn, R., & Evers, S.M. (2015). Economic evaluation of schema therapy and clarification-oriented psychotherapy for personality disorders: A multicenter, randomized controlled trial. *Journal of Clinical Psychiatry, 76*(11), E1432–E1440.

Battle, C.L., Shea, M.T., Johnson, D.M., Yen, S., Zlotnick, C., Zanarini, M.C., … & Morey, L.C. (2004). Childhood maltreatment associated with adult personality disorders: Findings from the Collaborative Longitudinal Personality Disorders Study. *Journal of Personality Disorders, 18*(2), 193–211. doi:10.1521/pedi.18.2.193.32777

Beck, A.T., & Deffenbacher, J. L. (2000). *Prisoners of hate: The cognitive basis of anger, hostility and violence.* Harper Collins Publishers, Inc.

Bellis, M.A., Hardcastle, K., Ford, K., Hughes, K., Ashton, K., Quigg, Z., & Butler, N. (2017). Does continuous trusted adult support in childhood impart life-course resilience against adverse childhood experiences – A retrospective study on adult health-harming behaviours and mental well-being. *BMC Psychiatry, 17*(1), 1–12.

Bernstein, D.P., Arntz, A., & Vos, M.D. (2007). Schema focused therapy in forensic settings: Theoretical model and recommendations for best clinical practice. *International Journal of Forensic Mental Health, 6*(2), 169–183. doi:10.1080/14999013.2007.10471261

Bernstein, D.P., Keulen-de Vos, M., Clercx, M., de Vogel, V., Kersten, G.C., Lancel, M., … & Arntz, A. (2021). Schema therapy for violent PD offenders: A randomized clinical trial. *Psychological Medicine,* 1–15. doi:10.1017/S0033291721001161

Bernstein, D.P., Keulen-de Vos, M., Jonkers, P., de Jonge, E., & Arntz, A. (2012). Schema therapy in forensic settings. In M. van Vreeswijk, J. Broersen & M. Nadort (Eds), *The Wiley-Blackwell handbook of schema therapy* (pp. 425–438). Routledge.

Bowlby, J. (1969/1982). *Attachment and loss: Vol. 1. Attachment.* New York: Basic Books.

Bowlby, J. (1988). Developmental psychiatry comes of age. *American Journal of Psychiatry, 145*(1), 1–10. doi:10.1176/ajp.145.1.1

Boyle, M., & Johnstone, L. (2020). *A straight talking introduction to the power threat meaning frame-work: An alternative to psychiatric diagnosis.* PCCS Books.

Briedis, J., & Startup, H. (2020). Somatic perspective in schema therapy: The role of the body in the awareness and transformation of modes and schemas. In G. Heath & H. Startup (Eds.), *Creative methods in schema therapy* (pp. 60–75). Routledge.

Briere, J., Hodges, M., & Godbout, N. (2010). Traumatic stress, affect dysregulation, and dys-functional avoidance: A structural equation model. *Journal of traumatic Stress, 23*(6), 767–774. doi:10.1002/jts.20578

Brown, B. (Host). (2021, May 5). Brené with Oprah Winfrey and Dr. Bruce D. Perry on trauma, resilience, and healing. [Audio podcast episode]. In *Unlocking Us with Brené Brown.* Parcast Network. Retrieved from https://brenebrown.com/podcast/brene-with-oprah-winfrey-and-dr-bruce-d-perry-on-trauma-resilience-and-healing/

Craig, J.M., Piquero, A.R., Farrington, D.P., & Ttofi, M.M. (2017). A little early risk goes a long bad way: Adverse childhood experiences and life-course offending in the Cambridge study. *Journal of Criminal Justice, 53,* 34–45. doi:10.1016/j.jcrimjus.2017.09.005

Dana, D. (2018). *The Polyvagal theory in therapy: Engaging the rhythm of regulation.* WW Norton & Company.

D'Andrea, W., Ford, J., Stolbach, B., Spinazzola, J., & van der Kolk, B.A. (2012). Understanding interpersonal trauma in children: Why we need a developmentally appropriate trauma diagnosis. *American Journal of Orthopsychiatry, 82*(2), 187–200. doi:10.1111/j.1939-0025.2012.01154.x

DeLisi, M., Drury, A.J., & Elbert, M.J. (2019). The etiology of antisocial personality disorder: The differential roles of adverse childhood experiences and childhood psychopathology. *Comprehensive Psychiatry, 92,* 1–6. doi:10.1016/j.comppsych.2019.04.001

Fazel, S., & Danesh, J. (2002). Serious mental disorder in 23 000 prisoners: A systematic review of 62 surveys. *The Lancet, 359*(9306), 545–550. doi:10.1016/S0140-6736(02)07740-1

Fonagy, P. (2003). Towards a developmental understanding of violence. *British Journal of Psychiatry, 183*(3), 190–192. doi:10.1192/bjp.183.3.190

Fonagy, P., Steele, M., Steele, H., Moran, G.S., & Higgitt, A.C. (1991). The capacity for understanding mental states: The reflective self in parent and child and its significance for security of attachment. *Infant Mental Health Journal, 12*(3), 201–218. doi:10.1002/1097-0355(199123)12:3<201::AID-IMHJ2280120307>3.0.CO;2-7

Heffernan, R., Wegerhoff, D., & Ward, T. (2019). Dynamic risk factors: Conceptualization, measurement, and evidence. *Aggression & Violent Behavior, 48,* 6–16. doi:10.1016/j.avb.2019.06.004

Hesse, E., & Main, M. (2000). Disorganized infant, child, and adult attachment: Collapse in behavioral and attentional strategies. *Journal of the American Psychoanalytic Association, 48*(4), 1097–1127. doi:10.1177/00030651000480041101

Howard, R., & McMurran, M. (2012). Whither research on 'high-harm' offenders with personality disorders? *Criminal Behaviour and Mental Health, 22*(3), 157–164. doi:10.1002/cbm.1834

Hudson, S.M., & Ward, T. (1997). Intimacy, loneliness, and attachment style in sexual offenders. *Journal of Interpersonal Violence, 12*(3), 323–339. doi:10.1177/088626097012003001

Kerig, P.K., Bennett, D.C., Thompson, M., & Becker, S.P. (2012). "Nothing really matters": Emotional numbing as a link between trauma exposure and callousness in delinquent youth. *Journal of Traumatic Stress, 25*(3), 272–279. doi:10.1002/jts.21700

Keulen-de Vos, M.E., Bernstein, D.P., Vanstipelen, S., de Vogel, V., Lucker, T.P., Slaats, … & Arntz, A. (2016). Schema modes in criminal and violent behaviour of forensic cluster B PD patients: A retrospective and prospective study. *Legal and Criminological Psychology, 21*(1), 56–76. doi:10.1111/lcrp.12047

Lam, D.C., Poplavskaya, E.V., Salkovskis, P.M., Hogg, L.I., & Panting, H. (2016). An experimental investigation of the impact of personality disorder diagnosis on clinicians: Can we see past the borderline? *Behavioural & Cognitive Psychotherapy, 44*(3), 361–373. doi:10.1017/S1352465815000351

Lamb, N., Sibbald, S., & Stirzaker, A. (2018). Shining lights in dark corners of people's lives: Reaching consensus for people with complex mental health difficulties who are given a diagnosis of personality disorder. *Criminal Behaviour and Mental Health, 28,* 1–4. doi:10.1002/cbm.2068

Livesley, W.J. (1998). Suggestions for a framework for an empirically based classification of personality disorder. *Canadian Journal of Psychiatry, 43*(2), 137–147. doi: 10.1177/070674379804300202

Luyten, P., Campbell, C., & Fonagy, P. (2020). Borderline personality disorder, complex trauma, and problems with self and identity: A social-communicative approach. *Journal of Personality, 88*(1), 88–105. doi:10.1111/jopy.12483

Lyons-Ruth, K. (1999). The two-person unconscious: Intersubjective dialogue, enactive relational representation, and the emergence of new forms of relational organization. *Psychoanalytic Inquiry, 19*(4), 576–617. doi:10.1080/07351699909534267

Moskowitz, A.K. (2004). Dissociative pathways to homicide: Clinical and forensic implications. *Journal of Trauma & Dissociation, 5*(3), 5–32. doi:10.1300/J229v05n03_02

Perry, B.D. (2006). The neurosequential model of therapeutics: Applying principles of neuroscience to clinical work with traumatized and maltreated children. In N. Boyd Webb (Ed.), *Working with traumatized youth in child welfare* (pp. 27–52). Guilford Press.

Perry, B.D. (2008). Child maltreatment: A neurodevelopmental perspective on the role of trauma and neglect in psychopathology. In T.P. Beauchaine & S.P. Hinshaw (Eds), *Child and adolescent psychopathology* (pp. 93–128). John Wiley & Sons Inc.

Perry, B.D., Pollard, R.A., Blakley, T.L., Baker, W.L., & Vigilante, D. (1995). Childhood trauma, the neurobiology of adaptation, and "use-dependent" development of the brain: How "states" become "traits". *Infant Mental Health Journal, 16*(4), 271–291. doi:10.1002/1097-0355(199524)16:4<271::AID-IMHJ2280160404>3.0.CO;2-B

Ramon, S., Castillo, H., & Morant, N. (2001). Experiencing personality disorder: A participative research. *International Journal of Social Psychiatry, 47*(4), 1–15. doi:10.1177/002076400104700401

Schore, A.N. (2003). Early relational trauma, disorganized attachment, and the development of a predisposition to violence. In D. Siegel & M. Solomon (Eds), *Healing trauma: Attachment, mind, body, and brain* (pp. 101–167). Norton.

Streeck-Fischer, A., & van der Kolk, B.A. (2000). Down will come baby, cradle and all: Diagnostic and therapeutic implications of chronic trauma on child development. *Australian and New Zealand Journal of Psychiatry, 34*(6), 903–918.

Tan, Y.M. (2015). *Schema therapy for borderline personality disorder: Patients' and therapists' perceptions* (Unpublished doctoral dissertation, Murdoch University).

Terr, L. C. (1981). "Forbidden games": Post-traumatic child's play. *Journal of the American Academy of Child Psychiatry, 20*(4), 741–760. doi:10.1097/00004583-198102000-00006

Tyrer, P. (2005). The problem of severity in the classification of personality disorder. *Journal of Personality Disorders, 19*(3), 309–314. doi:10.1521/pedi.2005.19.3.309

Tyrka, A.R., Wyche, M.C., Kelly, M.M., Price, L.H., & Carpenter, L.L. (2009). Childhood maltreatment and adult personality disorder symptoms: influence of maltreatment type. *Psychiatry Research, 165*(3), 281–287. doi:10.1016/j.psychres.2007.10.017

van der Kolk, B. (2014). *The body keeps the score: Mind, brain and body in the transformation of trauma.* Penguin UK.

Walji, I. (2015). *Narrative identities and self-constructs of individuals with histories of sexual and violent offences* (Unpublished doctoral thesis, Lancaster University).

Ward, T. (2016). Dynamic risk factors: Scientific kinds or predictive constructs. *Psychology, Crime & Law, 22*(1-2), 2–16. doi:10.1080/1068316X.2015.1109094

Ward, T., & Stewart, C. (2003). Criminogenic needs and human needs: A theoretical model. *Psychology, Crime & Law, 9*(2), 125–143. doi:10.1080/1068316031000116247

Young, J.E., Klosko, J.S., & Weishaar, M.E. (2003). *Schema therapy: A practitioner's guide.* Guilford Press.

PART II

Vulnerable Groups

5

FROM CARE TO CUSTODY?

Elizabeth Utting and Tamara Woodall

In 2020 there were over 80,000 young people being looked after in some form of care in England, including residential homes, foster care, short-term placements, and secure homes. For the majority of these young people, this is to *protect* them from neglect or abuse, while a small number of young people in care (approximately 2%) are looked after due to their criminal or "socially unacceptable" behaviours (Department for Education, 2020). While some of these young people may have been in contact with the Criminal Justice System (CJS) due to their behaviours, most will have been victims of, or witnessed, criminal offences. Despite the fact that trauma and adversity is ubiquitous for care-experienced young people, stigma follows them throughout society and these facts are often forgotten. But why is this relevant?

It is estimated that over 25% of young offenders and more than 50% of individuals in secure children's centres are care-experienced (Youth Justice Board, 2020). Care-experienced people are more likely to be found in young offender and adult facilities (both male and female) than in the community (Farmer, 2017). The Laming review (Prison Reform Trust, 2016) was set up to address the over-representation of young people with experience of care in the CJS. It highlighted that young people's early life experiences have a significant impact on their development and future life chances. As a result of their experiences before and during care, care-experienced young people are at greater risk of entering the youth justice system than their peers. Care-experienced young people are also more likely to be exposed to the risk factors established in research as associated with the onset of youth offending than the general population of young people (Schofield et al., 2012).

Sadly, care-experienced young people are at increased risk of negative outcomes. They are 10 times more likely to be excluded from school; 12 times more likely to leave school with no qualifications; 4 times more likely to be unemployed; 60 times more likely to become homeless; 50 times more likely to be sent to prison; and 66 times more likely to have children who themselves need public care (McSherry, Malet, & Weatherall, 2016). Furthermore, they are more vulnerable to mental, emotional and behavioural, and physical health difficulties (Dixon, 2008; McCann, James, Wilson, & Dunn, 1996; McCarthy, Janeway, & Geddes, 2003), alongside low self-esteem and self-concept (Ackerman & Dozier, 2005).

DOI: 10.4324/9781003120766-8

A sizeable volume of literature has highlighted the relationship between childhood trauma and offending (Skowyra & Cocozza, 2007; Smith, Chamberlain, & Deblinger, 2012; Widom & Maxfield, 2001). Neglect, abuse, poverty, and witnessing violence are some of the most common risk factors for post-traumatic reactions – aggression and antisocial behaviour (Dong et al., 2004; Finkelhor, 2008; Hussey, Chang, & Kotch, 2006).

As discussed in Chapter 1, several different patterns of childhood adversity have been found to be common among young people and adults involved in the CJS. However, research is lacking as to the role of social care, specifically, trauma and adversity from *being* in care and trauma that occurs *while* in care.

The Social Care System's Role in Trauma

The most common type of initial care placement is foster care (either *kinship* foster care which involves living with family members and *non-kinship* foster care with non-family members, if family members are unavailable or deemed unsuitable) (NSPCC, 2021). Residential group care placements (where young people live together in a shared accommodation) are subsequently sought for young people with more complex emotional and behavioural needs, or whose foster placements have broken down. Secure care placements (e.g., youth offending, mental health hospitals) tend to fall towards the end of young people's care pathways if they require enhanced care and risk management. More recently, placement type has been regarded as less of a priority than basing a young person's living requirements on their individual needs.

The key goal for child welfare systems internationally for over 40 years has been achieving *permanency* for young people in care (Biehal, 2014). Permanency is a multi-faceted concept that includes a young person having a stable family environment, a sense of belonging, secure relationships, and self-concept (Moran, McGregor, & Devaney, 2020). In particular, the notion of *felt security* within care and relational permanency has been described as fundamental for young people's development and positive outcomes (Cashmore & Paxman, 2006).

Experiences of Young People in Care

There is little research that captures the lived experiences of young people in the social care system. We have reflected on the most common issues relating to the social care system's role in trauma, based on research and our experience in practice. We discussed these with a number of care-experienced individuals. Themes from these discussions are described below.

- Retraumatisation of difficulties and issues for young people through navigating the current social care processes (such as repeated rejection (placement moves perceived as continual rejection by individuals and society, alienation and stigma, lack of stability and consistency).

- Young people falling through gaps in services (for example, there is a need for more understanding of developmental trauma in mental health and social care by a variety of staff, more specialist professionals needed for early prevention).
- Becoming "stuck" in the system. The message received by young people from the social care system appears to be that they are intrinsically a "problem", rather than a recognition that their difficulties or behaviours are a response to what has happened to them.
- Being treated differently to non-care-experienced young people. "Moving on the problem" through placement breakdowns. This creates a loss of trust and sense of control after each move. A young person can act in negative ways to re-gain that sense of control.
- Frequent exposure to further trauma within a care home or by individuals they meet in the care system. For example, young people can be vulnerable to exposure of more risky behaviours, environments, people, and attitudes. Care-experienced young people can be exposed to negative peers and risk-taking behaviours and may not be responded to or supported in the same way as young people in a family or foster environment.
- The social care system can often treat care-experienced young people as riskier than they are. The system can be highly sensitive to "risks" and have limited availability of professionals with the expertise to understand or respond to the complex nature of risk, resulting in a very reactive system, to the detriment of the young person.
- Multi-disciplinary information-sharing can be scarce, in addition to limited available resources for risk assessments/mental health assessments. This can create a disjointed experience for the care-experienced young person.

Permanency and Placement Instability

Care-experienced young people often experience multiple placement moves throughout their care pathway. Although some placement endings occur in the best interest of the young person, the majority happen unexpectedly and without consideration of the young person's voice or experience. In recent years, this issue has been well-documented as a serious public health concern across England. The Stability Index was introduced by the Children's Commissioner in 2017 to measure the annual stability of the lives of young people in care, in response to concerns about the high rates of instability experienced. The Children's Commissioner (2020) identified that between 2018 and 2019, one in four young people in care experienced two or more placement moves. Older young people were more likely to experience more placement moves, reflecting the greater social, emotional, and mental health needs of this group, and their vulnerability to child sexual exploitation and gang membership. Older young people included those who entered care later and those with a history of multiple placement breakdowns.

Young people are more likely to require secure or specialist care placements following multiple placement moves. The Stability Index highlighted young people who had once lived in a secure or specialist residential children's home had a disproportionately higher number of placement moves. Sallnäs, Vinnerljung, and Kyhle Westermark (2004) reported that Swedish teenagers displaying antisocial behaviour (criminal or violent conduct, alcohol/drug abuse) prior to placement are significantly more likely than others to experience breakdown in all forms of care. Placement moves are significant, given a history of placement breakdown is a common precursor to subsequent placement breakdowns and poor future outcomes (Leve et al., 2012; Oosterman, Schuengel, Slot, Bullens, & Doreleijers, 2007; Rock, Michelson, Thomson, & Day, 2015). It is concerning that Children's Commissioner's statistics highlight how environmental and relational loss have become the norm for many care-experienced young people. This confirms that the notion of *permanency* is currently far from being achieved for care-experienced young people (Department for Education, 2016).

What does the continual movement around the system and instability really mean for the young person? A lack of family relationships, separation of siblings, difficulty maintaining friendships, strained – if not completely lacking – education provision to name a few consequences. As one care-experienced young person explained, the labels applied to a young person can be internalised when experienced by an individual. When experienced by a whole system, the young person internalises those labels and are then applicable relating to every responsible adult in that system.

In recent years, the rates of young people being placed out of area has increased, causing disruptions to support mechanisms (i.e., school, family, peers) and ties to specialist care providers (e.g., mental health services). As a last resort, some young people under the age of 18 have been placed in unregulated accommodation, including semi-independent and independent accommodation because of a lack of available space in children's homes. In the most concerning cases, young people have even been placed in hostels and bed and breakfast accommodation. Consequently, young people's vulnerability to falling through the gaps in society increases, as does our ability to safeguard them from abuse or criminal exploitation.

> Every day I hear from "pinball kids" who are being pinged around the care system when all they really want is to be settled and to get on with normal life. These children need stability yet far too many are living unstable lives, in particular children entering care in their early teens. This puts them at greater risk of falling through the gaps in the education system and opens them up to exploitation by gangs or to abuse.
>
> *Anne Longfield, Children's Commissioner, cited in Weale (2018)*

Moving around the care system can have a significant detrimental impact on all aspects of a young person's development and future outcomes. This includes but is not limited to:

• Feeling unwanted and worthless by individuals and by society
• Loss of belonging and security which increases their vulnerability to the draw of gang involvement or experiencing Child Sexual Exploitation (CSE)

- Loss of trust
- Reliance on themselves to survive
- Internal working model/core beliefs development – a lack of communication and transparency results in young people internalising placement endings as their fault, reinforcing pre-existing negative beliefs about the self
- Impact on the formation of identity
- Impact on brain development
- Difficulties with education
- Feeling unsafe and viewing the world as a hostile place
- Problems with connection and attachment

All this is occurring at a crucial developmental stage for our young people who are susceptible to influence from a variety of people and organisations. Although there is limited research into this area, we are aware of how important the above is for young people and how crucial it is for us as a society to do something about it.

The "Care" Environment

The social care environment itself can increase the risk of re-traumatisation for young people. Despite most young people in care being looked after for their own protection following early trauma, many are later exposed to further trauma within their care placements, in particular residential or secure care settings. Young people typically warrant these forms of placements due to an increased level of need and accompanying risky behavioural and emotional difficulties. They may be exposed to antisocial peers and risk-taking behaviours (e.g., aggressive and violent behaviour towards self/staff, self-harm, bullying, substance misuse). These experiences may increase the risk of young people developing antisocial attitudes or may reinforce pre-existing attitudes developed through exposure to early (pre-care) trauma. Care homes themselves have been labelled as "criminogenic environments", particularly for older teenagers, as they often present a set of risks that tend to reinforce offending behaviour (Hayden, 2010). Additionally, adverse experiences within the care home may trigger a young person's trauma symptomatology resulting in them feeling unsafe in a chaotic and unpredictable environment. For some, this will inadvertently mirror their early familial experiences.

Johnson, Browne, and Hamilton-Giachritsis (2006) proposed that even apparently "good" institutional care can impact on a young person's ability to form relationships in later life, due to a lack of opportunity to form selective attachments compared to young people who are not care-experienced. Attachment security may be hindered, especially in environments with large groups of young people, low staffing levels, and a lack of consistency through shift work and staff rotation.

Care-experienced young people highlight themes of a loss of control, powerlessness, and difficulty in responding to ever-changing boundaries and rules (Woodall, 2022). Although the care system is governed by rules and regulations to uphold safeguarding practice, young people can find these environments overly restrictive and punitive compared to a family environment. Given the high rates of young people experiencing childhood abuse and attachment difficulties, it is likely that prior to care, many did not receive consistent or sensitive caregiving or adequate boundaries (National Institute for Health & Care Excellence, 2015). Consequently, young people may experience rules in care as a means of exerting control over their lives and may fight against them if they do not trust in the relationship or understand that these are enforced for their best interest. Furthermore, care-experienced young people commonly express feeling alienated from their non-care-experienced peers because of their perceived lack of freedom. Young people may develop unhelpful ways to re-exert control over their lives whilst in care. They may also become prone to risk-taking behaviours if they reach independence and feel automatically disconnected from the high supervision and structure previously placed around them.

What Can Be Done to Prevent a Trajectory from Care to Custody? "What Happened to You and How Can We Help You Moving Forward?"

Understanding Trauma Across and Throughout the System

In recent years, the child welfare system has advocated for the implementation of trauma-informed care (TIC). There is a growing body of research exploring the usefulness of TIC and seeking to capture young peoples' and professionals' experiences of these approaches (Hickle, 2020). TIC involves organisational practice and policy to be evidence-based and informed by trauma-focused research to ensure care is matched to the young person's individual needs (Brend & Sprang, 2020).

The National Child Traumatic Stress Network (2013) emphasise "understanding how a potentially traumatised child experienced a traumatic event is the first step in finding out how best to meet that child's needs in the immediate and long-term" (cited in Buckley, Lotty, & Meldon, 2016; p.35). In practice, this requires an understanding of "the relationship between a child's lifetime trauma history; his or her behaviour and responses; and identifying, the impact of trauma on child development and brain development" (Buckley et al.; p.35). Awareness of a young person's pre-care history can aid professionals' understanding and expectations of how they will interpret their care experiences, given the two are interlinked (Moran, McGregor, & Devaney, 2020). Some have argued that the sequelae of exposure to childhood victimisation or interpersonal trauma should constitute a distinct new psychiatric diagnosis or framework within which to research this topic. Further research would be needed to systematically develop and test the validity and clinical utility of a new diagnosis. It has been argued that diagnosis based upon exposure to developmentally adverse interpersonal trauma, victimisation, and neglect during childhood has the potential to alert clinicians to the influential role of childhood trauma in psychopathology (D'Andrea, Ford, Stolbach, Spinazzola, & van der Kolk, 2012).

Alternatively, given the ubiquitous nature of childhood trauma within the care-experienced population, complex behaviours can be best understood as young peoples' survival strategies. This information can encourage professionals to view young people's behaviour "through a trauma lens" and understand their presentation in the context of their early trauma (Sharda, 2013). This requires professionals to reframe their questioning of a young person's experiences from "what is wrong with you?" to "what has happened to you?". This fits well with the Power Threat Meaning Framework (Johnstone & Boyle et al., 2018) which focuses on the interplay between psychosocial factors, such as abuse or poverty, and adaptive threat responses. Rather than labelling behaviours as "antisocial" or "dysfunctional" and moving towards diagnosis, young people's behaviours can be seen as having been once adaptive and functional in the context of their trauma environment, "a set of learned responses to perceived threat, or as survival strategies for keeping physically and psychologically safe in interpersonal environments that are seen by the individual as dangerous, hostile, abusive, or neglectful" (Willmot & Evershed, 2018; p.340).

Physiological Responses to Trauma

Young people's behaviours may develop because of the psychological and physiological responses to developmental trauma. Traumatic stress is a natural response to adversity which can have long lasting implications for healthy brain development (Bremner, 2006). Living in early chaotic and hostile environments can result in a young person's *social monitoring system* becoming "hardwired" and prepared for danger. Consequently, they may remain in a defensive survival state, constantly anticipating threat and becoming hypersensitive to rejection, anger, or neglect (Golding, 2014). This trauma response can cause young people to misinterpret neutral facial cues, expressions, and others' body language as threatening, which can trigger a set of automatic survival responses (i.e., fight, flight, or freeze).

Attachment Responses to Trauma

Early traumatic relational experiences characterised by fear and conditional care can lead young people to develop mistrust in the first year of life (Golding, 2014). Young people's mistrust within relationships can become heightened through their experiences in care. Unfamiliar care environments, fear and anxiety following unexpected placement moves, and loss of relationships with professionals may reinforce negative perceptions of the unavailability and safety of others and may reinforce a need to remain in a hypersensitive survival state. Woodall (2022) described young people's responses to a lack of trust as instinctive and a maladaptive coping mechanism to fight against others and fend for themselves. Instability and loss of relationships appeared to create a cycle of self-fulfilling prophecy. Young people perceived their unworthiness of love or being cared for, leading to a reliance on unhealthy defensive strategies throughout their care experiences. As a result of persistent and pervasive mistrust, alongside feeling let down by the system, young people may start to resist authority and reject convention, especially where nurture feels novel to them. Instead, young people develop controlling behaviours to ensure their own safety in situations where it is safer to be in control than influenced by another (Golding, 2014).

Social Learning of Abusive Behaviour (The Cycle of Violence)

Through exposure to abusive and frightening experiences, children may develop negative attitudes and normalise violent beliefs, leading to a display of aggression or violence. In the *cycle of violence*, victimisation and offending appear inexorably linked to one another and can explain the interrelated nature of abuse for some children (Widom, 1989).

Shame Responses (The Shield of Shame)

Shame is a complex emotion that can result from complex trauma and can underlie children's dysfunctional behaviours (Golding, 2014). Shame is closely related to the emotion of guilt. However, it is distinct in that shame relates to a sense of self as bad and guilt to a sense that one's behaviour is bad. In the continual absence of relationship repair, children begin to internalise shame as part of their core identity; "I am a bad/shameful child". This toxic shame can become overwhelming and can result in a child being unable to regulate this emotion and think rationally, control their impulses, or respond flexibly. The child may therefore develop defences (the *shield of shame*) to protect themselves. This can involve behaviours such as lying, blaming others, and minimising. If shame becomes overwhelming, the child may respond with rage, chronic anger, and controlling behaviours to avoid acknowledgement of their defective self (Golding, 2014). As a population, care-experienced young people often internalise the perceived stigma of being in care and feeling different to their peers. Society can often label these individuals as "difficult" and "problem children", rather than acknowledging their vulnerabilities and victimisation. As such, young people's perceptions of shame and worthlessness are reinforced and can risk them feeling even more ostracised. This causes their *shield of shame* to strengthen the intensity and frequency of maladaptive survival responses. Children's experiences of unregulated shame are especially significant, since shame has been found to mediate pathways to offending within adult populations (Svensson, Weerman, Pauwels, Bruinsma, & Bernasco, 2013).

Misconstruing Young People's Behaviour

Without understanding of the impact of experiences and trauma on an individual, professionals may (and often do) misconstrue young people's behaviours. For example, aggression, violence, and property damage may be misinterpreted as purposely threatening, manipulative, and coercive, rather than as indication of distress or a response to perceived threat. A trauma-informed approach supports professionals to acknowledge young people's behaviours as adaptive, since they enabled young people to survive abusive and neglectful early caregiving experiences where their emotional and physical needs were unmet. Young people can remain reliant on these strategies once in care to overcome feelings of powerlessness, anxiety, and fear. This can be as a direct response to restrictive caregiving environments, loss of control, and uncertainty about placement and relational stability.

By focusing solely on the young people's behaviours, professionals may have difficulty showing empathy, acceptance, and understanding towards the young people – thus, increasing the risk of further tension and disconnect within the relationship. The risk of relationships breaking down and placements ending is then increased, further propelling young people into another cycle of loss, anxiety, and uncertainty as they move through the system. Rather than understanding young people, we are contributing to their difficulty and trauma – each move likely to reinforce and compound previous issues, creating more damage to already vulnerable young people. Of course, sometimes moves are necessary for the well-being and/or safety of the young person, the staff team, or the local community. However, we make a call here to thoroughly formulate as a multi-disciplinary team, so that placement moves become a last resort rather than a convenient resolution to a particular difficulty.

In parallel with adult forensic institutions, young people in the care system are required to learn to navigate systemic processes. Those with a self-protective strategy to fend for themselves will likely utilise strategies to fight against or sabotage boundaries and rules set for them if they do not feel safe and listened to. Professionals should focus on the underlying needs driving young people's behaviours in order to avoid pathologising and stigmatising responses, connect with young people's emotional experiences, and validate their pre-care and in-care trauma experiences.

Environmental Structure

Attachment to family is an important factor in preventing reoffending (Brunton-Smith & McCarthy, 2016) and points to why so many people within the CJS have had involvement with the social care system. A stable and secure family base can provide support with finances, education, and employment, overcoming adverse experiences and emotional support, which are recognised as important protective factors against involvement in crime and violence (de Vries Robbé, Vogel, & Douglas, 2013). Broad consensus among experts working with young people impacted by complex, or interpersonal trauma, is that the most effective therapeutic responses occur within culturally relevant, secure interpersonal relationships (Blaustein & Kinniburgh, 2018; Courtois & Ford, 2013).

Healthy childhood development exists within the context of secure attachment relationships (Bowlby, 1988). Young people who experience complex trauma have difficulty with their capacity to integrate traumatic self-states and events and require subsequent secure caregivers to facilitate typical development (Blaustein & Kinniburgh, 2018). Therefore, professionals who care for young people placed in residential settings are in key positions to act as their secure bases. Residential care workers have a unique capacity to serve as potential professional attachment figures for these children. Thorough consideration of this is required when placement matching young people and placement matching should include appropriate cultural matching to allow access to like-minded individuals which is essential in order to support our young people. There is currently very little training, financial or social recognition for the role of residential care worker. While this role is an extremely important and challenging (yet rewarding) profession, this is not reflected in the professional expectations required for such responsibility. It is imperative that we have the right people in this role, with the trauma-informed care training they need and deserve, to provide the care for our young people that they deserve. This can only be achieved by changes to policy regarding the training requirements and availability suitable for the role, in addition to appropriate working contracts and social recognition. Staff well-being plays a fundamental role in care and support we can offer our young people in care, and although outside the scope of this chapter to explore in detail, is important to raise and call for further research and exploration.

Embedded Knowledge and Training

Without training in trauma-informed care, staff in the social care system can struggle to provide effective management and interventions to address these problems (Bazalgette, Rahilly, & Trevelyan, 2015). Enhanced training and competency requirements for all staff involved in the system (from policy makers and directors to social workers and care staff) are essential in order to affect lasting change. Not only is this important for recognising best approaches for support, but in order to manage the conflict between the compassionate and empowering approaches needed and risk management. For example, Bronfenbrenner's ecological systems model speaks to making changes to the whole system around a young person, placing the young person at the heart of all decision-making (Bronfenbrenner, 1979). A trauma-informed approach must pervade all systems and maintain the well-being and resilience of the staff team.

There needs to be an acknowledgement that young people involved in crime are themselves victims. The proportion of young people entering the CJS for more serious and violent offences is increasing, with possession of weapons and robbery on the rise. In particular, the high rate of knife crime is significantly impacting families and communities. According to the Youth Justice Board for England and Wales (2019), in 2018, young people committed 21% of all knife and offensive weapon offences. There has been an increase in gangs and organised crime groups who use county lines[1] to exploit those young people who are particularly vulnerable or at a crisis point in their lives. These young people frequently experience family breakdown, intervention by social services, looked after status, frequent missing episodes, behavioural and developmental disorders, and exclusion from mainstream schooling. They have all too often been the victims of crime themselves, and, because of this, are deliberately targeted. Having an informed and well-trained understanding of the risks of certain behaviours and presentations across the service (staff *and* policies) is vital to changing one of the biggest challenges when working in this field – managing the anxiety of the systems surrounding the young people which are responsible for their care and well-being. Much of the anxiety experienced by individual professionals and systems in the social care arena is due to a limited understanding of the evidence base around behaviours such as sexually inappropriate behaviours, fire setting, violence and aggression, gang involvement, vulnerability to exploitation or weapon use. This lack of understanding can result in emotionally reactive responses, which can be damaging and harmful when supporting our care-experienced young people. There is a risk of pathologising and stigmatising young people within the social care system, a tendency to be risk adverse and to respond restrictively and punitively. Labelling young people as "risky" can trigger a complex social process of stigma that often results in reduced opportunities in life and self-development. Some care-experienced young people we have spoken to have felt that the system can make adolescence itself a risk. Deakin, Fox, and Matos (2020) call for a reconceptualisation of stigma, to include reference to young people's reactions and responses: alienation and marginalisation, anger and resistance, empathy and generativity. They argue that this stigma generally inhibits young people's engagement with wider society. Although, it was acknowledged that for some young people who are able to resist the label, resistance can be generative and enabling.

At times, the context of young people's behaviours can be overlooked. This in turn can have a consequence of reinforcing these young people's mistrust of professionals and systems. Enhancing the systems' understanding and response to these complexities could go a long way to assisting care-experienced young people to develop skills to help overcome the stigma and adversities.

Young People's Voices

Central to the role of professionals working in the social care system is consideration not only of the experiences and context of the young person's behaviours, but also appropriately capturing the young person's "voice". However, lack of time, resources, and training mean that often assessments can be inadequately thought out, completed by untrained professionals, and can fail to consider the needs and perspective of the young person or fail to identify appropriate support. Robust formulation to understand the trajectory of development of attitudes, beliefs, and behaviours is essential, and is incomplete without due understanding and appreciation of the young person's perspective. We *must* ask the young person. Formulation is best developed collaboratively, using accessible language, constructed reflectively and best understood in terms of *usefulness* rather than *truth* (British Psychological Society, 2011). It is our experience that children actively want to be involved in decision-making about their care pathways.

Addressing Behaviours

Young people within the social care system are generally not required to complete work to address risky, problematic, or offending behaviours as they would be in the CJS. Addressing offending is not the primary objective of social care (as many have not committed offences), but rather keeping the young person safe, supporting them to overcome adversity and to live well-adjusted lives. It is the authors' perspective that the youth justice and social care systems in fact have the same goal (see Table 5.1). Providing opportunity for support through joined-up working and improved communication with young people, transitional and adult services could help to provide timely interventions and support in areas such as identity development and emotional resilience, areas focussed on throughout interventions in the Youth Justice System (YJS). Taking strength-based approaches with our young people in a *trauma-informed*

Table 5.1 YJB child first principles

See children as children	Ensure the best interests of children are prioritised. Acknowledge their needs, rights, potential, and capacity. Support and intervention should recognise individual and structural barriers, be developmentally informed and ensure it meets the responsibilities held towards children.
Develop pro-social identity for positive child outcomes	Children's individual strengths and capabilities should be promoted to help develop their pro-social identity. This should lead to reduced number of victims and better impact on the community. Work should be focussed on the future and built on relationships which support and empower children to make positive contributions to society and achieve their potential.
Collaboration with children	Promote active participation from children to engage, including with wider society. Any work should be a collaboration between children and their carers/ supportive individuals.
Promote diversion	Prioritise pre-emptive prevention, minimal intervention with a goal of diversion from the justice system. Work and engagement should strive to minimise stigma that arises from contact with the system.

social care system could address these areas of challenge for our young people, providing a message of investment, worthiness, and hope so significantly lacking for our care-experienced young people. Often, care-experienced young people are marginalised or excluded from opportunities due to issues such as background checks, gaps in education and employment, and difficulty in gaining employability skills. The social care system needs to focus on supporting care-experienced young people in these areas, which are essential to preventing a trajectory into offending and secure/forensic services. Pre-emptive prevention using the concept of *Positive Youth Development* principles (Butts, Bazemore, & Saa Meroe, 2010) to inform the *Positive Youth Justice Model* could maximise young peoples' strengths, capacities, and potentials whilst simultaneously reduce offending. This focuses on interconnected factors such as number and strength of pro-social relationships, participation in extra-curricular activities, education, and readiness for employment.

Support for Leaving Care

Young adults can be especially vulnerable to a trajectory into criminal behaviours and potentially secure services, and when they do, are more likely to reoffend (Ministry of Justice, 2015). The National Offender Management Service (2015) identified distinct challenges, priority needs, and specific ways to help for young adults (aged 18–20). Key to their strategy is the evidence that young adults are still maturing. Although individuals generally reach physical maturity during mid-adolescence, and intellectual maturity by age 18, emotional and social maturity continues into the mid-20s (Prior et al., 2011). The strategy also stresses the importance of assisting young adults who engage in criminal behaviour to move away from criminal behaviour and increase planning for longer-term, pro-social goals (van Gelder, Hershfield, & Nordgren, 2013). Other priorities identified in the strategy included enabling resistance to peer influence; developing self-sufficiency and independence; building skills in managing emotions and impulses; strengthening bonds with family and other close relationships; and education and employment training. Given the evidence for the effectiveness of these interventions, and high rates of criminal justice involvement among care-experienced young people, services and interventions should focus on these areas from much earlier in the lives of care-experienced young people.

Leaving care at 16 or 17 poses particular challenges. Young people who are not care-experienced are generally not expected to cut ties with their support network and attachment relationships beyond 16–17 years old. Unfortunately, once our care-experienced young people reach this age, any positive professional relationships are sadly ended and the loss of these relationships can put significant stressors on young people that can exacerbate their existing socio-structural disadvantage (Kersley, Estep, & Leadley, 2014). This can be a difficult transition period, and local authorities should provide personal advisory support (at the child or young person's discretion) until care-experienced young people reach 25 years old (Department for Education, 2018). Kersley et al. (2014) explored the efficacy of mentoring and befriending schemes to fill this gap and reported that it helped children feel better about themselves and their lives, improved their experience of care and their outcomes on leaving care. Organisations such as Leeds Youth Justice and the Care Leavers Association do excellent work providing mentors for care leavers by individuals with lived experience. This provides young people with an independent, consistent advocate throughout their transition.

Finally, recent research has identified adolescence as a second window of opportunity for healthy brain development (UNICEF, 2017). This reinforces the significance of focusing resources and intervention on this crucial developmental period, to potentially reverse harm from early trauma and provide new opportunities and support for a young person's future. These insights can provide hope and encouragement to all those involved in the social care system and empower them to strive towards better future outcomes for this vulnerable population. Whilst there are pockets of excellent work and support across the country, we must work to develop our systems from the top down and bottom up in unison in order to achieve this for our young people, and strive to have an ethical, nurturing, and ultimately effective system we can be proud of.

Summary of Recommendations

- Work to ensure the system recognises that these are *young people* – individuals who experience and internalise language used. It is essential we move away from language and processes which may indicate to the young person they are "faulty" and can be experienced as dehumanising.

- Minimising placement moves. Ensuring policy and processes support consideration of a placement move as a final option. This is with an aim of fostering a sense of safety and belonging.
- Thought and planning into suitable placement matching by properly trained and experienced individuals, taking into consideration the needs of the young person (and those within the environment in which they are being considered).
- Recognise that current processes are often restrictive, creating a punitive environment that parallels the CJS. Developing of systems and language that provide the boundaries and safeguarding restrictions necessary while allowing for young people to develop.
- Normalising adolescent behaviour and understanding what is 'risk' vs 'typical adolescent behaviour'.
- Preparation for future /transition work. More focus on transition from care to avoid an intergenerational cycle of offending "back to what they know". A focus on building a young person's sense of identity and independence (emotional and practical skills).
- Increased recognition of diversity such as race/ethnicity/sexuality – access to likeminded people and appropriate matching as much as possible.
- Support and services to be available at key critical times in development and retrajectory with offending (e.g., support 17–21+).
- Enhancing societies' perception of care. Young people are stigmatised when it is not their behaviours that have resulted in care. This is most likely achievable by developing a system we are proud of.
- A priority focus on staff well-being and resilience in working with trauma and adversity.
- Comprehensive assessment at key points so young people's needs are identified promptly.
- Research into mentoring/positive role models for care-experienced young people. Such as Leeds Youth Justice and Care Leavers Association who created a group of mentor care leavers (CARE: Challenge and Raise Expectations) – the value of lived experience.

Note

1 County lines is a term used in the UK to describe a form of criminal activity where illegal drugs are transported from one area to another, often across Police and Local Authority boundaries. Usually young and/or vulnerable individuals are used to carry, store, and distribute drugs.

Further Reading

Blumenthal, S., Wood, H. & Williams, A. (2018). *Assessing risk: A relational approach*. Routledge. Presents a comprehensive model of risk that highlights the importance of childhood development, complex interpersonal processes, drawing on empirical research, threat assessment, developmental psychopathology, attachment theory, and a relational model derived from psychoanalysis.

Brierley, A. (2021). *Connecting with young people in trouble: Risk, relationships and lived experience.* Waterside Press. Highly recommended for anyone working within the care or secure/criminal behaviour field, written by an author with lived experience of care and custody.

Perry, B. D., & Szalavitz, M. (2017). *The boy who was raised as a dog: And other stories from a child psychiatrist's notebook-What traumatized children can teach us about loss, love, and healing.* Hachette UK.

Treisman, K. (2016). *Working with relational and developmental trauma in children and adolescents.* Taylor & Francis.

Winfrey, O. (2021). *What happened to you? Conversations on trauma, resilience and healing.* Bluebird.

References

Ackerman, J. P., & Dozier, M. (2005). The influence of foster parent investment on children's representations of self and attachment figures. *Journal of Applied Developmental Psychology, 26*(5), 507–520. doi:10.1016/j.appdev.2005.06.003.

Bazalgette, L., Rahilly, T., & Trevelyan, G. (2015). *Achieving emotional wellbeing for looked after children.* National Society for the Prevention of Cruelty to Children.

Biehal, N (2014). A sense of belonging: Meanings of family and home in long-term foster care. *British Journal of Social Work, 44,* 955–971. doi:10.1093/bjsw/bcs177

Blaustein, M., & Kinniburgh, K. (2018). *Treating traumatic stress in children and adolescents: How to foster resilience through attachment, self-regulation, and competency, Second Edition.* Guilford Press.

Bowlby, J. (1988). Developmental psychiatry comes of age. *American Journal of Psychiatry. 145*(1), 1–10. doi:10.1176/ajp.145.1.1

Bremner, J. D. (2006). Traumatic stress: Effects on the brain. *Dialogues in Clinical Neuroscience, 8*(4), 445–461. doi:10.31887/DCNS.2006.8.4/jbremner

Brend, D. M., & Sprang, G. (2020). Trauma-informed care in child welfare: An imperative for residential childcare workers. *International Journal of Child and Adolescent Resilience, 7*(1), 154–165. doi:10.7202/1072595ar

British Psychological Society. (2011). *Good practice guidelines on the use of psychological formulation.* British Psychological Society.

Bronfenbrenner, U. (1979). *The ecology of human development: Experiments by nature and design.* Harvard University Press.

Brunton-Smith, I., & McCarthy, D. (2016). The effects of prisoner attachment to family on re-entry outcomes: A longitudinal assessment. *British Journal of Criminology. 57*(2), 463–482. doi:10.1093/bjc/azv129.

Buckley, A. M., Lotty, M., & Meldon, S. (2016). What happened to me? Responding to the impact of trauma on children in care: Trauma informed practice in foster care. *The Irish Social Worker, Spring 2016,* 35–40.

Butts, J. A., Bazemore, G., & Saa Meroe, S. (2010). *Positive youth justice–framing justice interventions using the concepts of positive youth development.* Coalition for Juvenile Justice.

Cashmore, J, & Paxman, M. (2006). Predicting after-care outcomes: The importance of 'felt' security. *Child & Family Social Work, 11*(3), 232–241. doi:10.1111/j.1365-2206.2006.00430.x

Children's Commissioner. (2020). *Stability index 2020.* Children's Commissioner for England.

Courtois, C. A., & Ford, J. D. (2013). *Treatment of complex trauma: A sequenced, relationship-based approach.* Guilford Press.

D'Andrea, W., Ford, J., Stolbach, B., Spinazzola, J., & van der Kolk, B. A. (2012). Understanding interpersonal trauma in children: Why we need a developmentally appropriate trauma diagnosis. *American Journal of Orthopsychiatry, 82*(2), 187–200. doi:10.1111/j.1939-0025.2012.01154

Deakin, J., Fox, C., & Matos, R. (2020). Labelled as 'risky' in an era of control: How young people experience and respond to the stigma of criminalized identities. *European Journal of Criminology,* doi:10.1177/1477370820916728

Department for Education. (2016). *Knowledge and skills statement for achieving permanence.* Department for Education.

Department for Education. (2018). *Extending personal advisor support to all care leavers to age 25: Statutory guidance for local authorities.* Department for Education.

Department for Education. (2020). *Children looked after in England including adoption: 2019 to 2020.* Department for Education.

de Vries Robbé, M., Vogel, V., & Douglas, K. (2013). Risk and protective factors: A two-sided dynamic approach to violence risk assessment. *Journal of Forensic Psychiatry and Psychology. 24.* 440–457. doi:10.1080/14789949.2013.818162

Dixon, J. (2008). Young people leaving care: Health, well-being and outcomes. *Child & Family Social Work, 13*(2), 207–217. doi:10.1111/j.1365-2206.2007.00538

Dong, M., Anda, R., Felitti, V., Dube, S., Williamson, D., Thompson, T., Loo, C., & Giles, W. (2004). The interrelatedness of multiple forms of childhood abuse, neglect, and household dysfunction. *Child Abuse and Neglect,* (28), 771–784. doi:10.1016/j.chiabu.2004.01.008

Farmer, M. (2017). *The importance of strengthening prisoners' family ties to prevent reoffending and reduce intergenerational crime.* Ministry of Justice.

Finkelhor, D. (2008). *Childhood victimization: Violence, crime, and abuse in the lives of young people.* Oxford University Press.

Golding, K. (2014). *Connection before correction. Supporting parents to meet the challenges of parenting children who have been traumatized within their early parenting environments.* Retrieved from https://mobilise.kyrateachingschool.com/assets/uploads/files/Connection-before-Correction-Kim-S-Golding.pdf

Hayden, C. (2010). Offending behaviour in care: Is children's residential care a 'criminogenic' environment? *Child & Family Social Work, 15,* 461–472. doi:10.1111/j.1365-2206.2010.00697

Hickle, K. (2020). Introducing a trauma-informed capability approach in youth services. *Children & Society, 34*(6), 537–551. doi:10.1111/chso.12388

Hussey, J. M., Chang, J. J., & Kotch, J. B. (2006). Child maltreatment in the United States: Prevalence, risk factors, and adolescent health consequences. *Pediatrics, 118,* 933–942. doi:10.1542/peds.2005-2452Johnson, R., Browne, K., & Hamilton-Giachritsis, C. (2006). Young children in institutional care at risk of harm. *Trauma, Violence, & Abuse,* 7(1), 34–60. doi:10.1177/1524838005283696

Johnstone, L., & Boyle, M. (2018). with Cromby, J., Dillon, J., Harper, D., Kinderman, P., Longden, E., Pilgrim, D., & Read, J. (2018). *The power threat meaning framework: Towards the identification of patterns in emotional distress, unusual experiences and troubled or troubling behaviour, as an alternative to functional psychiatric diagnosis.* British Psychological Society.

Kersley, H., Estep, B., & Leadley, J. (2014). *Relationships for children in care: The value of mentoring and befriending.* New Economics Foundation (NEF).

Leve, L. D., Harold, G. T., Chamberlain, P., Landsverk, J. A., Fisher, P. A., & Vostanis, P. (2012). Practitioner review: Children in foster care-Vulnerabilities and evidence-based interventions that promote resilience processes. *Journal of Child Psychology and Psychiatry, 53,* 1197–1211. doi:10.1111/j.1469-7610.2012.02594.x

McCann, J. B., James, A., Wilson, S., & Dunn, G. (1996). Prevalence of psychiatric disorders in young people in the care system. *BMJ, 313,* 1526. doi:10.1136/bmj.313.7071.1529

McCarthy, G., Janeway, J., & Geddes, A. (2003). The impact of emotional and behavioural problems on the lives of children growing up in the care system. *Adoption & Fostering, 27*(3), 14–19. doi:10.1177/030857590302700305

McSherry, D., Malet, M. F., & Weatherall, K. (2016). Comparing long-term placements for young children in care: Does placement type really matter? *Children and Youth Services Review, 69,* 56–66. doi:10.1016/j.childyouth.2016.07.021

Ministry of Justice. (2015). *2010 to 2015 government policy: Young offenders.* Ministry of Justice. Retrieved from www.gov.uk/government/publications/2010-to-2015-government-policy-young-offenders/

Moran, L., McGregor, C., & Devaney, C. (2020). Exploring the multi-dimensionality of permanence and stability: Emotions, experiences and temporality in young people's discourses about long-term foster care in Ireland. *Qualitative Social Work, 19*(5-6), doi:10.1177/1473325019871607

National Child Traumatic Stress Network. (2013). Child welfare trauma training toolkit. Retrieved from www.NCTSN.org

National Institute for Health & Care Excellence. (2015). *Children's attachment: Attachment in children and young people who are adopted from care, in care or at high risk of going into care.* Retrieved from www.ncbi.nlm.nih.gov/books/NBK338143/

National Offender Management Service. (2015). *Better outcomes for young adult men: Evidence based commissioning principles.* National Offender Management Service.

NSPCC. (2021). Statistics briefing: Looked after children. Retrieved from https://learning.nspcc.org.uk/media/1622/statistics-briefing-looked-after-children.pdf

Oosterman, M., Schuengel, C., Slot, N.W., Bullens, R.A., & Doreleijers, T.A. (2007). Disruptions in foster care: A review and meta-analysis. *Children and Youth Services Review, 29*(1), 53–76. doi:10.1016/j.childyouth.2006.07.003

Prior, D., Farrow, K., Hughes, N., Kelly, G., Manders, G., White, S., & Wilkinson, B. (2011). *Maturity, young adults and criminal justice: A literature review.* University of Birmingham.

Prison Reform Trust. (2016). In care, out of trouble. Retrieved from www.prisonreformtrust.org.uk/Portals/0/Documents/In%20care%20out%20of%20trouble%20summary.pdf

Rock, S., Michelson, D., Thomson, S., & Day, C. (2015). Understanding foster placement instability for looked after children: A systematic review and narrative synthesis of quantitative and qualitative evidence. *British Journal of Social Work, 45*(1), 177–203. doi:10.1093/bjsw/bct084

Sallnäs, M., Vinnerljung, B., & Kyhle Westermark, P. (2004). Breakdown of teenage placements in Swedish foster and residential care. *Child & Family Social Work, 9*(2), 141–152. doi:10.1111/j.1365-2206.2004.00309

Schofield, G., Ward, E., Biggart, L., Scaife, V., Dodsworth, J., Larsson, B., ... & Stone, N. (2012). *Looked after children and offending: Reducing risk and promoting resilience.* UEA.

Sharda, L. (2013). Giving a trauma Lens to Resource Parents *CW360° Winter 2013, 19.*

Skowyra, K., & Cocozza, J. (2007). *A blueprint for change: Improving the system response to youth with mental health needs involved with the juvenile justice system.* National Centre for Mental Health and Juvenile Justice Policy Research Associates Inc.

Smith, D. K., Chamberlain, P., & Deblinger, E. (2012). Adapting multidimensional treatment foster care for the treatment of co-occurring trauma and delinquency in adolescent girls. *Journal of Child and Adolescent Trauma, 5*(3), 224–238.

Svensson, R., Weerman, F. M., Pauwels, L. J., Bruinsma, G. J., & Bernasco, W. (2013). Moral emotions and offending: Do feelings of anticipated shame and guilt mediate the effect of socialization on offending? *European Journal of Criminology, 10*(1), 22–39. doi:10.1177/1477370812454393

UNICEF. (2017). *The adolescent brain: A second window of opportunity.* Retrieved from https://reliefweb.int/sites/reliefweb.int/files/resources/adolescent_brain_a_second_window_of_opportunity_a_compendium.pdf

van Gelder, J. L., Hershfield, H. E., & Nordgren, L. F. (2013). Vividness of the future self predicts delinquency. *Psychological Science, 24,* 974–980. doi:10.1177/0956797612465197

Weale, S. (2018, June 1). Children in care being 'pinged' around schools and homes, says report. *The Guardian.* https://www.theguardian.com/society/2018/jun/01/children-in-care-being-pinged-around-schools-and-homes-says-report

Widom, C. S. (1989). The cycle of violence. *Science, 244,* 160–166. doi:10.1126/science.2704995

Widom, C. S., & Maxfield, M. G. (2001). *An update on the "cycle of violence"* (NIJ Research in Brief). US Department of Justice, Office of Justice Programs, National Institute of Justice.

Willmot, P., & Evershed, S. (2018). Interviewing people given a diagnosis of personality disorder in forensic settings. *International Journal of Forensic Mental Health, 17*(4), 338–350. doi:10.1080/14999013.2018.1508097

Woodall, T. G. (2022). "An exploration of young people's experiences relating to stability and permanence throughout their care journey." Manuscript submitted for publication.

Youth Justice Board, Ministry of Justice & the Office of National Statistics. (2020, January 30). Retrieved from https://assets.publishing.service.gov.uk/government/uploads/system/uploads/attachment_data/file/862078/youth-justice-statistics-bulletin-march-2019.pdf

Youth Justice Board for England and Wales. (2019). *Strategic plan 2019-2022*. Retrieved from https://assets.publishing.service.gov.uk/government/uploads/system/uploads/attachment_data/file/802702/YJB_Strategic_Plan_2019_to_2022.pdf

6

TRAUMA AND INTELLECTUAL DISABILITY

Emma Longfellow and Rachel Hicks

Introduction

Several contextual issues impact on our understanding of trauma within forensic Intellectual Disability (ID) populations. One of the most critical is the base issue of identifying who and where the ID population are, as there is immense variation in prevalence of ID in forensic settings noted in existing studies as well as inconsistency in ID definition (Hellenbach, Karatzias, & Brown, 2017; Murphy, Harnett, & Holland, 1995). This fundamental issue in understanding who this group are also limits our understanding of the prevalence and experience of trauma in this population. Although the data are flawed, it is largely accepted that individuals with ID are over-represented in forensic settings (Hayes, Shackell, Mottram, & Lancaster, 2007; Heaton & Murphy, 2013; Hellenbach et al., 2017). We also know that ID populations are more vulnerable than non-ID populations to experiencing trauma, have resiliency deficits (van der Put, Asscher, Wissink, & Stams, 2014), and are at a heightened risk of developing post-traumatic stress disorder (PTSD) (Daveney, Hassiotis, Katona, Matcham, & Sen, 2019). It is therefore reasonable to assume that trauma prevalence in forensic ID populations is likely to be high. This is likely to be further compounded by the trauma of receiving an ID diagnosis itself, or conversely from ID being undiagnosed and unrecognised (García-Largo, Martí-Agustí, Martin-Fumadó, & Gómez-Durán, 2020). Despite limitations in the literature there is a clear need to consider trauma and its sequelae when caring for individuals with ID.

Defining Intellectual Disability and Trauma

An Intellectual Disability is principally defined by three core criteria: a significantly reduced ability to understand new or complex information in learning new skills (evident in lower intellectual ability), reduced ability to cope independently (evident in impaired adaptive functioning), and that these difficulties started before adulthood and had a lasting effect on development (British Psychological Society, 2015). Individuals with ID are not a homogeneous group, which is evident in varied

DOI: 10.4324/9781003120766-9

cognitive and adaptive functioning, co-occurring neurodevelopmental difficulties, personality, environmental stressors (Emerson & Hatton, 2007), and attachments (Smith, 2009). To capture the varying degrees of functioning displayed, ID has been further subcategorised into mild, moderate, severe, and profound to support in identifying individual support needs (Department of Health, 2001).

As well as understanding what we mean by ID, it is important to clarify what we mean by trauma in ID populations. Based on the available literature and drawing from the authors' clinical experience we have identified two types of trauma for an individual with ID: the trauma associated with having an ID (both recognised and unrecognised) and the broader trauma of adverse life events (whether single or multiple traumas across the life course). These in reality do not exist in silos and regularly co-occur.

There have been several studies over the past 50 years that have explored the impact of diagnostic labels on an individual. In relation to cognitive abilities, labels have been found to have a negative impact on the perception of critical others – such as teachers, carers, and parents – and on self-perception (Daley & Rappolt-Schlichtmann, 2018). Labels associated with special educational needs and ID were noted to be perceived as "shameful", isolating, impacting on future placements, creating self-doubt, and learned helplessness (Daley & Rappolt-Schlichtmann). Ho (2004) argued that pathologising and labelling individuals based on their intellectual difference was counterproductive and unnecessary. They noted that inclusion was dependent on understanding the range of contexts that influence an individual's cognitive abilities and learning. They suggested starting from the presumption that all individuals are unique and that, in turn, we should be flexible in our approaches. Pathologising ID can create an "out group" and raises the issue of othering and micro-aggressions in ID populations. One of the critical elements associated with othering is the idea that the dominant group is distant from the other "lesser" group and can dehumanise, discriminate, and marginalise further (Staszak, 2008). In many cases this can occur subconsciously and can become easily embedded in institutions and complex systems. Peternelj-Taylor (2004) noted this as commonplace in forensic psychiatric settings, evident in the use of depersonalising language. This can manifest as micro-aggressions centred on "us" and "them" using blanket statements, being condescending (using a baby voice) and assuming ID means intellectual inability. Conversely those with ID who are not identified or recognised can experience similar difficulties due to a lack of understanding or reasonable adjustment contributing to decreased self-esteem, isolation, and exclusion (Peternelj-Taylor, 2004). García-Largo et al. (2020) note that not identifying those with ID within forensic settings impacts on provision and contributes to re-traumatisation of an already marginalised and vulnerable population.

People with an ID have been found to be more likely to experience traumatic events and negative life events than individuals who do not have an ID (Catani & Sossalla, 2015; Wigham, Taylor, & Hatton, 2014). Impaired intellectual ability generally is associated with increased risk of exposure to adverse events and development of PTSD (Breslau, Lucia, & Alvarado, 2006; Macklin et al., 1998; Tureck, Matson, Cervantes, & Konst, 2014). The increased likelihood of being exposed to environmental stressors, including issues such as poverty (Wigham & Emerson, 2015), contributes to people with ID being at a higher risk of having their resilience compromised and developing mental health difficulties. Children with an ID are significantly more at risk of experiencing physical and verbal violence (Jones et al., 2012), emotional abuse (Sullivan & Knutson, 2000), and neglect (Miller & Brown, 2014) than children without an ID. They experience significantly more disruptions in attachment and caregiver bonding as they are less likely to remain with their biological families after birth (Milligan & Stevens, 2006; Smith, 2009), and more likely to be placed on the *at-risk* register (Spencer et al., 2005), to enter the care system and to struggle to find long-term foster placements. This results in a reliance on carers and systems and contributes to high prevalence of carer perpetrated violence in institutional settings (Wigham & Emerson, 2015). People with an ID are more at risk of exposure to other types of trauma such as systematic abuse and neglect over long periods of time (Hatton & Emerson, 2004; Sobsey & Doe, 1991) compounded further by difficulties in recognising and reporting.

Trauma Prevalence

Brackenridge and Morrissey (2010) published a service evaluation within the National High Secure Learning Disability Service at Rampton Hospital exploring trauma experiences and post-trauma symptoms. They assessed for experiences of multiple types of abuse, including physical, psychological, sexual, institutional, discriminatory, financial and neglect, using information gathered from file information, self- and observer-report. This was repeated by Longfellow and Hicks (2020) who reviewed available file information and existing assessments that identified trauma presence or absence for each patient. Trauma was defined as any experience of physical or sexual violence, psychological or emotional trauma across lifetime and contexts. From this review 98% of patients were identified as having experienced some form of trauma. Eighty-six per cent experienced psychological or emotional trauma, 84% experienced physical violence, and 80% experienced sexual violence. Of the 98% who experienced some form of trauma, all experienced multiple (four or more separate types) forms of trauma suggesting complex chronic trauma experiences within the population.

In a recent meta-analysis, the weighted pooled prevalence of PTSD in people with ID who had accessed non-forensic services was found to be 10% based on 1,381 participants from seven included studies (Daveney et al., 2019). The estimated prevalence rates in the general population have ranged from five to ten per cent (Kessler, Chiu, Demler, & Walters, 2005; Shalev, Liberzon, & Marmar, 2017). This would place the estimated prevalence for individuals with an ID towards the upper limit, indicating that there may be a heightened risk of developing PTSD for individuals with ID (Daveney et al., 2019). However, the quality of studies included in the review was low and there was large heterogeneity in the estimates, with a 95% confidence interval of 0.4 to 19.5 per cent (Daveney et al., 2019). Despite its limitations, this study highlights the importance of considering trauma and its sequelae when caring for individuals with ID.

Reason for Under-Representation

There are several factors that contribute to why trauma prevalence is less known in ID populations. Formal diagnosis of trauma-specific difficulties remains rare within the ID population despite evidence to suggest that individuals with ID are likely to be susceptible to the full range of trauma associated psychiatric disorders (Dosen, 2007). Psychiatric assessment of ID is inherently problematic. Impairments in receptive and expressive language make it difficult for individuals with ID to understand and respond to clinicians who typically rely on the person's identification and description of his or her experiences and emotional states, especially as the level of intellectual functioning declines (Fletcher, Beasley, & Jacobson, 1999; Fletcher, Loschen, Stavrakaki, & First, 2007). Where symptoms and behaviours are observed, diagnostic overshadowing can contribute to the over-attribution of this to ID itself, contributing to a failure to adequately understand or address trauma needs. Moreover, psychiatric symptoms are often expressed differently in persons with ID compared to those without ID (Fletcher, Lyon, Fuchs, & Barnes, 2018). Additionally, there are difficulties for those with ID in recognising the behaviour of others as harmful or neglectful, further compounding any communication of events or impact.

It has been previously noted that trauma understanding, assessment, and interventions for the ID population are limited compared to the general population (Hastings, 2013; Wigham & Emerson, 2015; Wigham, Hatton, & Taylor, 2011) and this is compounded further in the forensic ID population. Failures to appropriately recognise and respond to trauma will likely impact on the length of residence within secure services as well as the inadequate and ineffective intervention for the individual. The Winterbourne View scandal which exposed physical and psychological abuse of people with learning disabilities at a private hospital in England in 2011, and further recent examples, highlights how individuals with ID are at a greater likelihood to be harmed within services that are supposed to be caring for them. This provided a catalyst for a range of subsequent policies, procedures, and guidance on working with ID from the Transforming Care Agenda, including the active closure and reduction in inpatient care settings and increased community placement. Commentary on the appropriateness of this agenda is beyond the scope of this chapter, although there has been much debate within the literature (Hollins, Lodge, & Lomax, 2019). However, to support individuals with ID who have offended or display behaviour that challenges to progress into less secure environments, reintegrate into the community, and live meaningful lives, the factors that contribute to behaviour that challenges and offending behaviour need to be understood to enable appropriate intervention and care. To neglect this is to further neglect an already marginalised and mistreated population (Taylor, McKinnon, Thorpe, & Gillmer 2017). Crucial to this aim is an increased knowledge of the impact of trauma and the consideration of trauma and its sequelae being priority targets for intervention (Lovell & Skellern, 2020; van der Put et al., 2014). Although a recent qualitative analysis of the views of learning disability nurses working in varying levels of secure psychiatric hospitals within the UK demonstrated anecdotal understanding of the significant impact of traumatic experiences on offending behaviour (Lovell & Skellern, 2020), there is still a lack of empirical enquiry.

Impact of Trauma on Behaviour in ID

The link between childhood maltreatment and offending is discussed in detail in Chapter 1. This highlighted that a minority of those exposed to childhood maltreatment will subsequently commit serious or violent offences, although the pathways are complex and not well understood. Despite the growing evidence base on the link between ID, trauma exposure, and over-representation in forensic settings, there is a paucity of research into the link between trauma and offending in those with ID. Research conducted using a sample of justice-involved juveniles in the US compared the history of maltreatment and abuse and the relationship between these experiences and subsequent offending behaviour for those with and without a formal diagnosis of ID (van der Put et al., 2014). As anticipated from the literature, juveniles with ID had a higher prevalence of adverse childhood experiences than those without an ID diagnosis. Furthermore, the relationship between being a victim of abuse and sexual offending was stronger for the juveniles with ID than those without, although for violent offending there was no significant difference between the ID and non-ID individuals. Although causality cannot be inferred because of the correlational nature of this research, this study supported the notion that trauma should be a core consideration when trying to understand the offending behaviour of individuals with ID.

Exploration of trauma and offending in ID populations can be more difficult than other populations. It has been found that individuals with ID are viewed as less accountable for their actions and that carers or staff in forensic services are reluctant to report behaviour to the police (Steans & Duff, 2020). Consequently, there can be a lack of formally recorded offending behaviour. It is therefore useful to consider *behaviour that challenges* and *behaviours of distress* when exploring the impact of trauma exposure (Rittmannsberger, Yanagida, Weber, & Lueger-Schuster, 2020). Those with ID who experience maltreatment and adverse events may present with behaviours that challenge at an elevated rate due to the nature of difficulties associated with ID, such as problems in emotion regulation, poorer problem-solving capacities, and difficulties in social communication (van der Put et al., 2014).

Significantly, the National Institute for Health and Care Excellence (NICE) does not formally consider the possibility for behaviour to represent manifestations of trauma responses in their published guidance (NICE, 2018a) for working with behaviour that challenges in individuals with ID (Morris, Webb, Parmar, Trundle, & McLean, 2020). In addition, NICE also neglects to consider individuals with developmental disorders as a population that are more at risk of exposure to adversity in their guidance for psychological trauma (NICE, 2018b), despite Morris, Shergill, and Beber (2019) highlighting that those with ID are disproportionately affected by adverse childhood events. Given that NICE have a key role in providing the guidelines for practice and quality standards for health and social care professionals in the National Health Service (NICE, 2021), these omissions can be considered to further exacerbate the vulnerability of individuals with ID. In doing so they fail to adequately capture the needs of individuals with ID or promote good practice to manage the impact of exposure to adversity within the services designed to care for them (Morris et al., 2020).

Trauma-Informed Care and ID

The concept of TIC was developed in the US in response to the increasing awareness that individuals entering human services have often experienced trauma, and that the services that they rely on for help could often inadvertently be re-traumatising (Fallot & Harris, 2008; Harris & Fallot, 2001; Keesler, 2016; Sweeney, Clement, Filson, & Kennedy, 2016). TIC is a philosophy to guide service culture, service delivery, and individual care with the principles of trustworthiness, empowerment, choice, safety, and collaboration to prevent re-traumatisation and support recovery (Fallot & Harris, 2008; Harris & Fallot, 2001). One core component of TIC is changing the narrative surrounding the individual's behaviour and preventing pathologising language by asking "what happened to you?" as opposed to "what is wrong with you?" (Harris & Fallot, 2001). This supports in reframing the understanding of the behaviour as being a survival strategy that developed in response to the context and enables clinicians to focus on the individual's underlying needs (Sweeney et al., 2016). TIC within hospital settings is discussed in more detail in Chapter 20.

Despite the increasing awareness that individuals with ID may be dispro-portionately exposed to adverse experiences compared to the general popula-tion and the fact that many individuals with ID are likely to have contact with support services (Keesler, 2014a), there has been little research into or imple-mentation of TIC within ID services (Keesler, 2014a; 2016). As discussed above, diagnostic overshadowing within ID populations can preclude the exploration of what happened to individuals and the consideration that current presenting behaviour may be the manifestation of previous trauma (Mevissen & De Jongh, 2010). This can be harmful for individuals as the response to the behaviour may fail to account for the potential for interventions to be re-traumatising and evoke the emotional and physiological experiences associated with the original event (Sweeney et al., 2016). If individuals continue to feel unsafe and re-experience trauma, they may continue to rely on the survival responses they developed to cope, such as self-harm or aggression (Sweeney et al., 2016). Practices that have the potential to trigger past trauma or create new trauma may occur within forensic and mental health settings, including restraint, seclusion, enforced medication, being the victim of violence from peers, and coercive practices (Butler, Critelli, & Rinfrette, 2011; Faccini & Allely, 2021; Goad, 2021; Keesler & Isham, 2017; Sweeney et al., 2016) and ultimately not having freedom. Therefore, adopting a TIC approach would support in identification of past trauma, potential triggers for this, and inform decisions on how to intervene when individuals display poten-tially harmful behaviour (Faccini & Allely, 2021).

Keesler (2014a) has outlined how TIC can be implemented within ID services. One component crucial to effective integration of TIC principles is the training of staff to increase their understanding of trauma and how this can impact on individuals (Keesler, 2014a, 2014b; Sweeney et al., 2016). In addition, Keesler (2014a) proposed that sensitive and consistent approaches, having clearly identified boundaries, adequate staffing resources, incorporating individuals' perspectives into their care planning, and focussing on individuals' strengths are all central to trauma-informed ID services.

One of the five TIC principles that has historically been problematic in ID services is *choice*, as staff assumptions that the presence of ID compromises an individual's ability to make an informed choice can exacerbate a sense of powerlessness (Keesler, 2014a; 2016). Essential to enabling choice and engendering a sense of empowerment will be a focus on supporting individuals' understanding of their available options and increase their ability to make their own informed choices (Keesler, 2014a). In a survey conducted with staff who support individuals with ID, Keesler (2020a) found that the collaboration principle was the least strongly endorsed by participants. This suggests that more needs to be done to ensure the voices of individuals with ID are heard and that their own preferences are at the core of decisions relating to support (Keesler & Isham, 2017).

Research conducted with non-ID populations has indicated that implementing TIC has had a positive impact, including a reduction in the use of restraint and seclusion in a psychiatric setting for children and adolescents (Azeem, Aujla, Rammerth, Binsfeld, & Jones, 2011). This would fit with the wider strategy for ID services in the UK to reduce the use of restrictive practices. Keesler and Isham (2017) presented the findings from the implementation of a new trauma-informed day service for individuals with ID who had recently exited institutions in the US. They found reductions in behaviours that challenge, aggression, and the use of medication, but an increase in least restrictive interventions that were used as an alternative. The use of TIC has also been found beneficial for staff working within support organisations, among whom there can also be a high level of trauma experiences (Keesler, 2018). A trauma-informed organisational culture in ID services has been found to be associated with increased psychological wellness and reduced burnout amongst staff (Keesler, 2020b). Therefore, TIC may support in staff well-being and retention, leading to greater consistency in the care of individuals with ID who use services which is seen as central in creating a safe environment (Keesler, 2014a).

Implementation of TIC within ID services is dependent on change in organisational culture and for all policies, procedures, and clinical practices to reflect the TIC principles by being sensitive to the trauma experiences that individuals may have been exposed to (Goad, 2021; Keesler, 2016). Organisations that support individuals with ID need to commit to adopting TIC (Keesler, 2020b; Rich, DiGregorio, & Strassle, 2020), which would enable access to interventions that consider trauma when attempting to understand current clinical presentation (Truesdale et al., 2019). Research suggests that staff view TIC as the most beneficial way to progress to ensure that services are effectively meeting the needs of adults with ID (Truesdale et al., 2019). The research base on TIC within the ID field is still in its infancy and studies conducted to date have failed to capture the views of those with ID or their carers. This should therefore be a focus of future research (Rich et al., 2020).

Case Example: Bob

We present an example of using a trauma-informed approach with an adult male diagnosed with ID. This highlights how the principles of TIC have informed his care since entering the service.

Bob was born in mainland Europe and was described as being an irritable baby who cried often. He is one of four children from his parents' relationship, with an older sister, a younger sister, and a younger brother. There is reference in his history to another sibling who sadly died suddenly in infancy, although Bob has never spoken about this. His mother was reported to have consumed up to 70cl of spirit alcohol daily during her pregnancy with Bob and there was some suggestion that he suffered from foetal alcohol syndrome. Bob demonstrated some developmental delay in his speech and was seen by a speech and language therapist from the age of four. He was noted to experience delays in creative play and difficulties interacting with other children. Bob received a diagnosis of Learning Disability and Attention Deficit Hyperactivity Disorder (ADHD) at the age of seven. He accessed a special school within his birth country.

Bob's family home was characterised by a lack of safety and he experienced multiple adverse childhood experiences. The level of care provided by his parents would have been considered to be neglectful, with Bob describing that he learned to look after himself and his younger siblings whilst his father was at work. Bob's father alleged that his mother spent time as a sex worker and would bring men back to the house, and that his mother also attempted to arrange for one of his sisters to have sex with men for money when she was nine years old. It is unclear whether Bob witnessed any of this or has any awareness that this occurred. The relationship between his parents was reportedly difficult and Bob witnessed domestic violence within the family home. His mother abused substances and was physically violent towards Bob. When his parent's relationship ended, Bob and his siblings initially stayed with their mother. However, Bob said that his mother wanted to place him, but not his siblings, in care because his behaviour was difficult to manage, and as a result, he felt unwanted and not part of the family.

Due to the difficulties in the relationship and the care provided by his mother, Bob went to live with his father when he was six years old. He remained in contact with his mother and said that he saw her approximately once or twice a week. Bob reported that his mother attempted to strangle him on one occasion and that, to protect himself, he threatened her with a knife. In response to this incident, Bob spent nine months in a psychiatric unit when he was six years old. Bob's father was also reportedly physically violent towards him, using this as punishment for unwanted behaviour from Bob. Bob also reported being the victim of unprovoked physical violence perpetrated by his aunt. The relationship between him and his siblings was also characterised by violence, with Bob reporting that on one occasion his older sister threw him down the stairs. He stated that he would retaliate with violence, and that sometimes he would also use violence towards his younger brother when he had become irritated by him.

Bob's behaviour at school was described as being extreme, including setting fires, which resulted in him twice being suspended from school and subsequently expelled for violent behaviour at the age of seven. After his expulsion, Bob was placed into a children's home where his education continued. Bob moved to the UK with his father and siblings when he was approximately ten years old and attended a mainstream high school. He reports that he experienced bullying within this high school and that one particular individual would make comments about his father and push him. Bob attempted to resolve this by telling teachers but said that he was not believed and therefore decided that he needed to take matters into his own hands. He was subsequently expelled from school for physical violence towards this individual and received one-to-one teaching for a short period of time.

In the UK, Bob's home life continued to be challenging. He came to the attention of his Local Authority when he was approximately 11 years old following a referral from the Child and Adolescent Mental Health Team. The next year, an investigation took place following statements made by Bob about touching his sisters in a sexually inappropriate manner. He was interviewed by the police and made disclosures about sexual behaviour, but his sisters wrote letters withdrawing the allegations. Shortly after this time, a child protection conference was held, and Bob and his siblings were made subject to a child protection plan. As there were continued concerns, Bob was placed into foster care when he was aged 13. Bob would often abscond so that he could visit his father and siblings as he wished to be reunited with them. His foster placement unfortunately broke down a year later due to reported aggressive behaviour by Bob. He was placed into a children's home and subsequently a residential unit for adolescents with emotional and behavioural disorders. Bob reported being the victim of bullying by other children. It was within this placement that he committed his index offence of sexual assault on a member of staff, resulting in his transfer to a CAMHS Unit and receiving a Hospital Order. Within hospital placements, Bob has demonstrated physical violence towards staff members and peers. This has resulted in transfers to higher levels of security and to his current placement.

Trauma-Informed Care and Bob

In accordance with the principles of TIC, the focus of attempts to understand Bob's past and current offending and behaviours of distress has been on gaining information on what has happened to him in his life and the meaning he has taken from this. Since entering the service he has been offered opportunities to report any traumatic experiences he may have had and receive validation and support with this.

Bob collaboratively developed a compassion-focussed formulation with his current therapist to explore the impact of his past experiences on his current behaviour. The diagrammatic format of this is presented in Figure 6.1. This highlights how the adverse childhood experiences contributed to a lack of experienced safety for Bob, leading him to develop survival strategies in the form of physical violence and hiding any form of vulnerability that he believes could be viewed as a weakness by other people. The frequent placement breakdowns and disruptions to his attachment relationships further exacerbated his lack of sense of safety and opportunities to feel cared for and valued, instead reinforcing his belief that he is unwanted and rejected by other people.

All staff in the National High Secure Learning Disability Service have received a one-day trauma awareness training package to support in their understanding of the impact of trauma and potential manifestation in current clinical presentations. In addition, Bob's therapist and Clinical Nurse Practitioner facilitated a reflective practice

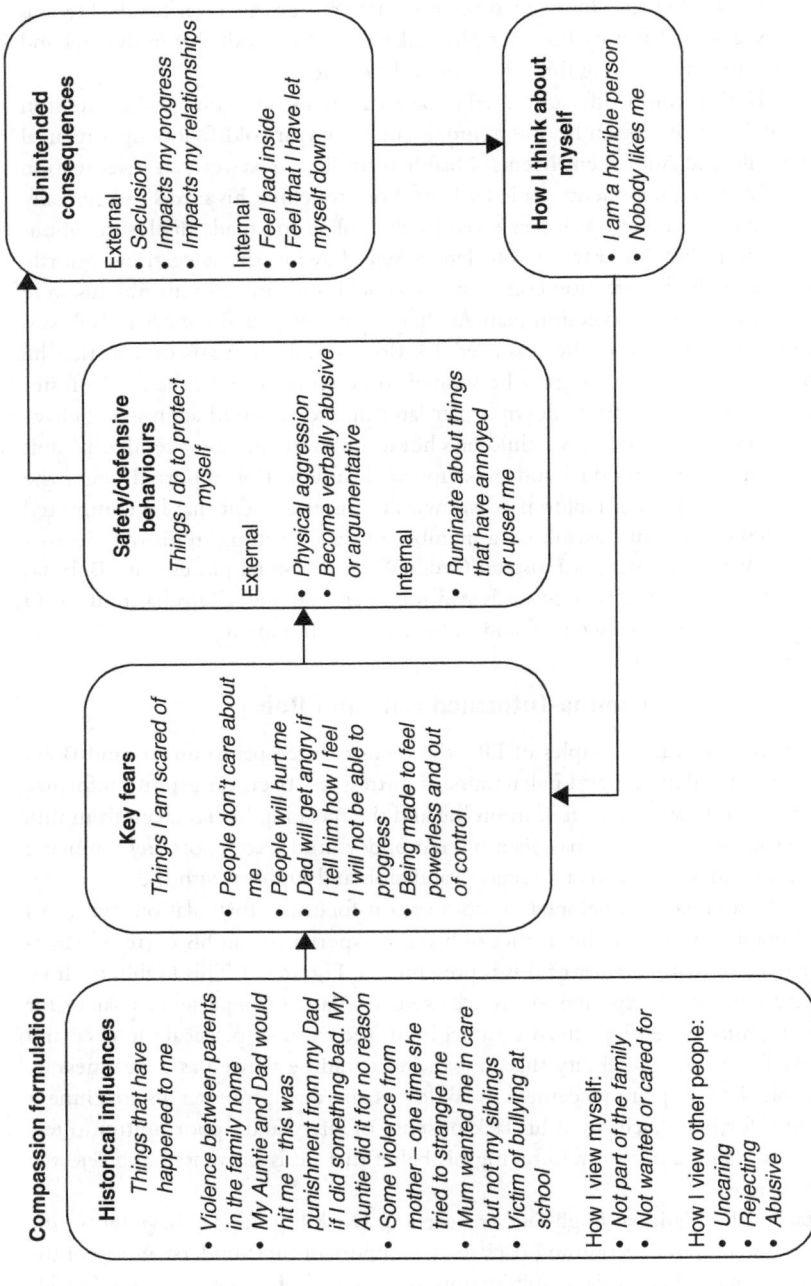

Figure 6.1 Collaboratively developed compassion formulation

day for members of his clinical team and nursing staff to share his life history and formulation. This space facilitated an enhanced awareness of the factors that could be contributing to his behaviour of distress to support staff in considering sensitive and least restrictive ways to support him with these. One factor that Bob identified as being triggering for him was the tone of voice of the person speaking to him as this could remind him of conflict between his parents. The knowledge gained from Bob has been used to inform his Positive Behaviour Support (PBS) plan (see Figure 6.2)

My Positive Behaviour Support (PBS) Plan

Name: Bob

A PBS plan is a way to help staff to get to know you, understand your behaviour, and support you to achieve your goals.

Staff can look at your PBS plan to know the best ways to help you to stay well. It will also let them know how to support you in positive ways when you are experiencing distress.

All About Me

This is where you can tell people the most important things about you. This could be about some of your favourite things, things that you don't like, your personality, or anything else that you think people should know.

I like to be busy and active.
I like to have jokes when I am feeling good.
I am very chatty.

My Goals

This is where you can share what you are currently hoping to achieve and what things you think you might need to change to help with this.

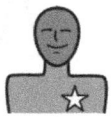

My goal is to move to a medium secure unit and out of hospital. I am doing my treatment.
I think I need to work on my anger – for example when I get told something not to react in an aggressive way and to sort it out in a positive way.

Figure 6.2 Collaboratively developed PBS plan for Bob. Pictures are from Widgit symbols © Widgit Software 2002–2021

When I am Well	
Things I will do and what people will see 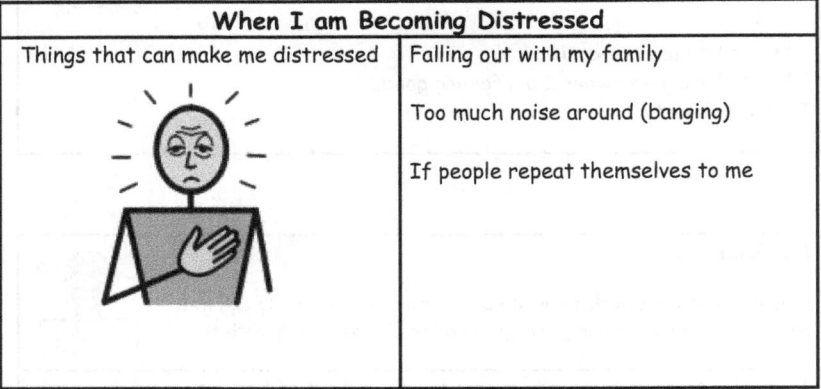	Doing loads of activities Speaking to people Interacting a lot Smiling a lot
Things that help me to feel well	Playing FIFA Football Board games (e.g. rummikub) Gym
What other people can do to support me to feel well	Encourage me to get off the ward as much as possible Tell me when I am doing well

When I am Becoming Distressed	
Things that can make me distressed	Falling out with my family Too much noise around (banging) If people repeat themselves to me

Figure 6.2 Continued

Things I will do and what people will see	Start wandering around a lot
	I disengage
	I sit quietly
	I stop doing my activities
What other people can do to support me to feel better	Have a chat with me – see if they can make me in a better mood
	Offer me things to do that might help – for example fresh air or music

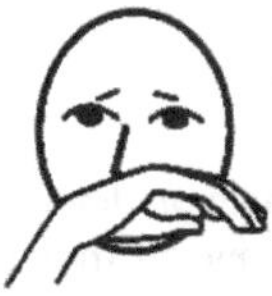

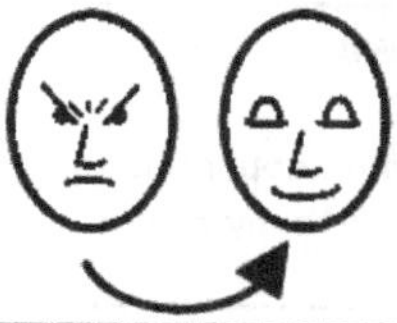

When I am Very Distressed	
Things that can make me very distressed	When people tell me what to do
	If people crowd around me – it makes me feel angry
	Having bad phone calls with family or friends
Things I will do and what people will see	I start fidgeting
	Play with my hair (twist it)
	I become rude
	I shout
	I won't listen

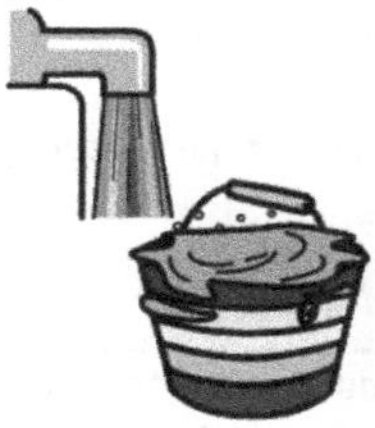

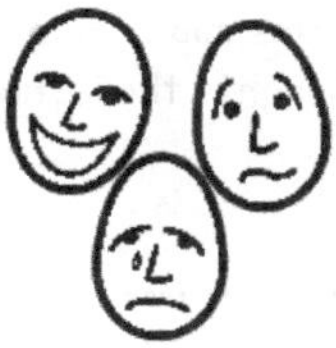

Figure 6.2 Continued

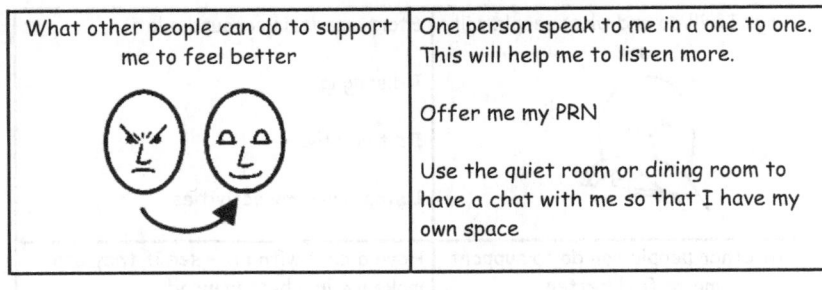

What other people can do to support me to feel better	One person speak to me in a one to one. This will help me to listen more. Offer me my PRN Use the quiet room or dining room to have a chat with me so that I have my own space

When I am Calming Down	
I am still not OK and I might go back to red if I am not supported to recover. Supporting me in the right way will help me to get back to my green.	
Things I will do and what people will see	I will be really quiet I feel sorry for myself I feel upset and sad – I think that I have let everyone down Sometimes I might take myself to my room
What other people can do to support me to get back to green	Staff can encourage me to go off ward to cheer me up or do things that will get me in a better mood Staff can offer to talk through what has happened - this might help me to challenge my thoughts that I have let everyone down

Figure 6.2 Continued

which informs staff of the most effective ways to support him at different phases of an emotional response. The implementation of plans that are informed by his trauma and his own preferences had a positive impact on his well-being and progress, with a significant reduction in the frequency and intensity of aggression displayed by Bob. This may represent an increased sense of safety and empowerment that has enabled him to relinquish his survival strategies.

My Skill Toolbox **All the skills I have learned to help me keep well**	
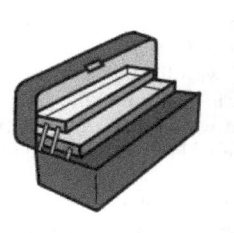	Listen to music Explain to people how I am feeling Use skills I have learned in therapy (such as cold water and paired muscle relaxation) Stop and think before acting on my urges

Figure 6.2 Continued

Moving forward, Bob is working on his goal to progress to less secure conditions and eventually return to the community. He is being supported to work towards this goal by his clinical team who are supporting him in accordance with his needs and incorporating his views and preferences within his care plans. Bob is currently engaged in adapted Dialectical Behaviour Therapy (I Can Feel Good; Ashworth, Brotherton, Ingamells, & Morrissey, 2018) to increase his capacity to cope with his emotional experiences. He will soon be commencing Compassion Focussed Therapy (CFT: Gilbert, 2005) to explore his offending in a trauma-informed way.

Conclusion

Progress has been made in the awareness of the increased victimisation and margin-alisation that can be experienced by individuals with ID, particularly the elevated trauma prevalence of those who have contact with forensic services. This still needs to fully translate into policy and systemic change to ensure that adverse experiences are identified and the impact for the individual can be understood. Central to this aim is empowering individuals with ID to have their voice and be heard by asking "what has happened to you?" rather than "what is wrong with you?". Although we are beginning to recognise and implement TIC within forensic ID services, there is a paucity of research evaluating the effectiveness of this. Available research indicates that successful TIC could reduce the need for restrictive practice and facilitate reinte-gration and maintenance in the community. This could support a better quality of life for those who have experienced contact with forensic services to be re-traumatising. For others, forensic settings represent stability, care, and safety that they were never able to experience in the community. What cannot go unnoticed is the ongoing need to reduce the victimisation, marginalisation, and stigma of this population way before they encounter forensic services.

Further Reading

Cowles, M., Medley, A., & Randle-Phillips, C. (2020). Compassion-focussed therapy for trauma in people with intellectual disabilities: A conceptual review. *Journal of Intellectual Disabilities, 24*(2) 212–232. For readers interested in the use of CFT with ID populations.

Goad, E. (2021). Working alongside people with intellectual disabilities who have had difficult experiences: Reflections on trauma-informed care within a service context. *Journal of Intellectual Disabilities*. For readers interested in the use of TIC with ID populations and systems.

Wiseman, P., & Watson, N. (2021). "Because I've got a learning disability, they don't take me seriously:" Violence, wellbeing, and devaluing people with learning disabilities. *Journal of Interpersonal Violence*. For readers interested in individuals with ID as their own narrators of their experiences.

References

Ashworth, S., Brotherton, N., Ingamells, B. and Morrissey, C. (2018). *I can feel good: DBT-informed skills training for people with intellectual disabilities and problems managing emotions* (2nd ed.). Hove: Pavilion Publishing.

Azeem, M. W., Aujla, A., Rammerth, M., Binsfeld, G., & Jones, R. B. (2011). Effectiveness of six core strategies based on trauma informed care in reducing seclusions and restraints at a child and adolescent psychiatric hospital. *Journal of Child and Adolescent Psychiatric Nursing, 24*(1), 11–15. doi:10.1111/j.1744-6171.2010.00262.x

Brackenridge, I., & Morrissey, C. (2010). Trauma and post-traumatic stress disorder (PTSD) in a high secure forensic learning disability population: Future directions for practice. *Advances in Mental Health and Intellectual Disabilities, 4*(3), 49–56. doi:10.5042/amhid.2010.0544

British Psychological Society. (2015). *Guidance on the assessment and diagnosis of intellectual disabilities in adulthood*. Leicester: British Psychological Society.

Breslau, N., Lucia, V. C., & Alvarado, G. F. (2006). Intelligence and other predisposing factors in exposure to trauma and posttraumatic stress disorder: A follow-up study at age 17 years. *Archives of General Psychiatry, 63*(11), 1238–1245. doi:10.1001/archpsyc.63.11.1238

Butler, L. D., Critelli, F. M., & Rinfrette, E. S. (2011). Trauma informed care and mental health. *Directions in Psychiatry, 31*(3), 197–209.

Catani, C., & Sossalla, I. M. (2015). Child abuse predicts adult PTSD symptoms among individuals diagnosed with intellectual disabilities. *Frontiers in Psychology, 6*, 1600. doi:10.3389/fpsyg.2015.01600

Daley, S. G., & Rappolt-Schlichtmann, G. (2018). Stigma consciousness among adolescents with learning disabilities: Considering individual experiences of being stereotyped. *Learning Disability Quarterly, 41*(4), 200–212. doi:10.1177/0731948718785565

Department of Health. (2001). *Valuing people: A new strategy for learning disability for the 21st century*. Stationery Office.

Daveney, J., Hassiotis, A., Katona, C., Matcham, F., & Sen, P. (2019). Ascertainment and prevalence of post-traumatic stress disorder (PTSD) in people with intellectual disabilities. *Journal of Mental Health Research in Intellectual Disabilities, 12*(3-4), 211–233. doi:10.1080/19315864.2019.1637979

Dosen, A. (2007). Integrative treatment in persons with intellectual disability and mental health problems. *Journal of Intellectual Disability Research, 51*(1), 66–74. doi:10.1111/j.1365-2788.2006.00868.x

Emerson, E., & Hatton, C. (2007). Mental health of children and adolescents with intellectual disabilities in Britain. *British Journal of Psychiatry, 191*(6), 493–499. doi:10.1192/bjp.bp.107.038729

Faccini, L., & Allely, C. S. (2021). Dealing with trauma in individuals with autism spectrum disorders: Trauma informed care, treatment, and forensic implications. *Journal of Aggression, Maltreatment & Trauma*, 1–11. doi:10.1080/10926771.2020.1853295

Fallot, R. D., & Harris, M. (2008). Trauma-informed approaches to systems of care. *Trauma Psychology Newsletter, 3*(1), 6–7.

Fletcher, J. M., Lyon, G. R., Fuchs, L. S., & Barnes, M. A. (2018). *Learning disabilities: From identification to intervention*. New York: Guilford Publications.

Fletcher, R., Loschen, E., Stavrakaki, C., & First, M. (Eds). (2007). *Diagnostic manual–intellectual disability: A textbook of diagnosis of mental disorders in persons with intellectual disability*. New York: National Association for the Dually Diagnosed.

Fletcher, R. J., Beasley, J., & Jacobson, J. W. (1999). Support service systems for People with dual diagnosis in the USA. In Bouras N. (Ed.) *Psychiatric and behavioural disorders in developmental disabilities and mental retardation* (pp.373–390). Cambridge University Press.

García-Largo, L. M., Martí-Agustí, G., Martin-Fumadó, C., & Gómez-Durán, E. L. (2020). Intellectual disability rates among male prison inmates. *International Journal of Law and Psychiatry, 70*, 101566. doi:10.1016/j.ijlp.2020.101566

Gilbert, P. (Ed.). (2005). *Compassion: Conceptualisations, research and use in psychotherapy*. Routledge.

Goad, E. (2021). Working alongside people with intellectual disabilities who have had difficult experiences: Reflections on trauma-informed care within a service context. *Journal of Intellectual Disabilities*. doi:10.1016/1744629520987717.

Harris, M., & Fallot, R. D. (Eds). (2001). *Using trauma theory to design service systems. New directions for mental health services*. Jossey-Bass.

Hastings, R. P. (2013). Running to catch up: Rapid generation of evidence for interventions in learning disability services. *British Journal of Psychiatry, 203*(4), 245–246. doi:10.1192/bjp.bp.113.127605

Hatton, C., & Emerson, E. (2004). The relationship between life events and psychopathology amongst children with intellectual disabilities. *Journal of Applied Research in Intellectual Disabilities, 17*(2), 109–117. doi:10.1111/j.1360-2322.2004.00188.x

Hayes, S., Shackell, P., Mottram, P., & Lancaster, R. (2007). The prevalence of intellectual disability in a major UK prison. *British Journal of Learning Disabilities, 35*(3), 162–167. doi:10.1111/j.1468-3156.2007.00461.x

Heaton, K. M., & Murphy, G. H. (2013). Men with intellectual disabilities who have attended sex offender treatment groups: A follow-up. *Journal of Applied Research in Intellectual Disabilities, 26*(5), 489–500. doi:10.1111/jar.12038

Hellenbach, M., Karatzias, T., & Brown, M. (2017). Intellectual disabilities among prisoners: Prevalence and mental and physical health comorbidities. *Journal of Applied Research in Intellectual Disabilities, 30*(2), 230–241. doi:10.1111/jar.12234

Ho, A. (2004). To be labelled, or not to be labelled: That is the question. *British Journal of Learning Disabilities, 32*(2), 86–92. doi:10.1111/j.1468-3156.2004.00284.x

Hollins, S., Lodge, K. M., & Lomax, P. (2019). The case for removing intellectual disability and autism from the Mental Health Act. *British Journal of Psychiatry, 215*(5), 633–635. doi:10.1192/bjp.2019.26

Jones, L., Bellis, M. A., Wood, S., Hughes, K., McCoy, E., Eckley, L., … & Officer, A. (2012). Prevalence and risk of violence against children with disabilities: A systematic review and meta-analysis of observational studies. *The Lancet, 380*(9845), 899–907. doi:10.1016/S0140-6736(12)60692-8

Keesler, J. M. (2014a). A call for the integration of trauma-informed care among intellectual and developmental disability organizations. *Journal of Policy and Practice in Intellectual Disabilities, 11*(1), 34–42. doi:10.1111/jppi.12071

Keesler, J. M. (2014b). Trauma through the lens of service coordinators: Exploring their awareness of adverse life events among adults with intellectual disabilities. *Advances in Mental Health and Intellectual Disabilities, 8*(3), 151–164. doi:10.1108/AMHID-04-2013-0028

Keesler, J. M. (2016). Trauma-informed day services for individuals with intellectual/developmental disabilities: Exploring staff understanding and perception within an innovative programme. *Journal of Applied Research in Intellectual Disabilities, 29*(5), 481–492. doi:10.1111/jar.12197

Keesler, J. M. (2018). Adverse childhood experiences among direct support professionals. *Intellectual and Developmental Disabilities, 56*(2), 119–132. doi:10.1352/1934-9556-56.2.119

Keesler, J. M. (2020a). From the DSP perspective: Exploring the use of practices that align with trauma-informed care in organizations serving people with intellectual and developmental disabilities. *Intellectual and Developmental Disabilities, 58*(3), 208–220. doi:10.1352/1934-9556-58.3.208

Keesler, J. M. (2020b). Promoting satisfaction and reducing fatigue: Understanding the impact of trauma-informed organizational culture on psychological wellness among direct service providers. *Journal of Applied Research in Intellectual Disabilities, 33*(5), 939–949. doi:10.1111/jar.12715

Keesler, J. M., & Isham, C. (2017). Trauma-informed day services: An initial conceptualization and preliminary assessment. *Journal of Policy and Practice in Intellectual Disabilities, 14*(2), 164–175. doi:10.1111/jppi.12206

Kessler, R. C., Chiu, W. T., Demler, O., & Walters, E. E. (2005). Prevalence, severity, and comorbidity of 12-month DSM-IV disorders in the National Comorbidity Survey Replication. *Archives of General Psychiatry, 62*(6), 617–627. doi:10.1001/archpsyc.62.6.617

Longfellow, E., & Hicks, R. (2020). Developmental trauma and learning disability. In Lawrence Jones (Ed.), *Trauma informed care in forensic settings*. Nottingham.

Lovell, A., & Skellern, J. (2020). Making sense of complexity: A qualitative investigation into forensic learning disability nurses' interpretation of the contribution of personal history to offending behaviour. *British Journal of Learning Disabilities, 48*(3), 242–250. doi:10.1111/bld.12325

Macklin, M. L., Metzger, L. J., Litz, B. T., McNally, R. J., Lasko, N. B., Orr, S. P., & Pitman, R. K. (1998). Lower precombat intelligence is a risk factor for posttraumatic stress disorder. *Journal of Consulting and Clinical Psychology, 66*(2), 323–326. doi:10.1037//0022-006x.66.2.323

Mevissen, L., & De Jongh, A. (2010). PTSD and its treatment in people with intellectual disabilities: A review of the literature. *Clinical Psychology Review, 30*(3), 308–316. doi:10.1016/j.cpr.2009.12.005

Miller, D., & Brown, J. (2014). 'We have the right to be safe': Protecting disabled children from abuse. Retrieved from www.nspcc.org.uk/preventing-abuse/research-and-resources/right-to-be-safe/

Milligan, I., & Stevens, I. (2006). Balancing rights and risk: the impact of health and safety regulations on the lives of children in residential care. *Journal of Social Work, 6*(3), 239–254. Doi.org/10.1177/1468017306071173

Morris, D. J., Shergill, S., & Beber, E. (2019). Developmental trauma in a forensic intellectual disability population. *Journal of Intellectual Disabilities and Offending Behaviour, 11*(1), 35–48. doi:10.1108/JIDOB-06-2019-0011

Morris, D. J., Webb, E. L., Parmar, E., Trundle, G., & McLean, A. (2020). Troubled beginnings: The adverse childhood experiences and placement histories of a detained adolescent population with developmental disorders. *Advances in Mental Health and Intellectual Disabilities, 14*(6), 181–197. doi:10.1108/AMHID-01-2020-0003

Murphy, G. H., Harnett, H., & Holland, A. J. (1995). A survey of intellectual disabilities amongst men on remand in prison. *Mental Handicap Research, 8*(2), 81–98. doi:10.1111/j.1468-3148.1995.tb00147.x

National Institute for Health and Care Excellence. (2018a). *Learning disabilities and behaviour that challenges: Service design and delivery [NG93]*. Retrieved from www.nice.org.uk/guidance/ng93

National Institute for Health and Care Excellence. (2018b). Post-traumatic stress disorder [NG116]. Retrieved from www.nice.org.uk/guidance/ng116

NICE. (2021). What we do. Retrieved from www.nice.org.uk/about/what-we-do

Peternelj-Taylor, C. (2004). An exploration of othering in forensic psychiatric and correctional nursing. *Canadian Journal of Nursing Research Archive, 36*(4), 130–146.

Rich, A. J., DiGregorio, N., & Strassle, C. (2020). Trauma-informed care in the context of intellectual and developmental disability services: Perceptions of service providers. *Journal of Intellectual Disabilities.* doi:10.1177/1744629520918086

Rittmannsberger, D., Yanagida, T., Weber, G., & Lueger-Schuster, B. (2020). The association between challenging behaviour and symptoms of post-traumatic stress disorder in people with intellectual disabilities: A Bayesian mediation analysis approach. *Journal of Intellectual Disability Research, 64*(7), 538–550. doi.org/10.1111/jir.12733

Shalev, A., Liberzon, I., & Marmar, C. (2017). Post-traumatic stress disorder. *New England Journal of Medicine, 376*(25), 2459–2469. doi:10.1056/NEJMra1612499

Smith, M. (2009). Working with disability in groups. *Group Analysis, 42*(1), 16–30. doi:10.1177/0533316408100930

Sobsey, D., & Doe, T. (1991). Patterns of sexual abuse and assault. *Sexuality and Disability, 9*(3), 243–259. doi:10.1007/BF01102395

Spencer, M. D., Gibson, R. J., Moorhead, T. W. J., Keston, P. M., Hoare, P., Best, J. J., ... & Johnstone, E. C. (2005). Qualitative assessment of brain anomalies in adolescents with mental retardation. *American Journal of Neuroradiology, 26*(10), 2691–2697.

Staszak, J. F. (2008). Other/otherness. *International Encyclopedia of Human Geography*, 43–47.

Steans, J., & Duff, S. (2020). Perceptions of sex offenders with intellectual disability: A comparison of forensic staff and the general public. *Journal of Applied Research in Intellectual Disabilities, 33*(4), 711–719. doi.org/10.1111/jar.12467

Sullivan, P. M., & Knutson, J. F. (2000). Maltreatment and disabilities: A population-based epidemiological study. *Child Abuse & Neglect, 24*(10), 1257–1273. doi:10.1016/S0145-2134(00)00190-3

Sweeney, A., Clement, S., Filson, B., & Kennedy, A. (2016). Trauma-informed mental healthcare in the UK: What is it and how can we further its development? *Mental Health Review Journal, 21*(3), 174–192. doi:10.1108/MHRJ-01-2015-0006

Taylor, J. L., McKinnon, I., Thorpe, I., & Gillmer, B. T. (2017). The impact of transforming care on the care and safety of patients with intellectual disabilities and forensic needs. *BJPsych Bulletin, 41*(4), 205–208. doi:10.1192/pb.bp.116.055095

Truesdale, M., Brown, M., Taggart, L., Bradley, A., Paterson, D., Sirisena, C., ... & Karatzias, T. (2019). Trauma-informed care: A qualitative study exploring the views and experiences of professionals in specialist health services for adults with intellectual disabilities. *Journal of Applied Research in Intellectual Disabilities, 32*(6), 1437–1445. doi:10.1111/jar.12634

Tureck, K., Matson, J. L., Cervantes, P., & Konst, M. J. (2014). An examination of the relationship between autism spectrum disorder, intellectual functioning, and comorbid symptoms in children. *Research in Developmental Disabilities, 35*(7), 1766–1772. doi:10.1016/j.ridd.2014.02.013

van der Put, C. E., Asscher, J. J., Wissink, I. B., & Stams, G. J. J. M. (2014). The relationship between maltreatment victimisation and sexual and violent offending: Differences between adolescent offenders with and without intellectual disability. *Journal of Intellectual Disability Research, 58*(11), 979–991. doi:10.1111/jir.12031

Wigham, S., & Emerson, E. (2015). Trauma and life events in adults with intellectual disability. *Current Developmental Disorders Reports, 2*(2), 93–99. doi:10.1007/s40474-015-0041-y

Wigham, S., Hatton, C., & Taylor, J. L. (2011). The effects of traumatizing life events on people with intellectual disabilities: A systematic review. *Journal of Mental Health Research in Intellectual Disabilities, 4*(1), 19–39. doi:10.1080/19315864.2010.534576

Wigham, S., Taylor, J. L., & Hatton, C. (2014). A prospective study of the relationship between adverse life events and trauma in adults with mild to moderate intellectual disabilities. *Journal of Intellectual Disability Research, 58*(12), 1131–1140. doi:10.1111/jir.12107

7

DEAFNESS AND TRAUMA

A Journey to Equitable Trauma-Informed Care

Sarah Todd

When I joined the National High Secure Deaf Service (NHSDS) as its psychological lead, I considered myself experienced both in forensic mental health and trauma, having developed knowledge and expertise throughout my forensic work for almost two decades. However, I soon discovered that the trauma-informed working I had invested so much in for a hearing population was vastly different with the Deaf population in prison and hospital. This unique, under-served, under-researched, and often misdiagnosed or misunderstood population was far from having trauma-informed pathways comparable to the rapidly developing pathways experienced by their hearing peers. In this chapter I will explore the unique relationship between Deafness and trauma, and how this is experienced by individuals within forensic services. This is a vast topic and I am unable to cover everything in depth. However, I hope to increase awareness and inspire further curiosity from the reader. I am also aware, as a hearing psychologist, that I am far from an expert on the isolation and discrimination Deaf people have endured (and still endure). However, through my own work and research I hope to speak as an advocate for increased understanding and equality in care. Although at present the service users in the NHSDS do not feel able to engage in sharing their experiences in this chapter for a number of reasons, I hope to help build a platform where they can safely share their voice and feel more empowered to do so.

Deafness and Hearing Loss

Within the UK, hearing loss affects 1 in 6 people (over 11 million), with approximately 900,000 experiencing severe/profound deafness (Royal National Institute for Deaf People, RNID, 2021). The Deaf and hard of hearing population represent a highly diverse continuum. Deafness can be classified by degree of hearing loss, age at onset of deafness, or by cultural and linguistic identity (Austen & Coleman, 2004).

DOI: 10.4324/9781003120766-10

Hearing loss is categorised from mild to profound by the World Health Organisation (2020). There is also an important distinction noted between the capital and small D/d used with the word D/deaf. Those who are predominantly prelingually Deaf, who do not recognise their deafness as a disability or medical diagnosis, who identify with the Deaf cultural and linguistic community identify with the use of a capital "D". For those who predominantly do not identify with the Deaf community, and most often have become deaf, the lowercase "d" is used.

The loss of hearing later in life is clearly traumatic. However, for the purposes of this chapter I will be focusing primarily upon the prelingually Deaf population and exploring what is needed to provide them with equitable trauma-informed care.

Trauma in the Deaf Population

Trauma has already been defined in earlier chapters of this book, and in relation to these definitions (complex, polyvictimisation, betrayal) the Deaf population not only experience a high prevalence of such childhood maltreatment but a greater one; with the rate of maltreatment estimated to be twice that of the hearing population (Tate, 2012). Vernon and Miller (2002) for example, suggested that up to 50% of Deaf children suffer childhood sexual abuse, compared to 10–25% of hearing children.

This pattern unfortunately remains throughout adulthood with Deaf people reporting nearly twice the rates of intimate partner violence and sexual assault (Anderson & Leigh, 2011), physical and emotional abuse (Øhre, Uthus, von Tetzchner, & Falkum, 2015), and ongoing communication abuse (causing harm through misuse or neglect of effective communication), compared to hearing people (Mastrocinque et al., 2015). It has been suggested that Deaf people may experience at least six types of unique trauma across their lifespan (Schild & Dalenberg, 2012a discussed below) which affect multiple domains of functioning, leading to higher levels of trauma responses such as mental health difficulties, anger, sexual issues, substance use, anger/frustration, and rates of suicide in adults compared with a hearing population. It is likely that these are an underestimation due to the vastly unmeasured experiences of Deaf people and, in my experience, there is much greater disparity and inequity in access to services, support, and treatment.

Deafness and Childhood Trauma

Childhood maltreatment can be experienced similarly in many ways across both a hearing and a Deaf population; however, Deaf children potentially experience trauma not commonly experienced by their hearing peers. Approximately 90% of Deaf children are born to hearing parents who have little or no experience of Deafness. For Deaf children this can mean parents' non-acceptance of Deafness, leading to obstructed communication; difficulties with attachment; isolation from families; memories of parents' grief and attempts to "cure" their deafness; as well as incurring developmental delays, language, and cultural deprivation (Brice & Adams, 2011). Longstanding beliefs that sign language prevents or delays development of spoken language (which can be more highly valued) has led to some Deaf children being deprived of all language due to their parents' attempts to "correct" their Deafness, and the development of their brain can be subsequently affected (Hall, 2017). Delayed language development and problems with theory of mind and challenging behaviour are also observed in Deaf children with hearing parents (Austen, 2010). Communication deprivation (the withholding of development of healthy communication methods and style), as described above, may be formulated as a unique form of neglect that has longstanding consequences for Deaf children.

Deaf children have been recognised as more susceptible to neglect and abandonment, are more vulnerable to early attachment disruptions, and there is evidence to suggest that Deaf children born to hearing parents are disciplined more harshly and with greater physical force (Knutson, Johnson, & Sullivan, 2004). Deaf children may be perceived as less likely to disclose maltreatment, to complain/resist less or to be naïve or overly trusting, all of which increases their vulnerability to maltreatment and abuse. Perpetrators may also assume that Deaf children are less likely to understand something is wrong, will find it harder to report abuse, and may be less likely to be believed if they do report abuse (Denmark, 1994). Overall, Deaf children potentially become more vulnerable in both the home and school environments.

Deaf children who attend mainstream school face potentially vast communication barriers, especially without adequate adaptation to support their learning style. Many mainstream schools still do not have sufficient access to British Sign Language (BSL) or assisted signing. Deaf children in mainstream schools are probably more vulnerable to isolation and bullying, and their educational and developmental needs are often left unmet (formulated as systemic neglect).

In my experience, Deaf children who stay in residential Deaf schools (a common experience) can suffer increased isolation and perceived abandonment by family. Placement in residential schools has been shown to increase the risk of sexual and physical abuse (Miller, Vernon, & Capella, 2005), leaving many Deaf children in these placements with little or no healthy understanding of sexual behaviour. Patients in NHSDS have spoken about communication deprivation (neglect) experienced in residential Deaf schools where their signing was prohibited to promote spoken voice. This included being physically forced to use their voice rather than sign by being made to sit on their hands or having their hands taped together or being beaten if they would/could not use their voice. Given the disconnection between themselves and the adults holding responsibility, Deaf children may forge deeper connection to peers with whom they are able to communicate, but who may not be able to model sophisticated coping skills. If such skills are absent, Deaf trauma survivors may develop more unhealthy survival strategies to cope, including strategies that potentially develop into offending (e.g., inappropriate sexual behaviour, substance use, aggression).

Ridgeway (1993) noted that many Deaf individuals believe that maltreatment (maybe perceived as care/normality) is simply "part of being Deaf" and this certainly seems to be the experience of some of the individuals I have worked with who accept their experience as "normal".

Based on the histories of patients in the NHSDS, alongside increased exposure to maltreatment, there is also vast inequality in access to information and education; awareness and knowledge regarding trauma; support, care, and services; and to opportunities to share experiences with others. Deaf people face limited access to incidental learning and have less opportunity to develop language relating to understanding what traumatic experience is and how it may affect them. This is known as the "fund-of-information deficit" and can represent a distinct limitation in a Deaf person's knowledge base due to being unable to access information compared to a hearing population, despite normal IQ and capability (Pollard, 1996). This can represent systemic neglect of Deaf people's needs.

Deaf people are over-represented in the prison population, both in the UK and in the USA, particularly for sexual offences (Williamson & Grubb, 2015). While there remains little research into why this is the case, high rates of ongoing trauma may well be a contributory factor. As already discussed, approximately 50% of Deaf children experience sexual abuse. Many Deaf children grow up with a limited knowledge of sexual boundaries and behaviour (Schild & Dalenberg, 2015). Deaf children in residential schools are more likely to experience sexual abuse. A number of patients in the NHSDS have described engaging in sexual activity in residential school with peers (either forced or as means of meeting their unmet needs) and had little understanding of their own boundaries/rights. Such school age experience seems also to be linked to attachment difficulties, a mistrust of adults and difficulties with self-esteem, identity, and relationships. Combined with the lack of culturally and linguistically accessible assessments and intervention at an early age for Deaf children, and limited or no access to health literature and sex education, all these factors could contribute to increased risk of sexual offending.

Of course, not all Deaf children go on to sexually offend, and although some researchers have proposed a "Deaf personality", characterised by impulsive, selfish, and aggressive behaviours (Miller, Vernon, & Capella, 2005), brain damage and intellectual disability may be additional factors (Williamson & Grubb, 2015), it is perhaps more useful to formulate a Deaf Individual's offending in the cultural, linguistic, and trauma-informed context of their life (including factors that influence their own resilience, protective/risk factors).

Unique Characteristics of Trauma in the Deaf Population

Like their hearing peers, Deaf people experience a full range of trauma responses. However, there are unique differences in what influences trauma experience that can have long-term implications for equity in care.

Language Deprivation and Disfluency

Glickman (2008) defines language disfluency as the inability to communicate fluently in any language. Language disfluency can be understood to have three general causes. The first two – physical causes and mental illness – are experienced by both hearing and Deaf individuals, while the third – language deprivation – is recognised as almost exclusively experienced in the Deaf population (Gulati, 2003). Language deprivation is the failure to develop fluency and refers to individuals with poor or no language skills in any language (spoken or sign). It is caused by insufficient exposure to language, leading to the child not acquiring language at the expected rate or developmental level (Glickman, 2008). It has been suggested that 75% of Deaf individuals receiving services in psychiatric hospitals have some level of language disfluency (Black, 2005) though the actual proportion is likely to be higher. I would suggest that in forensic populations the population is greater still, and this is certainly the case in NHSDS.

Language deprivation is common in Deaf people due to hearing families holding beliefs that learning sign language could prevent the development of spoken word, or the delay in learning a language due to the seeking of surgical/cochlear implant as a way of "fixing" Deafness. These are potentially examples of neglect of a child's core language, communication, and emotional needs. Similarly, failure to recognise and rectify when a Deaf child of normal intelligence is not at the same developmental stage as hearing peers in schools and other areas could be formulated as systemic neglect (Gulati, 2003). Without language, a Deaf child could potentially suffer isolation unlike anything a hearing peer may have to experience, and without language it may be very difficult for them to become aware that they have experienced trauma, or to access services/support that they may not even know exist and that are predominantly language-based.

Øhre et al. (2015) highlight that communication and language form the basis for the conceptual and emotional processing of stressful events and therefore play a crucial role in preventing subsequent traumatisation and in facilitating recovery. Therefore, its absence can put Deaf people at a disadvantage when processing trauma. Hall (2017) found that a fully accessible language is a protective factor for healthy development, and language disfluency and deprivation are key in understanding the impact of traumatic events, the internalising of misunderstood traumatic experience, managing trauma responses, and providing support for recovery for the Deaf population. In my experience without language and effective communication to facilitate processing traumatic experiences, Deaf people may be more likely to develop survival responses – often conceptualised by the individual as "helping" – such as dissociation, substance use, and behavioural methods of communicating need or expression such as aggression and challenging/offending behaviour.

Information Deficit Trauma (IDT)

Schild and Dalenberg (2012a) define IDT as an event that is experienced as traumatic (or more traumatic) because information about the event is limited or not available. The lack of information increases the impact of factors such as unpredictability, suddenness, and uncontrollability. When a lack of information is associated with a traumatic event, this is likely to exacerbate the traumatic experience in a way that may not be experienced by someone without this deficit. IDT is probably more common in Deaf individuals and is an important factor in understanding their unique traumatic experiences. Øhre et al. (2015) add that Deafness can interfere with the interpretation of verbal information and consequently with the appraisal of situations. Deaf people may perceive events as traumatic that hearing individuals do not. Anecdotally, Deaf people may be over-protected by families (not told details about relatives' deaths or not communicated to about something that has happened to them), as information is often not overtly offered in a way that can be understood, and this form of information deprivation (formulated as neglect) can worsen a person's reaction to a situation and heighten the traumatic response, as well as perpetuate survival strategies.

Assessment

Many researchers warn that achieving validity and reliability in diagnosing disorders in the Deaf population is extremely difficult, and it requires specialist knowledge, experience, and skill. Inaccurate assessment often leads to this population being misdiagnosed and mistreated at a much greater rate than hearing peers (Du Feu, 2017). This is particularly the case for trauma. Du Feu emphasises the importance of specialist assessments when it comes to mental health examinations of Deaf individuals to minimise any over- or under-emphasis of the impact of a person's Deafness on their mental health difficulties. Furthermore, she states that any assessment should be done with support from an appropriately qualified and registered sign language interpreter (RSLI) who has experience of working in mental health settings. Inaccurate diagnosis may stem from misunderstandings of cultural and linguistic differences and variations in manifestations and expressions of traumatic responses. All assessments for mental health and trauma are normed on hearing populations, and therefore not culturally or linguistically valid for Deaf people (including ICD classifications). Accurate clinical decisions and formulation require knowledge and understanding of cultural and linguistic information and appropriate adaptions to assessment methods. In my experience, cultural differences in labelling affect or behavioural states may influence measures of both mental health and trauma, and somatic presentations are much more likely in the Deaf population that many cognitively orientated assessments would not capture.

Assessments and classifications also need to explore traumas unique to the Deaf population, as well as generalised to both hearing and Deaf. Studies exploring trauma assessment tools have noted that Deaf people were more likely to score highly on "other traumas", highlighting that their experience is not captured equally (Schild & Dalenberg, 2012a). They also concluded that the psychometric properties of the Trauma Symptom Inventory (TSI) and the Clinician administered PTSD checklist (CAPS) are excellent for both Deaf and hearing populations.

When assessments, clinical opinion, and formulation are not rooted in cultural and linguistic understanding, do not facilitate shared language, meaning, and understanding or are not communicated effectively, then the Deaf person is at a significant disadvantage for trauma recovery and the barriers for developing protective factors remain. The same issues are relevant for risk assessment. Anecdotally, this is more likely for those Deaf individuals in the criminal justice system (CJS) where specialist assessment and care is sparse or non-existent. In my experience this is another example of ongoing systemic neglect where Deaf people, who have offended, face the ongoing adversity of inequitable care.

PTSD

Schild and Dalenberg (2012b) suggest that Deaf individuals are more likely to develop PTSD than their hearing peers, but their research also found lower prevalence rates than expected, different predictors of PTSD, and different symptom constellation. They questioned whether the current definition of PTSD is appropriate for Deaf people, since expressions of trauma often displayed in Deaf people, such as avoidance/ numbing, internalisation of expression, hyperarousal, and re-experiencing symptoms internally (Gulati, 2003), may not be captured. Schild and Dalenberg explored the importance of how Deaf people express trauma responses, concluding that, as in hearing samples, dissociation (both psychoform and somatoform) was significantly related to PTSD symptoms but that psychoform dissociation was significantly more common in Deaf adults than in hearing adults. In addition, those with dissociative PTSD displayed significantly more symptoms of depression, anger, impaired self-reference, tension reduction behaviour, and somatoform dissociation than did the non-dissociative PTSD group. Therefore, scales of assessment normed on hearing people may underestimate trauma experience in Deaf people (which of course has implications for recovery and care).

PTSD classification focuses on short-term impact of trauma and "in the moment" expressions of distress. However, Deaf people are more likely to internalise their experiences with limited ways/ability/language to express them externally. Anecdotally, Deaf people's experiences of trauma are also more likely to be pervasively experienced throughout the lifetime; therefore, focusing on the immediate short-term impact of a traumatic event is incomplete. Even when a Deaf individual experiences trauma in adulthood, this is often on top of trauma already experienced. Therefore, PTSD criteria/classification will probably miss Deaf people's experiences and present as another ongoing barrier to receiving equitable trauma care.

Dissociation

Dissociation is highly correlated with PTSD in the hearing population and is widely recognised to be a trauma-related avoidance strategy (Briere, 1995). Schild and Dalenberg (2012b) highlighted that despite the recognition that the Deaf population experience high rates of traumatic experience, little is studied relating to dissociation. They noted that both Deafness and dissociation disconnect an individual from certain aspects of their external environment and, as a population that is at a greater risk of not being able to share experiences with others and express reflections using shared language skills or experience an information deficit, they are more likely to internalise their experiences and dissociation is more likely to be a trauma response (Freyd, 1994). Schild and Dalenberg also add that by closing their eyes, a deaf person can more fully, consciously, or unconsciously refuse to know. The use of the body to consciously avoid knowledge and/or experience may be an alternative to or an antecedent of dissociation (Stern, 1997) that serves a similar purpose. I have often witnessed this in NHSDS; what might be perceived as "being dismissive" or "ignoring" could in fact be a trauma response.

Isolation throughout a Deaf person's lifetime is also more likely to perpetuate dissociative experiences (such as derealisation, "spacing out", detachment from feelings) as survival strategies. Potentially when a Deaf person is already prevented from accessing information, support or shared experience, trauma responses may not be as obvious to the assessor (perhaps even looking like there is little effect, with the Deaf individual seeming resilient in their self-management). Therefore, it is important that the Deaf individual is assessed and formulated in a trauma-informed way that allows their differences in trauma response to be considered, and that any assessment of PTSD highlights the importance of evaluating dissociation (Schild & Dalenberg, 2012b).

Psychosis

Deaf individuals are equally likely to experience psychosis, thought disorder, mania, and depression as trauma responses (Du Feu, 2017). In my experience Deaf people can experience auditory hallucinations, but they can be difficult to identify accurately. Some Deaf people may be classified as "delusional" or "thought disordered" when in fact they just have difficulty with placement in time and place, have little access to information to clarify, struggle to understand interactions around them, or difficulties in interpreting thoughts and feelings. Hallucinations and delusions are both culturally influenced. In NHSDS, I formulate psychosis within the cultural and linguistic context of their experience, often developing a shared meaning using the individual's preferred communication to facilitate a shared understanding of trauma at the onset of their care.

Resilience

Of course, I cannot talk about trauma without talking about resilience, and this is no different in the Deaf population. In my experience the ability to adapt and survive in the face of adversity is clearly a trait of Deaf people. However, in the forensic environment it may have come at a higher cost to themselves and others. The Deaf community's strong identity and cultural roots probably offer the opportunity to make connections and to feel a sense of belonging and identity without having to express need or "adapt" to a less open hearing population. Johnson, Cawthon, Fink, Wendall, and Schoffstall (2018) studied resilience in a Deaf population and found that resilience is formed and utilised in similar ways to hearing populations. Additionally, five themes were identified as crucial protective factors in the resilience process for Deaf people: individual assets (personal characteristics viewed as having positive value e.g., self-awareness, motivation, purpose in life, sense of humour), identity development, access to language and communication, access to information, and supportive networks. These are clearly important factors that need to be in place to enable Deaf people to understand and process their trauma experiences, to recover, and to build healthy protective responses. Unfortunately, when Deaf people are placed in a forensic service without contact with other Deaf people or any community, and where there is little Deaf awareness, let alone adapted assessments, treatments, and limited access to basic human needs (communication, healthcare, supports), there are far too many barriers to the facilitation of resilience. To provide equal trauma-informed care for Deaf people in forensic services, we need to not only understand the unique nature and presentation of their traumatisation but also provide equal access to recovery. The resilience literature tells us that without these key features it will be harder for these individuals to manage their mental health, personality, and risk.

Johnson et al. (2018) helpfully reframe resilience as a product of living life as a Deaf person. Where being Deaf is a resilience- and resourcefulness-promoting characteristic, we should utilise it in our care and treatment of Deaf people who have offended. Johnson et al. show how Deaf identity (if understood, valued, and encouraged/supported) can be held internally as a protective factor and utilised to promote recovery from trauma – a useful concept to bear in mind for all trauma-informed care in Deaf services.

Being Deaf in the Criminal Justice System (CJS): Isolated Inside

In my experience from initial contact with the CJS, there is an ongoing theme of being disadvantaged. Deaf Prisoners serving indeterminate sentences are often long over tariff and seem to easily become the forgotten population, scattered across prison systems with little support for their specific needs. The NHSDS's prison in-reach programmes have found it very difficult to even identify where Deaf prisoners are located (hearing level is not routinely screened or recorded and many Deaf people would not class or record their Deafness as a disability), let alone offer access to specialist support.

As Race, Todd, Kaler, Dobson, and Lowe (In press) summarise in their review of the NHSDS's in-reach programme, Deaf prisoners are more likely to become socially isolated due to communication barriers and lack of access to support networks and the cultural benefits of the Deaf community. Some have described this as a "prison within a prison" (HEARD, 2018). This is often exacerbated by having limited available healthy coping strategies or protective factors. Not only are these prisoners socially isolated within the prison but also in relation to external support, due to complex systems and procedures, and barriers to using telephones. A further example that highlights the need for greater awareness of the needs of this population comes from the British Deaf Association (2015) report which described a failure to provide counselling services to Deaf prisoners, despite a large proportion of them expressing suicidal intent. Even when there are available specialist Deaf services or prison in-reach, because this resource is so scarce it often results in the Deaf prisoner being located a long way from family/community support. In addition, there is limited access to educational and health support, exacerbated by limited access to RSLIs. Thus, survival strategies are not only in response to traumatic experience in early life but are adaptions to ongoing adversity.

Gibbon and Doyle (2011) also highlight that social isolation and lack of access to appropriate communication also place Deaf prisoners at increased risk of developing mental health difficulties once in prisons. In fact, it is suggested that while some Deaf people who have offended enter the CJS with anxiety or mild mental health difficulties, many will experience dissociation, paranoia, psychosis or PTSD once incarcerated (Tate, 2012) indicating that stronger trauma survival strategies may be required for surviving the prison environment.

It is not uncommon for Deaf people who have offended to be labelled as isolative, disobedient, intimidating, or aggressive. It is often acceptable in the Deaf community to be very straightforward, blunt, and "say it as it is". This can lead hearing people to misinterpret a Deaf person's behaviour as rude, blunt, or dismissive, and in prison settings that may be seen as challenging and incur punishment.

Gahir (2007) describes how aggression and violence may be a language substitute to communicate unmet needs and frustration when communication barriers are extensive and inequity apparent. Without being Deaf-aware, skilled in communicating fluently in sign language or having access to RSLIs, it is harder to read indicators of anger/frustration which may be missed or misunderstood, leading to frustration that can escalate to violence. In prison, where there is little or no access to interpreters or signing staff, Deaf prisoners can become frustrated in not being able to communicate, and then face punitive and re-traumatising consequences for the resulting behaviour (which may have been avoided if adequate communication was facilitated). This seems to correlate with Deaf prisoners not achieving parole, spending more time in isolation, and being unable to access support and treatment programmes.

By the time Deaf people first come into contact with the CJS, their vulnerability to traumatisation is great and their survival strategies are often misunderstood and entrenched. The NHSDS's Prison in-reach programme represents an attempt to provide an equitable trauma-informed service for Deaf prisoners, offering specialist assessment and intervention, training, education, and consultation. However, we are far from being able to offer a trauma-informed specialist Deaf service to all Deaf people who have offended in the UK.

What Is Needed to Achieve Equity in Trauma Care for Deaf People in Forensic Services?

Trauma-informed care should represent a shift from focusing solely on disease/symptoms and risk to include an individual's self-determined focus, empowering Deaf people who have offended and giving them equal access to what they need to achieve recovery. Resilience research shows us that we need to attend to individual assets, including identity development, ensuring access to language and communication, and access to information and support (Johnson et al., 2018). We can look at the need for adaptions in two ways. Firstly, in the individual tools/models and processes we use to assess and treat trauma and secondly in the systemic changes needed to ensure an equitable trauma-informed care model.

Initially, a trauma-informed model needs to be evidence-based and include Deaf perspectives and experience in the research evidence, which is currently lacking. Investment and research are needed so Deaf people who have offended can access culturally and linguistically appropriate trauma care and risk reducing treatment programmes. However there has been a stark lack of Deaf experience represented in research. Anderson, Glickman, Mistler, and Gonzalez (2016) explored the barriers that prevented Deaf trauma survivors from being involved in health research and found that a need for communication access, empathy, respect, strict confidentiality procedures, trust, and transparency of the research process were key themes. They also found that, unlike other minority groups, the inclusion of Deaf individuals in research trials was uniquely difficult due to Deaf people's sensory and linguistic characteristics that needed to be adapted for research methodologies. Problems in other research were use of inaccessible recruitment, sampling, and data collection procedures and no adaptations for information processing, understanding, culture, and linguistic. If we are to improve trauma care for Deaf people, we need to account for such barriers.

It is vital that in all stages of the CJS, awareness and training is provided to help identify and meet the needs of any offender who has hearing impairment or is Deaf. This should also include specific safeguarding standards that allow staff to utilise linguistically accessible tools to measure individual Deaf people's opinions, experiences, and feedback to be utilised to attend to re-traumatisation and to develop and maintain standards of equitable care. We need to develop and evaluate empirically validated tools that will allow early trauma screening and clinical assessments that are accessible and will allow early identification of trauma experience for Deaf individuals (the earlier the better!). Training in Deaf awareness and trauma are essential. This should include information on the manifestation of trauma in Deaf people and how to signpost/assess them reliably using trained clinicians and RSLIs. Awareness training relating to language disfluency and deprivation is also important, as is a compassion-focused approach in working with people who have offended. Finally, it is imperative that accessible information about trauma and how to access help are readily available to all Deaf people who have offended, throughout both the Deaf community and in forensic and mental health services.

In my experience like many minority communities that have faced oppression and discrimination, the Deaf community can hold negative beliefs about mental health issues and services, and it can be difficult for a Deaf individual to overcome these to seek support, especially in prisons. Prisons need to develop and disseminate stigma reduction strategies to help Deaf individuals with trauma experiences to access the treatment they need.

Consistent access to specialist RSLIs, and ensuring institutions recognise the importance of this at every stage of the CJS, is imperative. Funding is clearly a barrier in many services; in fact most funding has resulted from litigation and lawsuits rather than thought-out needs analysis. Deaf people need to be involved in research, analysis, planning, development, and delivery of trauma-informed care, though forensic services are far from this at present. Research is needed into identifying not only the mental and physical costs to both individuals and society of not providing accessible trauma care, but also the costs of Deaf prisoners serving indeterminate sentences being detained past tariff.

Tate (2012) highlighted the need for competent, culturally appropriate health professionals and peer support with demonstrated knowledge and experience in Deaf culture and trauma assessments/treatments. The current forensic workforce does not appear to meet this need, particularly in the prison service. Deaf staff who understand Deaf trauma are invaluable in spreading awareness and training other staff to be able to identify barriers. It is also essential that specialist Deaf services are known and made accessible to provide training, consultancy, signposting, and support.

Trauma Treatments

It is accepted that the complexity of working with Deaf people who have offended increases the time required to comprehensively complete assessment and treatment. In addition, many Deaf people who have offended need a longer, individualised "pre-treatment" phase in their treatment pathway. Most require preparatory work which may include health, emotional and sexual literacy, trauma understanding, the development of a shared understanding of meaning and vocabulary for complex concepts and a basic understanding of the links between thoughts, feelings, and behaviour prior to any trauma work commencing. In NHSDS each patient has different linguistic ability, each using varying levels of BSL, signed English, self-taught sign, and communication through alternative means. Visual images are used alongside language, and roleplays and experiential/kinaesthetic work are facilitated to develop a shared understanding. Often a timeline mapping process is used to assist in developing a collaborative understanding of what may have happened in a person's life, as well as exploring cultural and linguistic identity/understanding between patient and clinician. This is time consuming but essential to facilitating recovery and risk reduction.

This pre-treatment stage also allows the individual to get used to working with the clinician and start to build trust in a therapeutic relationship. Mistrust is a common theme within any marginalised or oppressed population and since many clinicians are hearing and represent prior inequity in interpersonal dynamics, we must attend to this in a culturally sensitive and compassionate way. At times there can be barriers to working collaboratively as many Deaf people who have offended have experienced little empowerment in their lives as seen in the "you're the boss" response (Anderson et al., 2016) where responsibility and power is always deferred to the clinician. This is especially so in forensic services where there is a clear division in authority between people who have offended and staff. We know that a sense of autonomy and self-determination is vital to promote resilience and trauma recovery, thus collaborative working is essential. The clinician must remain self-reflective throughout and be aware of the ongoing dynamic of privilege and discrimination that could play out when the hearing clinician is trying to work with a Deaf offender. It is important to adapt and remain aware of an individual's cultural and linguistic needs that even with an experienced RSLI may not be enough to meet fully.

Culturally and linguistically accessible trauma-specific treatments based on empirical research with the Deaf population are still sparse. Many standard therapies used to treat trauma are not accessible for Deaf people. Most therapies rely on abstract concepts, use metaphors/analogies, are spoken language, and are cognitively driven. Therefore, adaptions are necessary to ensure Deaf people receive culturally and linguistically valid and reliable Trauma treatment.

There is a strong need for somatic and sensory working with a Deaf offender population whose traumatic experiences may have occurred prior to or without access to language, and/or language surrounding the trauma may have been visual and linked strongly to felt experience. Trauma is often stored and re-experienced somatically in the body rather than linguistically or cognitively, and Deaf people who have offended experience vast difficulties in accessing cognitive therapies and other language-based therapies. As such, sensorimotor psychotherapy for trauma is a useful component of a trauma-informed care pathway.

In NHSDS, Schema Therapy (Young, Klosko, & Weishaar, 2003) allows a collaborative approach to understanding each Deaf individual in the context of their life experience, highlighting trauma experienced and how it impacts upon their development of survival strategies (schema modes). It allows clinicians to incorporate trauma experience, manifestation, expression, and responses and link them to both protective factors/resilience and risk management. We do not focus upon the language used in schema therapy but adapt the schema mode way of working to individuals' own linguistic, cultural, and learning needs. An example is the formulation of survival strategies for one patient using masks that we were able to visually create together to show the function of survival responses and how to adapt and manage them in a healthier way to help the facilitation of core emotional needs. The masks in Figure 7.1 represent an understanding of their different survival strategies: (a) avoidant detachment, (b) daydreaming, (c) anger and violence, (d) predatory offending behaviour, (e) over-controlling through striving for perfectionism/order and (f) through suspiciousness/hypervigilance for threat, (g) the vulnerable sadness and isolation that is felt underneath, and (h) the healthy part that is working hard to manage these presentations and finding new healthy ways to meet needs and recover from traumatisation. The experiential and flexible nature of schema work allows us to find shared understanding, language, communication, and meaning and therefore use visual and roleplay methods to drive understanding, recovery, and change.

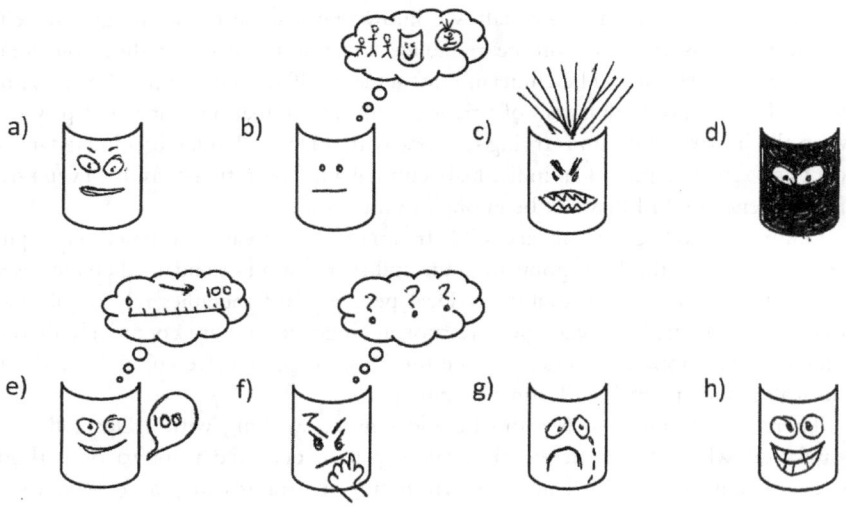

Figure 7.1 Visual masks that represent a shared understanding of different survival strategies

In NHSDS we also use Eye Movement Desensitisation and Reprocessing (EMDR; Shapiro, 1995) adapted with the Deaf population. For Deaf people who have offended, trauma may have occurred preverbally or be nonverbal, thus visual and somatic flashbacks are common. EMDR allows the processing of visual and kinaesthetic sensory experiences without the need for complex language. The option to use a body scan to attend to trauma responses felt in the body (without a need to verbalise) allows the Deaf person's processing to be focused and for the clinician to assess change (as clenched hands, sweating palms, fast heart rate or tension in the body can all be measured nonverbally). The standard protocol may not be completed in its entirety; appraisals of distress (SUDS) or validity of positive feelings (VOC) can be replaced with visual images that better facilitate meaning for the individual (these are developed collaboratively so they have meaning for the individual such as emoji-like simple facial expressions). These can also be adapted for the individual's developmental level. EMDR already positions the clinician in a less verbal or directive role which focuses more on identifying needs rather than "talking" through issues. In fact, the therapist does not need to know all the details of the trauma to assist in EMDR processing. An adaption of the bilateral stimulation modality may be needed; eye movements, self-tapping, and the use of buzzers can be used with success. Acceptance that we may not fully "know" if all channels are processed is needed, but experience indicates that enough of the trauma appears to be processed for the trauma responses to lessen and more adaptive changes to be noticed.

As well as adapting treatment modalities, the role of skilled RSLIs in bridging the communication gap in the delivery of trauma therapy for myself as a hearing trauma clinician has been vital! Many Deaf people in forensic services have no awareness of the word "trauma" (and have no sign for it), nor of words like recovery, trigger, trauma response, or survival strategy. In fact, many of the trauma-informed (and empowering) words, phrases, and understandings that facilitate recovery (used intrinsically in this book) have no meaning for many Deaf people. It is also worth reflecting that if they have never heard of these words, they are unlikely to have ever been asked to meaningfully share their experiences. In our service each patient has a different linguistic ability and communication style and, without experienced specialist RSLIs bridging the complex gap, we would not be able to meet their communication needs. For trauma-informed working I would suggest that these RSLIs are not easily replaced by bank interpreters and as the quality of RSLIs can vary widely. Training RSLIs in clinical and forensic trauma-informed language is a vital component to delivering equitable trauma-informed care.

We must also be aware of the risk of vicarious trauma. An RSLI's role is to not only witness the traumatic experience of an individual as a therapist does, but often to express it for them in the first person. This puts an interpreter at greater risk of absorbing someone else's trauma and others' responses to it, as, due to the expressive nature of BSL, they often act out or embody the experience to communicate it. In a forensic environment this can include interpreting an individual's own trauma and offending behaviour, as well as experiencing the transferential dynamics present in therapeutic interactions. Vicarious trauma can be linked to greater levels of stress, compassion fatigue and burnout, mental health difficulties, and impact upon relationships. A trauma-informed service must provide support and supervision for its RSLIs to allow them to work in a safe and supported way, thus ensuring their efficacy and meeting ethical responsibilities. Interpreters may at times be overlooked because their job is often to "not be there as themselves", so we must hold their experience in mind.

Summary

With vast experience of traumatisation throughout their lifespan and vast barriers to protective factors and support, it is little surprise that Deaf individuals are overrepresented (and often stuck) in forensic services. But when trauma is so intricately linked to offending, and with many forensic services' focus on retribution, diagnosis, risk, and rehabilitation continues to re-traumatise, we must find a way of achieving balance to promote resilience, empowerment, and recovery for Deaf people in forensic services. This cannot be done without equality in research, strategy, delivery, and evaluation. The answer cannot just be trauma-informed practice; it must be trauma-informed care equitable to all! It will no doubt require systemic change on many levels, but Deaf experience must be included.

Further Reading

Department of Health. (2002). *Sign of the times: Modernising mental health services for people who are deaf.* Retrieved from www.nimhe.org.uk/downloads/signoftimes.pdf. For readers who are curious about Deafness and the difficulties Deaf people had endured, this is recognised as core to the changes that followed.

References

Anderson, M.L., & Leigh, I.W. (2011). Intimate partner violence against deaf female college students. *Violence Against Women, 17*, 822–824. doi:10.1177/1077801211412544

Anderson, M.L., Glickman, N.S., Mistler, L.S., & Gonzalez, M. (2016). Working therapeutically with deaf people recovering from trauma and addiction. *Psychiatric Rehabilitation Journal, 39*(1), 27–32. doi:10.1037/prj0000146

Austen, S. (2010). Challenging behaviour in deaf children. *Educational and Child Psychology, 27*(2), 33–40.

Austen, S., & Coleman, E. (2004). Controversy in deafness: Animal farm meets brave new world. In S. Austen & S. R. Crocker (Eds), *Deafness in mind: Working psychologically with deaf people across the lifespan* (pp.3–20). Whurr Publishers. Black, P. (2005). *Language dysfluency in the deaf inpatient population.* Unpublished doctoral dissertation, Fielding Graduate University: Santa Barbara, CA. Brice, P.J., & Adams, E.B. (2011). Developing a concept of self and other: Risk and protective factors. In D.H. Zand & K.J. Pierce (Eds), *Resilience in deaf children.* Springer. doi:10.1007/978-1-4419-7796-0_5

Briere, J. (1995). *Trauma symptom inventory: Professional manual.* Psychological Assessment Resources, Inc.

British Deaf Association. (2015). *What is deaf culture?* British Deaf Association. Retrieved from https://bda.org.uk/what-is-deaf-culture/. Accessed 26 May, 2020.

Denmark, J. (1994). *Deafness and mental health.* Jessica Kingsley Publishers.

Du Feu, M. (2017). Deaf people: What every clinician needs to know. *BJPsych Advances, 23*(2), 89–94. doi:10.1192/apt.bp.116.016154

Freyd, J.J. (1994). Betrayal trauma: Traumatic amnesia as an adaptive response to childhood abuse. *Ethics & Behavior, 4*(4), 307–329. doi:10.1207/s15327019eb0404_1

Gahir, M. (2007). High secure care for deaf people in England and Wales. In S. Austen & D. Jeffery (Eds), *Deafness and challenging behaviour: The 360 perspective* (pp.275–291). John Wiley & Sons.

Gibbon, S., & Doyle, C. (2011). The development and future of deaf forensic mental health services. *British Journal of Forensic Practice, 13* (3), 191–196. doi:10.1108/14636641111157832

Glickman, N. (2008). *Cognitive-behavioral therapy for deaf and hearing persons with language and learning challenges.* Routledge.

Gulati, S. (2003). Psychiatric care of culturally deaf people. In N. Glickman & S. Gulati (Eds), *Mental health care of deaf people: A culturally affirmative approach* (pp.33–107). Mahwah, NJ: Lawrence Earlbaum Associates.

Hall, W.C. (2017). What you don't know can hurt you: The risk of language deprivation by impairing sign language development in deaf children. *Maternal & Child Health Journal, 21*(5), 961–965. doi:10.1007/s10995-017-2287-y

HEARD (2018). *Face file on deaf prisoners.* Retrieved from https://behearddc.org/wp-content/uploads/2018/11/DeafInPrison-Fact-Sheet-.pdf Accessed January 2021

Johnson, P., Cawthon, S., Fink, B., Wendall, E., & Schoffstall, S. (2018). Trauma and resilience among deaf individuals. *Journal of Deaf Studies & Deaf Education, 23*(4), 317–330. doi:10.1093/deafed/eny024

Knutson, J., Johnson, C., & Sullivan, P. (2004). Disciplinary choices of mothers of deaf children and mothers of normally hearing children. *Child Abuse & Neglect, 28*, 925–937. http://dx.doi.org/10.1016/j.chiabu.2004.04.005

Mastrocinque, J.M., Thew, D., Cerulli, C., Raimondi, C., Pollard, R.Q. Jr., & Chin, N.P. (2015). Deaf victims' experiences with intimate partner violence: The need for integration and innovation. *Journal of Interpersonal Violence.* Advance online publication, *32*(24), 3753–3777. doi:10.1177/0886260515602896

Miller, K.R., Vernon, M. & Capella, M.E. (2005). Violent offenders in a deaf prison population. *Journal of Deaf Studies and Deaf Education, 10*(4), 417–425. doi:10.1093/deafed/eni039

Øhre, B., Uthus, M.P., von Tetzchner, S., & Falkum, E. (2015). Traumatization in deaf and hard-of-hearing adult psychiatric outpatients. *Journal of Deaf Studies and Deaf Education, 20*(3), 296–308, doi:10.1093/deafed/env013

Pollard, R. (1996). Professional psychology and deaf people: The emergence of a discipline. *American Psychologist, 51*, 389–396. doi:10.1037/0003-066X.51.4.389

Race, L., Todd, S., Kaler, G., Dobson, J., & Lowe, J. (In Press). Deaf inside: Service evaluation of the deaf prison in-reach service provided by the National High Secure Deaf Service at Rampton Hospital. Submitted to *International Journal of Mental Health and Deafness.*

Ridgeway, S.M. (1993). Abuse and deaf children: Some factors to consider. *Child Abuse Review, 2*(3), 166–173. doi:10.1002/car.2380020306

Royal National Institute for Deaf People (RNID). *Facts and figures.* https://rnid.org.uk/about-us/research-and-policy/facts-and-figures/ Accessed 30 July, 2021.

Schild, S., & Dalenberg, C.J. (2012a). Trauma exposure and traumatic symptoms in deaf adults. *Psychological Trauma: Theory, Research, Practice, and Policy, 4*, 117–127. doi:10.1037/a0021578

Schild, S., & Dalenberg, C.J. (2012b). Psychoform and somatoform dissociation and PTSD in deaf adults. *Journal of Trauma & Dissociation, 13*(3), 361–376. doi:10.1080/15299732.2011.641711

Schild, S., & Dalenberg, C.J. (2015). Consequences of child and adult sexual and physical trauma among deaf adults. *Journal of Aggression, Maltreatment and Trauma, 24*(3), 237–256. doi:10.1080/10926771.2015.1002654

Shapiro, F. (1995). *Eye movement desensitization and reprocessing: Basic principles, protocols and procedures* (1st ed.). Guilford Press.

Stern, D.B. (1997). *Unformulated experience: From dissociation to imagination inpsychoanalysis.* Hillsdale, NJ: Analytic Press.

Tate, C. (2012). *Trauma in the deaf population: Definition, experience, and services.* National Association of State Mental Health Program Directors.

Sarah Todd

Sarah Todd

Sarah Todd

Vernon, M., & Miller, K.R. (2002). Issues in the sexual molestation of deaf youth. *Americans Annals of the Deaf, 147*(5), 28–36. doi:10.1353/aad.2012.0218

Williamson, L.H., & Grubb, A.R. (2015). An analysis of the relationship between being deaf and sexual offending. *Journal of Sexual Aggression, 21*(2), 224–243. doi:10.1080/13552600.2013.842001

World Health Organisation. (2020). *Deafness and hearing loss.* Retrieved from www.who.int/news-room/fact-sheets/detail/deafness-and-hearing-loss

Young, J.E., Klosko, J.S., & Weishaar, M.E. (2003). *Schema therapy: A practitioner's guide.* Guilford Press.

8

TRAUMA AND OFFENDING IN UK MILITARY VETERANS

Jane Jones

The Armed Forces have an excellent track record of deterring their personnel from offending behaviour, yet military veterans represent the largest occupational group in UK prisons (Phillips 2014; Wainwright, Lennox, McDonnell, Shaw, & Senior, 2017). Offences by ex-military personnel are most commonly violent offences (MacManus et al., 2019), though sexual offences are also common (Wainwright et al., 2017).

Despite the acknowledged high number of ex-military personnel in prison this number is accepted to be a gross underestimate. This is partly because ex-military personnel are often reluctant to disclose their veteran status, and partly because the long-term fate of ex-military personnel is a relatively new area of concern (Phillips, 2014). Certainly, those who were incarcerated prior to The Armed Forces Covenant (Ministry of Defence, 2011) would not have been asked about military history and relevance to offending behaviour.

The Armed Forces Covenant pledges a moral obligation by government, on behalf of the nation, to ensure that military and ex-military personnel, and their families, are not disadvantaged as a consequence of military service. The Armed Forces Act (2011) intended to secure the core principles of the Covenant in Law. This followed widespread recognition throughout the UK that armed forces personnel and their families are significantly disadvantaged in terms of housing, employment, children's education, and healthcare. Despite the covenant addressing these disadvantages, not all local councils or healthcare services have honoured it adding distress to already complex situations.

This chapter presents an overview of aspects of life in military service in an attempt to understand potential links between military-related trauma and offending behaviour. All the issues detailed are issues brought to the attention of the author by veterans involved in the Criminal Justice System (CJS).

People who enter military service go on to have a broader range of experiences compared to the general public. These experiences are influenced by role, rank, and service dates. Some experiences are unquestionably life enhancing, others damaging.

DOI: 10.4324/9781003120766-11

However, not all damaging experiences result in harm to the individual. For those who do go on to have psychological struggles the multiple elements of military life combined with non-military experiences more often than not result in difficult to identify and complex presentations.

Most people joining the military have been raised in optimal conditions and attain or exceed personal potential. A significant number however do come from backgrounds of adversity, childhood trauma, abuse, neglect, or social deprivation (Busittil, Hacker-Hughes, & Kitchiner, 2017). For this group, the military can offer much in comparison to civilian life: a home, respected employment, and a sense of belonging, encompassing psychological safety and physical protection. For many with adverse backgrounds, the military provides sufficient stability to channel mental resilience, enabling them to mature and lead productive lives. For others, childhood experiences continue to impact. Such vulnerability can naturally oscillate between dormant and active causing occasional problems during service. However, the close attachment fostered within the military family is such that, so long as behaviours are kept within "military acceptable" limits the family remains tight. Indeed, some behaviours, for example excessive risk taking, are actively rewarded when it benefits "the greater good". This can mean that "problem behaviours" are often tolerated beyond the "greater good" for fear of losing the benefit. Take, for example, a recruit with anger problems often getting into physical fights. His anger-driven behaviours may well be an advantage on the battlefield and so his aggressive behaviour is left unchecked. Consequently, behaviours not compatible with civilian life become entrenched in the behavioural responses of vulnerable recruits.

Most recruits into the forces join straight from school, so childhood development is bound to have a considerable impact on individuals' behaviour and personal interactions. It is now understood that the human brain continues to develop rapidly throughout the teenage years and into the mid-twenties (Johnson, Blum, & Giedd, 2009). The armed forces therefore become the environment that shapes the adult brain of the young recruit.

Once recruited into the forces, military personnel continue to be exposed to the same life adversities as the rest of the general population. In addition, they are exposed to far greater adversity and more frequent life-threatening situations. While other groups, such as emergency service personnel, are also exposed to frequent life threatening and adverse situations, within the military, physical and mental capacity can often be stretched to and beyond personal limits. Military personnel are committed to risk their own lives for the protection of others. They are deployed far away from family and friends and exposed to multiple stressors, including having to adapt quickly to extreme climate changes, alien cultures and languages, deprivation, war, and death.

Military personnel can be exposed to intense and unrelentingly distressing circumstances over weeks and months during combat and live exercise. It is to be noted that live exercise can be as life threatening as actual combat. Fatalities and injuries do occur. The wounded and their families must face the consequences of potentially life-changing injuries. Death leaves survivors and families behind to cope with the psychological and practical impact. Military Personnel are frequently exposed to conflicts and disasters around the world. They can be called upon at a moment's notice, creating a "stand-by stress" even in times of relative peace.

The stresses of military life affect not only service personnel but also their families, who are subject to postings around the UK and overseas. Housing, schooling, employment, healthcare, social network all change with each posting, making the service life practically, socially, and emotionally unpredictable.

On top of all these stresses, military personnel are markedly more at risk than other groups of losing employment, usually as a result of reduced mental or physical wellness. However, everyone eventually leaves the military; most are still of working age and need to adapt to non-military employment. Even where leaving is a choice, few find the transition into civilian life to be straightforward. The vast majority of ex-service men and women and their families report unexpected struggles when leaving the forces (Naval, Army, and RAF Families Federation, 2018).

To make sense of why so many ex-servicemen and women struggle on leaving the forces it is necessary to understand that military service is far more than just a job. It is a way of life that has powerful emotional attachments and practical implications not comparable to other work-life situations. In the beginning, like any celebration that accompanies a new addition into a family, the new recruit is welcomed into full military service with huge pomp and ceremony. The passing out parade is a public affair where family and friends celebrate the accomplishment of each person and their graduation from basic training. Already the recruit has started to develop a new way of thinking that differs from their family of origin. The term *basic training* belies the reality of the whole person impact. While the public may perceive basic training to be about honing excellent physical fitness and psychological focus, a much deeper psychological transition is taking place where the "military family" becomes embedded into the identity of serving personnel.

From day one in basic training and throughout military service the "military family" adopts individuals who in turn provide protection and who are protected by this living bond. It has long been known that in dangerous situations, such as combat, instinctive attachment to others is an innate human response that increases the chances of survival (Ein-Dor, 2014). In a similar way the families of serving personnel form equally close-knit bonds, supporting each other when their partners are deployed, during postings and moves of home both in the UK and abroad. The military community as a whole identifies with the military family. Going into a military Family Centre for a social evening could not be more different from most other community social events. Husbands, wives, babies, children, teenagers are all present. Sporting events and weekend socials are enthusiastically attended by all, reinforcing the sense of an extended military family. Just as families protect their closed and special status via unique use of language, nicknames, and behavioural interactions so does the military family. With language for example, asking for a "NATO brew" in the armed forces will get you a cup of tea with milk and two sugars. The depth of attachment formed is a force that is arguably a necessary enabling contributor to successful military action.

Of course, joining the armed forces comes with an understanding that part of the service might involve warfare. Armed combat is one of the most traumatic experiences a human being must endure. No matter that the men and women who are deployed into combat situations are trained to do so, no training fully prepares for the emotional experience of combat. As you might expect, military training does focus on combat resilience and psychologically preparing individuals for the task ahead. It is recognised that the psychological states of military personnel involved in combat is as important to the battle as weapons, logistics, or tactics. Yet despite the intense preparation military personnel go through, combat remains an adverse experience regardless of training, expectation, or expertise.

The psychological impact of combat is internationally recognised and much has been recorded academically and via narratives of lived experience and by those who offer support (Osório et al., 2018; Wang et al., 2018). Combat equally involves those who provide the intelligence behind operations that will almost certainly lead to death, and those not in face-to-face battle who tend to the injured and the dead and the administration of the same.

Military Service Psychological and Behavioural Impact

While offending behaviour is by no means a given outcome of combat-related psychological problems (Wainwright et al., 2017), the disproportionate number of ex-military personnel serving prison sentences with previous combat experience calls for a better understanding. A review of offending leading to conviction by UK military personnel deployed to Iraq and Afghanistan concluded that those deployed into a combat role were at increased risk of violent offending, and that risk increased depending on frequency of exposure to traumatic events (MacManus et al., 2013). Offending behaviour was strongly associated with post-traumatic stress disorder (PTSD), anger, and alcohol misuse. Subsequent reviews have validated these findings reinforcing the need for healthcare services to develop assessment and interventions that better fit the need of military and ex-military personnel (Taylor et al., 2020).

Bashford, Hasan, Evans-Jones, and Patel (2020), in a study commissioned to inform trauma services being developed by the NHS, found that veterans reported a number of common experiences including: intense anxiety and fear, especially in crowded settings; poor sleep patterns with frequent nightmares; rapidly fluctuating moods including guilt, remorse, and depression; feelings of powerlessness and inability to cope; feeling overwhelmed with anger and rage; and acts of self-harm and suicide. They also identified common social and interpersonal issues including relationship breakdowns, loss of employment, financial problems, homelessness, offending, excessive alcohol use, and experience of discrimination and prejudice. While Bashford et al. acknowledge bias, given that all participants in their study had sought help, their study is a fair representation of the difficulties expressed by the majority of veterans who find themselves involved in the CJS. The difficulties described can be associated with various psychological problems but are strongly representative of the re-experiencing, avoidance and hyperarousal symptoms identified with PTSD. In particular, they are representative of complex post-traumatic stress disorder (CPTSD) as defined in ICD-11 (World Health Organization, 2018).

Both ICD-11 and DSM-V (American Psychiatric Association, 2013) include PTSD in their diagnostic criteria. DSM-V defines PTSD in terms of 20 symptoms, four symptom clusters, and a subtype for dissociation. The ICD-11 has organised the characteristics of PTSD into two distinct disorders, PTSD and CPTSD. CPTSD differs from PTSD by including symptoms in the domains of emotion regulation, self-identity, and relational capacities. These three domains are relevant to many who have significant ongoing struggles when they leave the armed forces.

Emotional complexity linked to emotional regulation is one area of increasing enquiry, in particular the impact of *moral injury*. Moral injury arises when a person acts, fails to act, witnesses, or learns about acts that transgress deeply held moral beliefs or expectations (Litz et al., 2009). Bryan et al. (2016) define three distinct categories of moral injury that make a clear association between military service and moral injury: perpetration (being unable to help civilians due to rules of engagement, and/or killing/injuring others), witnessing (witnessing mistreatment of others), and betrayal (friendly fire/fatality during combat or otherwise). While there is currently no consensus on whether or not moral injury is a symptom of or a source of PTSD/CPTSD (Molendijk, Kramer, & Verweij, 2018), there is no doubt that the emotional consequences of these experiences can be extremely distressing. Those who suffer can experience pervasive and intrusive levels of disgust, shame, guilt, and anger leading to major behavioural, life, and relationship problems.

Moral injury as a consequence of military service in the UK is a relatively new field of enquiry. It is identified as having significant presentation in ex-military personnel seeking psychological help in the community (Williamson, Greenberg, & Murphy, 2019). It is difficult to recognise when a person's moral codes have been violated, not least because, with age and experience, ethical values can shift over time. Take for example a young soldier who, in time of conflict, fatally wounds an enemy soldier of a similar age. He goes onto have a family and, when his son reaches the age of 18, he becomes wracked with guilt, as if he had killed the other person as the 48-year-old man he now is, rather than as the 18-year-old he was at the time. Others torment themselves from the moment of experience, blaming their action or lack of action as the cause of another's fate. Others talk about fighting wars that contradict their own belief system, going as far as to describe themselves as a conscientious objector. Even where no one gets hurt, being the person who must repeatedly make decisions about deploying others can leave a chronic sense of anxiety. One veteran described the situation as "playing God" deciding "who lives and who dies".

In my experience, a high percentage of those seeking psychological intervention for military-related problems in prison struggle with one or more of the above complaints. The media often refers to PTSD when discussing military personnel who experience psychological difficulties. The intention of this reporting is generally good and ensures ongoing public support for the armed forces. However, this assumption can be misleading, underrepresenting equally distressing symptoms of depression, anxiety, and psychosis, all of which have strong associations with trauma. This can be confusing for individuals who are struggling with these conditions, leading to frustration in trying to articulate their experiences and the feeling that they are not understood. The result can lead to interventions not best suited to the problem and ultimately the person concluding that they cannot be helped.

Lack of understanding can also lead those who have not experienced live combat to underestimate the impact of different military experiences. The military way of life is littered with adverse circumstances. Institutional bullying, for example, within the military has been the subject of many investigations where accusations of bullying have not only been upheld but recognised as the cause of such extreme distress that individuals have suffered symptoms of PTSD and some committed suicide (Blake, 2006).

As a contribution to this chapter a focus group of ex-military personnel representing the RAF, Army, and Royal Navy discussed their own experience of bullying in the military. All acknowledged that, in hindsight, bullying occurred throughout their service which lasted between 4 and 32 years. Whilst all said they had been the subject of bullying, only one had made a complaint and, although this was investigated, he felt he had no choice but to leave the service. Another left because he could not cope with what he described as "ongoing humiliation".

All participants said that they were aware that bullying behaviours took place. However, all were drawn to describe this with positive language such as "character building" and "learning to man-up". "Beastings" (referring to intense and prolonged physical exercise often used as a punishment) although not at first glance a positive term was discussed in association with achievement. All participants were familiar with the threat of being "taken around the back of the guardroom" (punishment by way of a physical beating), and the common occurrence of the "kangaroo courts" (ad hoc courts that do not adhere to common law or justice). One person described the hatred he and his peers unanimously felt towards certain Non-Commissioned Officers who used bullying and threatening behaviours throughout their training. He described how the recruits, then in their teens or early twenties were deeply united by their experiences of being subject to or witnessing this bullying. However, he went on to describe how this bond, born out of adversity, served them well in their military careers. He even said he believed that it saved their lives when they fought together in combat. Of course, it could be argued that this person's recollection is a reflection of his own ability to make meaning out of adversity. However, his narrative upholds the commonly recounted belief that within the armed forces, individuals need to be "broken down" and "rebuilt".

Research into attachment conducted by Ein-Dor and Hirschberger (2016) supports the theory that group traumatisation can create a group bond which optimises the chances of survival. It is this group bond that creates efficiency in fighting forces. However, bullying behaviours cause significant harm, border on criminal behaviour, and have no place in our modern armed forces.

Discrimination is equally unacceptable in any workplace. The 2010 Equalities Act describes discrimination as treating someone unfairly based on nine characteristics which include sexual orientation and gender reassignment. Before 2,000 people who identified as gay, lesbian, bisexual, or transgender (LGBTQ+) were banned from serving in the UK military. Many who identified as LGBTQ+ would still join up but hid their sexual or gender identity. Homophobic language, which was commonly used in the military, contributed to a hostile environment which was perpetrated throughout the ranks. Individuals who were identified as LGBTQ+ would be subject to an internal investigation which frequently resulted in discharge on administrative grounds, predominately based on the perceived security risk that they presented. Others were subjected to a court martial, often resulting in a custodial sentence before being dishonourably discharged. Personnel would routinely have to endure the ignominy of having their medals or long service awards torn or cut from their uniforms as they were stripped of their military honours. Humiliation of this sort in any field should be regarded as traumatic (Lindner, 2001).

After a long-fought campaign, in February 2000, the ban on individuals who identify as LGBTQ+ serving in the UK military was lifted. Subsequently, but not until 2014, people who identify as transgender can now openly serve. However, it took until February 2021 for the Ministry of Defence (MoD) to announce that veterans who had been stripped of their military honours could apply to have them restored. The MoD has described its past actions regarding personnel who identified as LGBTQ+ as "deeply regrettable" (Ministry of Defence, 2021). Despite the lifting of the ban, it is still believed that many serving personnel continue to hide their sexual or gender identity for fear of discrimination.

The Impact of Transition from the Military to Civilian Life

Regardless of postings, combat, live exercise, bullying, and discrimination, continued service in the AFs reduces the likelihood of convictions for offending behaviour (Short, Dickson, Greenberg, & MacManus, 2018). The focus of attention is therefore drawn to the transition from military service to civilian life. Few military personnel say the transition back into the civilian way of life is straightforward, irrespective of rank, length of service, and whether or not they left the military through choice. Many describe the transition as having a severe impact on their view of themselves, others and the world – an impact so contrary to their expectations that it can lead to acute and chronic distress, with individuals describing their inability to be "a civvy". Palmer, Rona, Fear, and Stevelink (2021) state that leaving the military introduces rupture across all levels. Loss is paramount, and because it affects all areas of a person's functioning – loss of family, community, belonging, home, employment, earnings, purpose, support, status, identity – it is pervasive. While the vast majority do adapt to the non-military way of life some continue to struggle and unsupported can go on to develop an adjustment disorder.

Adjustment disorder is primarily a short-term condition that is the consequence of a stressful life event such as ill health, financial or marital problems. DSM-5 determines that an adjustment disorder will generally occur within three months of the event and will usually be resolved within six months. Members of the armed forces are more likely to seek help for adjustment disorder than the general population (NHS, 2020). This is no surprise given the transient lifestyle of military personnel. However, the ultimate transition back into civilian life may result in much longer-term adjustment difficulties than DSM-5 suggests.

A potential contributor to extended adjustment disorder may well be lack of help seeking which is a longstanding and recognised problem for military personnel (Rafferty, Wessely, Stevelink, & Greenberg, 2019). Lack of professional support can ultimately lead to self-management via maladaptive behaviours (Bashford et al., 2020).

Among armed forces personnel, rates of excessive alcohol use are high; service personnel are twice as likely as the general population to drink hazardous amounts of alcohol (Ministry of Defence, 2017). Historically, alcohol has played a significant role in the armed forces. It has long been used to foster a sense of belonging and unity. Up until 1970 naval ratings received a daily tot of rum, which was eventually replaced with the option to draw three half-pint cans of beer a day. Alcohol in military bars is much cheaper than other licenced premises. Alcohol is used as an incentive, for example in preparation for an inspection, as a reward for sporting triumph or as a sign of gratitude from senior personnel. It is reliably reported that Prime Minister Margaret Thatcher rewarded the 28 man SAS team with 400 cans of lager to share as a celebration immediately following the Iranian Embassy Siege in 1980. More recently, not with the blessing of the armed forces, the misuse of prescription medication, such as benzodiazepines and illicit substances, has risen steadily. According to the Ministry figures released by the Ministry of Defence, 660 army personnel were dismissed after failing a drug test in 2019, the most widely detected substance being cocaine followed by cannabis and ecstasy (Busby, 2020).

While the armed forces now have well-established alcohol and substance misuse training programmes in conjunction with strict alcohol and drug testing protocols, the problem remains. Armed services personnel and veterans are known to use alcohol and substance misuse to enable them to deal with the negative impact military service has had on their mental and physical health. Continued use of what can be regarded as avoidant behaviour can have a marked impact on both the individuals physical and mental health whilst exposing them to the risks associated with addiction. Although some decline is reported, it remains that up to 11.4% of serving personnel and 15.1% of service leavers could have a significant problem with alcohol misuse (Armed Forces Network, 2020).

There is no doubt that military service can for some lead to psychological injury, resulting in maladaptive coping and behavioural change. The following narratives detail two veterans' personal perspectives of how they believe military service shaped their thinking and behaviours ultimately resulting in offending behaviour.

Peter's Story

I left the army with an exemplary service record of 14 years. I've been out longer than I was in. But not a day has gone by when I haven't thought about my time in the army.

In March 1978 I arrived for basic training and for 18 weeks we were thrown together, isolated from the outside world, screamed and shouted at; kept busy, exhausted and always in a position where we had to work together as a group. With hindsight, I suppose I can look back and see this was all part of the brainwashing necessary to create a fighting machine, but at the time all I knew was that this is what I'd been born for.

My first posting was a cushty number in Gibraltar. Next it was Northern Ireland on a 5-month emergency tour. That wasn't great. I was terrified. I had postings and detachments all over the world, from Germany to the Falklands, but I always seemed to end up back in Northern Ireland. Eventually you can't live in a constant state of terror so it's like your mind switches off and you don't give a shit; you accept it, you stop worrying. You distance yourself with a dark sense of humour, diluting the terror with laughter. Like the time I was escorting engineers working in Sniper Country; Forkhill, South Armagh, and because of the drilling we hadn't heard a sniper shooting at us. A panic-stricken bloke ran to tell us, and I'll never forget the look on his face when we all just cracked up laughing.

R&R (Rest & Recuperation) seemed to make things harder; the real world becomes an alien world full of civvies who don't have a clue. So, you drink, and you fight and then you go back on duty where you know where you stand.

I spent two years as a "Brigadier's Sandbag" in Londonderry. Two years putting myself in a position where they'd have to kill me, not the Brigadier. I never questioned it; it was just a laugh really. You don't question it in the army; you just get on with it. You do what you're told.

I knew my time in the army was coming to an end in 1988, two days before Christmas, I was on duty at The Maze prison watching in disbelief as they let the prisoners out for a holiday. My wife was pregnant then; I'd have quite liked a Christmas holiday myself.

At the end of yet another three-year posting to Northern Ireland, I'd had enough and decided my army days were over. I bottled out of my own leaving do and flew out of Belfast City Airport feeling like it was the last day of my life, gutted. But by the time we landed my spirits had lifted. I felt set free and positive about my future as a civilian; and it seemed like my feeling was spot on when I breezed straight into a job. How wrong was I?

This first job turned out to be a cold lesson on the difference between being a soldier and being a civilian at work. I was used to orders and getting on with the task as quickly as possible, to the best of my ability and, while this is appreciated by your colleagues in the army, it's not appreciated by your colleagues in a factory. Not when management start to wonder why everyone can't graft as hard as you can. So, I was called a blackleg and I was alienated.

I walked out and got another job which meant frequent trips between Manchester and London. I started taking detours on these London trips, to my old army camp to see my mates. These detours became what I lived for; a brief respite in the nightmare world of civvy street. Eventually, of course, my mates had less and less time for me each time I stopped off; after all, they had their lives to live as soldiers. I felt more and more isolated, but I couldn't stop these detours, even if it was only to drive past the camp. On one occasion I went into the mess, gave my old number and ordered a meal. Just to be back in a world where I could breathe. Back home, my life was starting to get out of control; I was drinking heavily, cheating on my wife and sparking off meaningless fights with groups of lads just to get myself a kicking. I knew my life was like a plane falling out of the sky, but I didn't know how to stop it crashing, and I definitely didn't know how to ask for help. Eventually I'd had enough of the job. I dumped the company car, hitched home and ended up in a row with my wife, which turned violent. Within a year of that night I'd been locked up for life. In a way it was a relief.

I don't blame the army for my offence; that was down to me and, who knows, maybe I was destined to end up in prison and maybe it was only the army that kept me out of serious trouble for the 14 years I was a soldier. The army turned me into a soldier but the things that made me a good soldier, made me a bad civilian; and that's probably true of a lot of veterans. When I was a soldier the army was the making of me, when I became a civilian, the army was the breaking of me. I didn't know how to be a civilian anymore. Now I'm in prison it's almost like I'm back in the army, with the rules and the structure and the regime, the getting told what to do and when to do it.

Sean's Story
Don't Steal My Chips

Iraq: Playing cards
(Sound of motar attack)
Thought – "If I move, they will take my (poker) chips"
(Sounds of attack gets closer)
No one moves
Who will be the first to move?
Body surging, heart going dum dum dum
Thought – "Whatever happens it doesn't matter so long as they don't take my chips"
First time you hear the alarm you panic, hearts beating 100 miles an hour, you put on your helmet and body armour and get under that coffin (bunk) and hope it doesn't land on you. You count the bangs as they are released and how many explode when they hit ground. That's what you are taught to do. This dwindles – looking back there is no way of telling how, or when it changed. Who decided first – mentally as a group, sub-consciously – if you could speak without words, "let's carry on and sit here and play cards"? You looked to the others to see who would be the first to move.

We took increasing risks, waiting longer and longer, you get addicted to the adrenalin, the rush. You start to think that coffin isn't going to save me.

Afghanistan: Operation Herrick

The front two soldiers would use the metal detectors to search for landmines. We played a game, a challenge "Falmer Barmer". Everyone knew about it apart from the officers. Who goes the longest without switching the machine on! One guy found an IED and then jumped on it to confirm that it wasn't a pressure plate. It's a different world out there but that's the mindset you get to. It gives you control of the situation, a way of being in control.

On patrol we would be fired at but couldn't see where it was coming from, where the enemy was. Someone had to take the risk, someone had to run. The officer would say, "I need you to run". You run and the moment they open fire we know where they are. I've stuck my head up plenty of times. You don't think or feel, it's just what you have to do. You have to understand for us it's not much of a risk because you know everyone is on the job. For us that was not so much of a risk you see you have to understand we have trained, drilled, together. I know them, I know they will see where the enemy is and take them out. I know they have my back.

We helped each other out. "Patrol bingo" was something we did. We were the same group, same checkpoint, same officer, in it together. Officers decide who does what day to day. After two weeks you can see the strain on the officer because he is deciding who lives and who dies. So, we put the names in a hat and pick out who will do what. It's a weight off the officer – it's risky, exciting and got you nervous. It was like tombola you might win or lose. But it had a purpose – the pressure was off the boss, the lads, it made life easier – what will be will be.

There were other reasons for me taking risks. I didn't care if I died. My life outside of the army was a nightmare so I was volunteering, putting myself forward. I was volunteering at every opportunity, the dangerous jobs. The more I did the less happened to me. I delayed my R&R because there was another operation I wanted to do, I tried to delay it again after that, but they wouldn't let me. I didn't want R&R I was getting addicted to the fight, being behind enemy lines. Being behind enemy lines is a dream come true for a soldier.

Respect for me went up, I was getting acknowledgment from all over the place and from the officers. I was a Kingsman, the lowest rank. But I was given some of the duties of the lance corporals. I got stepped up in everyone's opinion because I was doing well. I kept my composure, I benefited from being the best. I was good at what I was doing but I was good because I wanted to die. I was considered to have true grit. The commanders were saying "get him there". It was good for my ego. Growing up, my reputation wasn't the best, I wasn't the brightest, never had the best clothes. For me this was recognition.

This is a section from my Performance Report:- "This soldier has an outstanding performance particularly during Operation Herrick. He was moved through a number of different CP (Control Points) when manpower shortages required, and he could be relied upon to fit in and work hard as soon as he arrived. He led from the front and was respected and trusted by all that he worked for and with. He takes things in his stride and can be relied upon to complete a task to a high standard. He should look to become a section commander. He has a bright future".

1000s have been on deployment but only 100s have been in combat situations. It's addictive, you can't live without the adrenalin. But it creates threats all over the place. I was on R&R, I wasn't right, wasn't seeing things the same way other people were, I was reacting. I called to take me back to camp but I didn't get there military training teaches a threat is a threat, regardless, if it's a man, woman or child. It's what's instilled, this makes the mind-set.

I was still in the forces when I committed my crime but I wasn't there if you know what I mean. I got arrested and went straight from one war zone to another. Prison is like a war zone, putting someone like me in with a lot of violent offenders is not good. I was in segregation for two and a half years when I first came to prison. I came straight from the military; I was never in civvy street.

I have to manage the negatives of the military especially the hypervigilance which presents as anxiety. Looking every day for the violent, the out of the ordinary. I have to control the adrenalin and not get involved. My adrenalin is rushing, it's back. I struggle not to get involved and have to swallow my pride. How do I walk away? Save the shame? I was an elite soldier – now you are telling me that I can't fight – how do I suppress the feelings of enjoyment. Outside you could supplement the enjoyment with something else like sky diving, driving too fast but in here nothing… I understand the transition now, but it's taken a long time. I was pumped, primed ready to rock and roll. An elite fighting machine!

I did well in the military, don't get me wrong. I have seen the world, had adventures, worked with horses, I've got skills, I've never missed a day's work, punctual, polite, respectful I've got all the military ethics. This makes jail easier for me than for most.

Family – There is no collaboration between the military and families. My family did not know what I was going through. I'd be saying I'm going on training for 4/5 weeks and my girlfriend would be upset that I'm going. She didn't realise that I needed support because this is the hardest thing I will do. I needed cuddles not moaning at because I hadn't phoned for two days. I was thrashed for days, weeks with minimal food and water I had no head space or time given to phone, it was hard – she doesn't know that.

Discussion

Despite these two narratives describing events worlds and years apart, both describe the close bonds, attachments, and camaraderie of serving personnel. Both evidence development of addictions, chronic distress, and a disconnect from the civilian world.

Sean describes making an unsuccessful attempt to seek help. He reported a lack of awareness regarding deterioration in his mental well-being, hitting a "too late" crisis point before seeking help. This experience reflects the findings of Rafferty, Wessely, Stevelink, and Greenberg (2019), who reported that help seeking often only occurred when the severity of symptoms takes the decision out of veterans' hands. For some, this can be many years after leaving service (Albertson, 2019).

There are many reasons why veterans are reluctant to seek help; fear of being seen as weak; feeling undeserving of help in the light of another's death or physical injury; fear that seeking help would jeopardise their career; shame at "letting the military down" (usually described in terms of having let the unit or military mates down); not knowing where to go; feeling that services do not understand military service; complicated referrals systems; lack of consistency; long waiting lists and confusion as to who provides what support. One veteran reported that he sought help, was then posted to a different area and had to start the referral process from scratch creating delay, frustration, and his eventual disengagement.

Recognising mental health difficulties in armed forces personnel is a positive influence on help seeking with engagement further strengthened by an appreciation of and knowledge of the unique military experience (Hurley, 2021; Rafferty et al., 2019; Stevelink et al., 2019). Nevertheless, knowing where to go does not guarantee access (Williamson, Greenberg, & Stevelink, 2019). Raised awareness and collaborative working between the MoD, NHS, and military-focused organisations including military charities is however proving to be a successful bridge to help seeking. Collaborative, military-experienced organisations are improving accessibility and engagement with services relevant to the needs of the armed forces community. Needs including housing, employment, finances, living independently, mental and physical health are all on the agenda. The Veterans Gateway provides a first point of contact connecting the armed forces population with the right support as soon as possible. Cobseo (2020) the confederation of service charities (www.cobseo.org. uk) provides a unified approach to government, private sectors, and the armed forces community. Services such as these working in collaboration with the MoD will serve to minimise stressors that can lead to offending behaviour.

The Ministry of Defence, NHS (2018) have formed a working partnership agreement to provide consistent healthcare for serving and ex-serving members of the armed forces. Op Courage provides specialist NHS care from healthcare staff working in collaboration with military charities to provide community and inpatient support and treatment for veterans. Offender Health and its enhanced complexity is now served by Liaison and Diversion experts. Specialist pathfinders such as *ReGroup*, a partnership between Offender Health Nottinghamshire Healthcare NHS Foundation Trust and veterans' charities *Care after Combat* and *Project Nova*, are working together throughout the CJS. ReGroup is based on three core principals *Care not Custody*, *Care in Custody*, and *Care post Custody*. Such pathfinders will provide the evidence base to inform a national NHS roll-out for healthcare and social support for veterans in the CJS. There is no doubt that the short- and long-term well-being of armed forces personnel and their families is currently high on the agenda for public services. It is paramount that this remains the case so that what is learnt can be embedded into consistent provision of care.

Summary

For the majority, service in the armed forces has many lifelong enhancing benefits. The extent, scope, and nature of the work of the armed forces means that service cannot be without adverse experience and, for a minority, links can be made between military-related experiences, the development of trauma responses, and offending behaviour.

This chapter focused on military-related experiences and the work in progress to minimise negative outcomes for armed forces personnel. During the collaborative work with veterans in the CJS, which gave rise to this chapter, veterans shared much about their experiences in the CJS. Giving this population a voice is a positive initial step towards understanding potential links between military service, offending behaviour, and the impact of the CJS. Such insights are integral to the partnership pathfinders focus of work.

Acknowledgements

Thanks to all who participated in the writing of this chapter. Thanks also to Simon Ralls, Clinical Specialist for Veterans, for valuable contributions and ongoing support.

Further Reading

Johnson, J. (2016). *The veteran's survival guide: Explaining combat-related PTSD for ex-servicemen and their families.* CPI Group: Croydon. For readers who want a veteran's perspective, recognising offending behaviour and offering support for veterans and their families.

References

Albertson, K. (2019). Relational legacies impacting on veteran transition from military to civilian life: Trajectories of acquisition, loss, and reformation of a sense of belonging. *Illness, Crisis & Loss, 27*(4), 255–273. doi:10.1177/1054137319834773

American Psychiatric Association. (2013). *Diagnostic and statistical manual of mental disorders: DSM-5.* American Psychiatric Publishing.

Armed Forces Act. (2011). c.18. www.legislation.gov.uk/ukpga/2011/18/contents

Armed Forces Network. (2020). *Mental health and the armed forces community factsheet.* Retrieved from https://sussexarmedforcesnetwork.nhs.uk/wp-content/uploads/2018/06/AFN-Mental-Health-Factsheet.pdf

Bashford, J., Hasan, S., Evans-Jones, G., & Patel, L. (2020). *Trauma in mind: Addressing high intensity needs of veterans and family members affected by mental health-related trauma.* Solent NHS Trust.

Blake, N. (2006). *The Deepcut review: A review of the circumstances surrounding the deaths of four soldiers at Princess Royal Barracks, Deepcut between 1995 and 2002.* The Stationery Office.

Bryan, C.J., Bryan, A.O., Anestis, M.D., Anetis, J.C., Green, B.A., Etienne, N., & Ray-Sannerud, B. (2016). Measuring moral injury: Psychometric properties of the moral injury events scale in two military samples. *Assessment, 23*(5), 557–570. doi:10.1177/1073191115590855

Busby, M. (2020). Rise in the number of British soldiers being sacked for drug use. *The Guardian.* Retrieved from www.theguardian.com/uk

Busittil, W., Hacker-Hughes, J., & Kitchiner, N. (2017). Introduction. In J. Hacker-Hughes (Ed.), *Military veteran psychological health and social care contemporary issues* (pp.3–13). Routledge.

Cobseo. (2020). *The confederation of service charities. Independent auditors report.* Invicta House: London.

Ein-Dor, T. (2014). Facing danger: How do people behave in times of need? The case of adult attachment styles. *Frontiers in Psychology, 5,* 1452. doi:10.3389/fpsyg.2014.01452

Ein-Dor, T., & Hirschberger, G. (2016). Rethinking attachment theory: From a theory of relationships to a theory of individual and group survival. *Current Directions in Psychological Science, 25*(4), 223–227. doi:10.1177%2F0963721416650684

Hurley, E.C. (2021). *A clinician's guide for treating active military and veteran population with EMDR therapy*. Springer Publishing Company.

Johnson, S.B., Blum, R.W., & Giedd, J.N. (2009). Adolescent maturity and the Brain: The promise and pitfalls of neuroscience research in adolescent health policy. *Journal of Adolescent Health, 45*(3), 216–221. doi:10.1016/j.jadohealth.2009.05.016

Lindner, E.G. (2001). Humiliation-trauma that has been overlooked: An analysis based on field-work in Germany, Rwanda/Burundi, and Somalia. *Traumatology, 7*(1), 43–68. doi:10.1177/153476560100700104

Litz, B.T., Stein, N., Delaney, E., Debowitz, L., Nash, W.P., Silva, C., & Maguen, S. (2009). Moral injury and moral repair in war veterans: A preliminary model and intervention strategy. *Clinical Psychology Review, 29*, 695–706. doi:10.1016/j.cpr.2009.07.003

MacManus, D., Dean, K., Jones, M., Rona, R.J., Greenberg, N., Hull, … & Fear, N.T. (2013). Violent offending by UK military personnel deployed to Iraq and Afghanistan: A data linkage cohort study. *Lancet, 381*(9870), 907–917. doi:10.1016/S0140-6736(13)60354-2

MacManus, D., Dickson, H., Short. R., Burdett, H., Kwan, J., Jones, M., Hull, L., … & Fear, N.T. (2019). Risk and protective factors for offending among UK armed forces personnel after they leave service: A data linkage study. *Psychological Medicine, 51*(2), 236–243. doi:10.1017/S0033291719003131

Ministry of Defence. (2011). *The armed forces covenant*. Ministry of Defence.

Ministry of Defence. (2017). *Alcohol usage in the UK armed forces 1 June 2016 – 31 May 2017*. Retrieved from https://assets.publishing.service.gov.uk/government/uploads/system/uploads/attachment_data/file/630184/20170718_Alcohol_Usage_bulletin__-_O.pdf

Ministry of Defence. (2021). Press release. Retrieved from www.gov.uk/government/news/former-personnel-discharged-over-sexuality-to-have-medals-restored

Ministry of Defence, NHS. (2018). *Partnership agreement between the Ministry of Defence and NHS England for the commissioning of health services for the armed forces*. NHS.

Molendijk, T., Kramer, E-H., Verweij, D. (2018). Moral aspects of "moral injury": Analyzing conceptualisations on the role of morality in military trauma. *Journal of Military Ethics, 17*(1), 36–53. doi:10.1080/15027570.2018.1483173

Naval, Army, and RAF Families Federation. (2018). *Lifting the lid on transition. The families' experience and the support they need. Forces in mind trust*. Retrieved from https://nff.org.uk/lifting-the-lid-on-transition/

NHS. (2020). *Mental health and the armed forces community factsheet, The Armed Forces Network*. NHS.

Osório, C., Jones, N., Jones, E., Robbins, I., Wessely, S., & Greenberg, N. (2018). Combat experiences and their relationship to post-traumatic stress disorder symptom clusters in UK military personnel deployed to Afghanistan. *Behavioral Medicine, 44*(2), 131–140. doi:10.1080/08964289.2017.1288606

Palmer, L., Rona, R.J., Fear, N.T., & Stevelink, A.M. (2021). *The evolution of post traumatic stress disorder in the UK armed forces: Traumatic exposures in Iraq and Afghanistan and responses of distress (TRIAD study)*. Kings College London.

Phillips, S. (2014). *Former members of the armed forces and the criminal justice system: A review on behalf of the Secretary of State of justice. Independent report*. Ministry of Justice.

Rafferty, L.A., Wessely, S., Stevelink, S.A.M., & Greenberg, N. (2019). The journey to pro-fessional mental health support: A qualitative exploration of the barriers and facilitators impacting military veterans' engagement with mental health treatment. *European Journal of Psychotraumatology, 10*(1), 1700613. doi:10.1080/20008198.2019.1700613

Short, R., Dickson, H., Greenberg, N., & MacManus, D. (2018). Offending behaviour, health and wellbeing of military veterans in the criminal justice system. *PLoS ONE, 13*(11), e0207282. doi:10.1371/journal.pone.0207282

Stevelink, S.A., Jones, N., Jones, M., Dyball, D., Khera, C.K., Pernet, D., … & Fear, N.T. (2019). Do serving and ex-serving personnel of the UK armed forces seek help for perceived stress, emotional or mental health problems? *European Journal of Psychotraumatology*, *10*(1), 1556552. doi:10.1080/20008198.2018.1556552

Taylor, E.N., Timko, C., Nash, A., Owens, M.D., Harris, A.H.S., & Fimlay, A.K. (2020). Posttraumatic stress disorder and justice involvement among military veterans: A systematic review and meta-analysis. *Journal of Traumatic Stress, 33*, 804–812. doi:10.1002/jts.22526

Wainwright,V., Lennox, C., McDonnell, S., Shaw, J., & Senior, J. (2017). Offending characteristics of male ex-armed forces personnel in prison. *Howard Journal of Crime and Justice, 56*(1), 19–33. doi:10.1111/hojo.12189

Wang, C., Rapp, P., Darmon, D., Trongnetrpunya, A., Costanzo, M.E., Nathean, D.E., … & Keyser, D. (2018). Utility of P300 ERP in monitoring post-trauma mental health: A longitudinal study in military personnel returning from combat deployment. *Journal of Psychiatric Research, 101*, 5–13. doi:10.1016/j.jpsychires.2018.02.027

Williamson, V., Greenberg, N., & Murphy, D. (2019). Moral injury in UK armed forces: A qualitative study. *European Journal of Psychotraumatology, 10*(1), 1562842, doi:10.1080/20008198,2018,1562842

Williamson,V., Greenberg, N., & Stevelink, S.A.M. (2019). Perceived stigma and barriers to care in UK armed forces personnel and veterans with and without probable mental disorders. *BMC Psychology, 7*, 75. doi:10.1186/s40359-019-0351-7

World Health Organization. (2018). *International classification of diseases for mortality and morbidity statistics*. World Health Organization.

PART III

Survival Responses

9

"WHEN YOU HAVE GOT LIKE TWENTY THOUSAND THOUGHTS IN YOUR HEAD, THAT ONE LITTLE THING CAN JUST MAKE IT ALL GO AWAY"

Trauma and Non-Suicidal Self-Injury in Forensic Settings

Rachel Beryl and Jessica Lewis

Introduction

Within forensic settings the management of those causing harm to themselves presents a significant challenge to the services that look after them, particularly in women's services (Uppal & McMurran, 2009). Trauma experiences, both in childhood and adulthood, and non-suicidal self-injury (NSSI) are highly correlated (Swannell et al., 2012) and the exact relationship between NSSI and trauma has been explored within the literature (see Serafini et al., 2017). This chapter will explore the relationship between trauma experiences and NSSI, and reflect on the responses within a high secure hospital setting to understanding, managing, and reducing the occurrence of NSSI, considering the impact of these on both staff and patients.[1] We advocate trauma-informed treatment responses for this population, to compassionately respond to the distress and challenge of NSSI.

The lived experience of trauma and NSSI is woven as a narrative throughout, with three women (we called them *Denise, Gina, and Emily*) contributing to our understanding by reflecting on their own NSSI, what they felt were the functions of

DOI: 10.4324/9781003120766-13

it, and how that might link to their traumatic experiences, commenting on staff and system responses to NSSI.

Non-Suicidal Self-Injury

The act of causing deliberate harm to oneself is given a number of labels such as NSSI, self-mutilation, or deliberate self-harm, and is viewed as a separate entity to suicidal behaviour. The definition of "intentionally causing physical harm to one's own body, without the intent to die" (Ford & Gómez, 2015) is used, as it covers the broad range of behaviours. NSSI is highly associated with suicidal risk, particularly in forensic settings (Hawton et al., 2014), and both behaviours can be present in some individuals. However, many studies view them as being distinct entities, in that each can exist without the other, with the clear defining characteristic being the presence or absence of the intent to die (Ford & Gómez, 2015). In this chapter we focus on NSSI, without an intent to die.

Trauma

This chapter will consider trauma in its broadest sense to encompass exposure to psychologically traumatising experiences such as early traumatic experiences, e.g., abuse and neglect; adult traumatic experiences, such as sexual violence; racial trauma, seen as the "cumulative traumatising impact of racism on racialised individuals" (Williams, Haeny, & Holmes, 2021); sexual minority trauma, including interpersonal violence, victimisation, and discriminatory events (House, van Horn, Coppeans, & Stepleman, 2011); and, within forensic populations, the potential traumatising impact of their offending, and detainment (Gunter, Chibnall, Antoniak, Philibert, & Hollenbeck, 2011).

Prevalence

The rate of NSSI varies greatly when considering a range of different populations, such as adolescents, and those with various psychiatric diagnoses (Cipriano, Cella, & Cotrufo, 2017). There is also evidence that childhood sexual abuse, and other forms of maltreatment, including severe family dysfunction are risk factors for NSSI for a range of age groups and populations (Maniglio, 2011).

NSSI can be a particular challenge for the prison estate, with yearly NSSI rates recorded at 5–6% of male prisoners, and 20–24% of female prisoners (Hawton et al., 2014). In the 12 months up to September 2020 the Safety in Custody Statistics (Ministry of Justice, 2021) recorded self-harm incidents of 595 per 1,000 for male prisoners, in contrast to a rate of 3,597 per 1,000 for female prisoners. Within prison, NSSI rates are strongly associated with residing in solitary confinement, having disciplinary infractions and experiencing physical or sexual victimisation whilst in prison, as well as experience of childhood abuse, particularly sexual abuse (Favril, Yu, Hawton, & Fazel, 2020).

Rates of NSSI are similarly high within forensic hospital settings. Within a High Secure Hospital over a 16-month period, 30.9% of all incidents were self-harm, with a staggering 54% of these carried out by the female patients who represented just 13.5% of the population. The rate of violence among female patients was also high, representing 36.2% of the hospital total (Uppal & McMurran, 2009). Longdon, Beryl, and Siddall (2020) reported that 98% of women in a high secure forensic population had experienced at least one form of childhood trauma, and 54% had experienced five forms of childhood trauma (physical, sexual, and psychological abuse, and physical and emotional neglect).

It is recognised that some populations are uniquely vulnerable to increased exposure to traumatic experiences, due to the long-term impact of systematic prejudice, discrimination, and targeting due to minority status (see Bhui et al., 2003; De Genna & Feske, 2013 for NSSI rates in different ethnic populations and House, van Horn, Coppeans, & Stepleman, 2011 for NSSI rates for gay, lesbian, bisexual, and/or transgender individuals).

Making Sense of the Links between Trauma and NSSI

The relationship between trauma and NSSI is complex and multifaceted, with many mediating variables, such as dissociation (Swannell et al., 2012; Ford & Gómez, 2015), alexithymia (Paivio & McCullock, 2004), and self-criticism (Glassman et al., 2007). Much of the existing literature is also cross-sectional in nature, further complicating the question of *whether*, and if so, *how*, trauma leads to NSSI (see Liu, Scopelliti, Pittman, & Zamora, 2018 for a review of the area). Throughout this section, the lived experience of individuals forms the narrative and provides opportunity for understanding the complexity of both the relationship between trauma and NSSI and NSSI and the individual. Yates's (2009) Organisational Developmental Pathway model helps to illustrate different pathways/trajectories from trauma exposure to NSSI. These pathways also help illustrate the various "functions" of NSSI, as well as pointing to different areas of focus for therapeutic interventions.

Yates (2009) proposes that there are three key pathways from trauma to self-injury: *regulatory, representational,* and *reactive*; these can operate in isolation, or in conjunction with one another. In the *regulatory* pathway towards self-injury, childhood maltreatment can impact on the development of integrative, symbolic, and reflective affect-processing capacities. The thwarting of these capacities thus renders the individual less able to integrate thoughts and feelings, and to "know what they feel and to feel what they know" (Yates, 2009; p.125). It also results in reduced capacities to symbolise affect through language (i.e., to use language to share and communicate internal states), or to reflect on the feeling states of oneself or others. In this context, self-injury can become a means of communicating and regulating affect. Early caregiving experiences also shape patterns in physiological reactivity, and child "maltreatment may initiate neurobiological alterations and physiological cascades that contribute to a *reactive* path towards NSSI" (Yates, 2009; p.118). Self-injury can therefore represent a tool to alter biological reactivity/arousal. Thus, trauma exposure can result in both trauma–induced changes in arousal (*reactive pathway*) as well as reduced regulating capacities (*regulatory pathway*), demonstrating the inter-related and interactional nature of the pathways. The *representational* pathway relates to the negative representations (of self, others, and relationships) that form as a consequence of maltreatment, and can lead to the enactment of NSSI (in isolation, or in co-existence with the other two pathways). The early caregiving milieu lays the foundation for a child's core beliefs about themselves, their expectations of others, and of relationships. In the context of child maltreatment, the child develops representations of self as defective, unlovable, or bad; of others as malevolent and untrustworthy; and of relationships as dangerous. NSSI can therefore become a means of self-soothing (in the absence of relational soothing resources), and/or a means of self-punishment. Indeed, "self-harm can provide a paradoxical function that involves both attacking the self while simultaneously offering a self-soothing response to distress" (Grocutt, 2009; p.103).

Yates's pathways can be viewed as synergistic and inter-related (Lang & Sharma-Patel, 2011), as can the functions and levels of meaning to a single act of NSSI. Our attempt to highlight some key themes in the functions NSSI is not to diminish the individualised and complex meanings of NSSI for a person, and indeed the reader is urged to hold in mind that "everyone self-harms for their own reason and they shouldn't always be put like into one bubble" *(Emily)*.

The Regulatory Pathway and Functions/Meanings of NSSI

Affect regulation is the most cited function of NSSI (Klonsky, 2007) garnering most empirical support and playing a prominent role in treatments for self-injury (Lang & Sharma-Patel, 2011). For some, NSSI offers a means of coping with emotional distress:"I've done it out of stress, anxiety to calm myself when I'm incredibly emotional/ upset" (Chandler, 2014). It is also described as a means of "releasing all that tension and stuff" *(Emily)*, and "feels good at the time and it makes them feel better" *(Gina)*.

The act of NSSI can help the individual to "forget about something" (Young, van Beinum, Sweeting, & West, 2007) *and* "to get relief from a terrible state of mind" (Boergers, Spirito, & Donaldson, 1998). NSSI can thus offer a sense of distraction from emotional pain:

> It just calms me down, like when you have got like 20,000 thoughts in your head, that one little thing can just make it all go away.
>
> *Emily*

This distraction can also offer a physical focus for pain, distracting from emotional pain:

> after I cut myself ... it starts to hurt a little bit ... and then I focus on that because it hurts. It's like, oh God, I've got this to focus on now. Thank goodness. So it also kind of gives me something else to focus on rather than everything else, some- thing surface.
>
> *Himber, 1994*

NSSI can represent an attempt to distance from emotional pain and "produce a feeling of numbness when my feelings are too strong" (Swannell, Martin, Scott, Gibbons, & Gifford, 2008).

It can also represent an attempt to *generate* feelings, to cope with the numbness brought about by a dissociative state (Klonsky & Muehlenkamp, 2007):

> it's a way of getting myself awake again, it's a wakening experience.
>
> *Himber, 1994*

> I feel numb—physically and emotionally. I can't feel my own skin. [after self-harming] I can physically feel again. My senses come back. I get a surge of energy and regain sensation.
>
> *Horne & Csipke, 2009*

Indeed, NSSI can be a means of *generating* feeling (Nock & Cha, 2009), when you "want to feel something else for a change" *(Gina)*, or want to disrupt a sense of derealisation or "psychic numbness" (Yates, 2009; p.30) and respond to or generate altered states of consciousness.

NSSI is also described as an *anti-suicide* survival strategy (Messner & Fremouw, 2008), where, for some people, NSSI can be a means of regulating intense emotional states and managing their risk of suicide (Edmondson, Brennan, & House, 2016): "I wouldn't be here today if this hadn't happened [self-harm]" (Demming, 2008).

The communicative function of NSSI is further acknowledged, where symbolic and reflective affect-processing are limited, such that acts of self-injury can be "a way of saying through gestures and acts of violence, that which cannot be put into words. Through self-harm the body speaks" (Motz, 2009; pp.21–22).

The Representational Pathway and Functions/Meanings of NSSI

The role of *self-criticism, negative self-image,* and *shame,* in the association between trauma and self-injury is well evidenced in the literature (Klonsky, Oltmanns, & Turkheimer, 2003); and in the voices of individuals:

> lack of self-esteem because that can play a big part for some people so if they don't like themselves ..., they might want ... to destroy their own bodies or something ... like if they hate themselves or people have made them feel shit about themselves over the years.
>
> *Denise*

Self-injury is also described as inducing further self-criticism:

> at the time you might think that you could feel better for a couple of minutes ..., but then when that feeling goes – and it will go – and you're just left feeling just as bad again or worse for like giving in to it, and you'll be disappointed in yourself and upset people that love you.
>
> *Gina*

Another related theme in the enactment of NSSI is the experience of self-blame and self-hatred. Trauma survivors may "blame themselves for what has happened in the past" *(Denise),* and develop representations of themselves as defective and bad (Yates, 2009). NSSI (especially in the form of cutting or bloodletting) is described by some as a means of "cleansing" or "letting out badness" (Edmondson et al., 2016):

> All the bad escapes in the blood and it's like you can physically watch every-thing just wash away.
>
> *Abrams & Gordon, 2003*

The *self-punishment* function of self-injury is also well documented in the literature (Klonsky & Muehlenkamp, 2007), and in service user accounts of their experience of NSSI (Edmondson et al., 2016).

In addition to negative *self*-representations, the negative representations of *others* and *relationships* are also evident in the various *interpersonal* functions of NSSI. Without other means of communicating needs for care and support, NSSI can "be a cry for help for some people, say like 'something's wrong and I don't know how to ask for help'" *(Denise).* Through acts of self-injury, a relational need can be met:

> Doing this [self-harm] I found … I received the warmth, love and attention I had been looking for.
>
> *Harris, 2000*

> if you have grown up like in a traumatic like home environment or grown up and not had the attention that you need like and the care and stuff, it might be the only way you have learnt to get that attention and …, even though it's negative, it could be the only way that you know how to get like your needs met.
>
> *Emily*

The description of "seeking attention" as a function of self-injury is not, however, endorsed by many (Gratz, 2003); the pejorative connotations of "self-harmers" being "attention seekers" may perhaps influence this. It is however recognised that NSSI can play a role in shaping one's environment and influencing others (Nock & Cha, 2009). It can also offer a means of regaining some sense of control in one's environment (Klonsky, 2007); and, in the context of secure/custodial settings, it can prompt a move in location (DeHart, Smith, & Kaminski, 2009). In forensic contexts, self-harm may further serve as a replacement for aggression (Daffern & Howells, 2009), and as an expression of aggression and revenge (Gallagher & Sheldon, 2010).

The long-term effects of NSSI on relationships is also acknowledged:

> It can have an impact on your relationships with people especially if they don't understand as to why you're doing it in the first place, then it can scare another person cos they don't know if that person's going to take it too far one day, and so instead of waiting for that to happen they might just reject 'em and that, cos it's easier to reject someone than to losing someone completely.
>
> *Denise*

Another proposed meaning of NSSI relates to the maintenance and exploration of boundaries (Edmondson et al., 2016), for instance "to create a symbolic boundary between myself and others" (Klonsky and Glenn, 2009). NSSI can also serve as a means of protection – both as self-protection, as well as protecting others from oneself. When NSSI serves to protect *from others*, this can manifest in making one's body unattractive to others "as a barrier against unwanted advances" (Edmondson et al., 2016; p.113):

> I've been cutting myself so that if someone does try anything they'll see my body and think what a freak, she's disgusting, she's ugly.
>
> *Parfitt, 2005*

When functioning for the protection *of others*, it can involve expressing fury at oneself rather than others (Motz, 2009; p.28). Indeed, some describe how they "would rather take it out on themselves rather than take it out on other people" *(Gina)*.

The Reactive Pathway and Functions/Meanings of NSSI

Repeated exposure to stress and maltreatment in childhood is known to stimulate the autonomic nervous system, and lead to alterations in physiological reactivity and the functioning of stress response systems (Yates, 2009). States of hyper- and hypo-arousal can be experienced with overwhelming rapid shifts and fluctuations, and NSSI can serve as a means of attempting to modulate this autonomic dysregulation. The arousal modulation model of the Window of Tolerance (Ogden, Pain, & Fisher, 2006; Siegel, 1999) offers a framework for understanding these biphasic reactions, and NSSI can be interpreted as a strategy to up- or down-regulate autonomic arousal. Therefore, when in a state of hyperarousal, NSSI may be enacted to soothe and lower arousal, and manage the intrusions of flashbacks and traumatic memories (Van der Kolk, Perry, & Herman, 1991), whereas, from a state of hypoarousal, NSSI may serve to reduce or interrupt feelings of numbness and flattened affect.

The role of the pleasure/reward systems in the enactment of NSSI is also note-worthy, as "the turmoil and destruction are nonetheless addictive, and offer a kind of pleasure" (Motz, 2009; p.25). NSSI is described by some as a means of generating excitement and exhilaration (Edmondson et al., 2016; Klonsky & Glenn, 2009), and the potential addictive quality of NSSI is noted, alongside a need to "escalate":

> You can get addicted to it.
>
> *Bennett & Moss, 2013*

> when you first start doing it you think 'this works' and then when it doesn't work anymore then you take it a step further, so then it becomes one big vicious cycle in the end.
>
> *Denise*

Another system that appears to be impacted by exposure to trauma is the sensory system, with evidence to suggest alterations to sensory processing in the aftermath of trauma (Schaan et al., 2019). Interoception (the sensing of internal bodily sensations, states, and experiences) appears to be impacted by trauma, and cultivating interoceptive awareness can be considered an important element of trauma recovery (van der Kolk, 1994). There is growing evidence regarding the role of interoception in understanding self-injury (e.g., Forkmann et al., 2019; Young, Davies, Freegard, & Benton, 2021), and interoception may represent an example of alterations to biological systems that may impact on pathways between trauma and self-injury, and offer new avenues for therapeutic interventions.

Responses to NSSI in Forensic Settings

It is recognised that within institutional settings, especially forensic settings, NSSI and aggression can co-exist (Hawton et al., 2014). This phenomenon, sometimes referred to as *dual harm* (Slade, 2019) is understood as a linked behaviour, with emotional regulation proposed as a shared function (Shafti, Taylor, Forrester, & Pratt, 2021). Within forensic settings there is therefore often a tension between safely managing risk, both to self and others, and avoiding overly restrictive interventions.

The impact of the use of *restrictive interventions* with female patients in a high secure setting when they engage in NSSI is explored through patient narrative. Restrictive interventions refer to physical, mechanical, or chemical restraint, seclusion and restricting access to risk items. For a broader discussion on restrictive interventions in forensic settings see Völlm and Nedopil (2016).

The reasons why people engage in NSSI are very individual and varied (e.g., Edmondson et al., 2016), and their response to the interventions used to prevent and stop NSSI can also be complex and unique (see Soininen, Konito, Joffe, & Putkonen, 2016). When staff are faced with a person who is engaging in NSSI they can experience strong and painful feelings (Aiyegbusi & Kelly, 2015), and the challenge is to respond in a calm and containing way, which increases the opportunity for the individual to respond positively, to minimise or stop their self-injurious behaviour, and to have a shared opportunity to explore the meaning and function.

> It's helpful if they don't panic because you're already distressed, that's why you are self-harming.
>
> *Emily*

> not judge you for doing it, just think that 'well she must have done it for a reason, let's try and find out what that reason is and see if we can help with it' because that's just the best way.
>
> *Gina*

Unfortunately, for a small minority of patients their severe emotional distress, combined with high risk, makes it hard for them to feel safe enough to respond to verbal de-escalation, and in the light of escalating risk it can be necessary to consider restrictive interventions in order to manage and contain the situation (Elcock & Lewis, 2016). For patients, staff, and organisations the use of restrictive interventions are recognised as interventions of 'last resort' to prevent life-threatening self-injury and minimise harm (Hui, 2016), and this is acknowledged by patients:

> I think that it's not nice for the person that has to have it but I think that it is needed sometimes, because they might not see it at the time but ... I think they'll be like 'yeah realised how serious it was' and that it's what was best for them at the time.
>
> *Gina*

> because if they are not stopped or something then they will just keep going until they are actually stopped, and that's a safety thing for them 'cos they can do what they need to do and then be stopped.
>
> *Denise*

Although restrictive interventions preserve life, they can produce a complex array of emotional and psychological responses in the patient (Soininen et al., 2016). The clear shift of power and control away from the patient, towards the staff and the system, can mirror previous traumatic experiences. The realisation, that attempts to prevent patients from hurting themselves, can in themselves be (re)traumatising (Frueh et al., 2005), can be a difficult concept to rationalise. Patients also describe a real ambivalence towards interventions such as physical restraint:

> for some people it does help because it gives them that bit of comfort like ... if they are being held then they know they are not going to go further than what they intend to ... but for some people it can be a difficult one, because of their past history.
>
> *Denise*

The linked nature of NSSI and violence sometimes seen in forensic settings means that a NSSI incident can shift into a more interpersonally violent presentation, and the containment response can be seclusion, which also triggered mixed views:

> Seclusion helps me because it just gives me that space, with the person outside like if I need to talk ... to like calm myself down, away from the ward environment where it's a bit quiet.
>
> *Emily*

> it might make them more distressed because you are putting them in a room with nothing.
>
> *Gina*

One identified theme is of the importance of the relationship the patient has with the staff members involved, their knowledge of the patient's experiences, and what is the most effective way of keeping them safe. Another theme identified is the importance of matching the restrictive intervention to the risk, to avoid any blanket use of interventions, so when removing risk items:

> I think for some people it is not needed ... once they've done it [NSSI] they feel better and they don't need to do it again ... but if they are still distressed then they'll try and find anything to use and they will probably regret it the next day ... so I think just taking that away for just a while, until they feel better ... is right.
>
> *Gina*

> It depends on what method of self-harm you've done, like if you have like ligated ... obviously shutting the wardrobe off and removing all those items that you can do that again with, but like say if someone has cut themselves, emptying their room of like photos and teddies ... doesn't help because that's like what they need.
>
> *Emily*

Equally the recognition that mechanical restraint should be viewed as the absolute last resort and just for life threatening NSSI e.g., occlusion, or life altering NSSI e.g., blinding oneself (Elcock & Lewis, 2016) is represented in patient views:

> I get why they use that 'cos obviously it's to save a person's life if it's to the extent of where they're actually almost going to kill themselves, but if it's for minor self-harming I don't agree with it because you can try and talk to that person first.
>
> *Denise*

Overall, the patient's experience of restrictive interventions being used to manage NSSI is mixed. Unsurprisingly there is a clear preference for compassionate interventions that seek to talk to the patient, understand their feelings, and respond in a calm and non-judgemental way. When restrictive interventions are used there is general acceptance of the need for them to preserve life, but a clear request that interventions are individually tailored, based on a thorough knowledge of the patient's traumatic experiences, their risk history and preferences for risk management. Additionally, explanations as to why an intervention is being used, and the availability of familiar staff can create a sense of safety (Kontio et al., 2014). It is therefore recognised that the trend towards patient involvement throughout the process is a benchmark for good practice (Soininen et al., 2016). Including patients in an open and transparent way in the clinical discussions around the use of restrictive interventions in response to their presenting risk helps the process be more predictable which can: reduce staff injuries (Hill & Spreat, 1987); lead to the patients experiencing some interventions as less restrictive (Carr, 2012); and help form part of advance decisions about their care (Elcock & Lewis, 2016).

Trauma-Informed Treatment

not everyone's the same ... everyone should be treated as an individual, everyone should have different care plans on how to help each individual in that situation.

Emily

The effectiveness of specific interventions to address NSSI has been described elsewhere within the literature (e.g., Hetrick, Robinson, Spittal, & Carter, 2016; Hawton et al., 2016). Given the significant distress and challenges associated with NSSI (for the individual and the wider system), the multiple pathways from trauma to NSSI, and the multifaceted complex meanings ascribed to these acts, it is therefore essential that treatment responses are also multifaceted, individualised, and formulation-driven. We propose that the treatment of NSSI should be viewed through a trauma lens, and that a whole-system approach is necessary to effectively support people engaging in NSSI, whilst responding to the challenges posed in relation to NSSI within forensic settings. An example of a service which aims to provide a trauma-informed whole systems approach to the management of NSSI is the Trauma and Self-Injury (TASI) Service, within the National High Secure Healthcare Service for Women (NHSHSW).

The TASI Service was founded to respond to the co-occurring high rates of trauma and self-injury within the patient population of the NHSHSW. Since its creation in 2007, the service has continually evolved, with patient-involvement central to all elements of service development. The TASI Service influences, and is influenced by, the wider context in which it is situated. The NHSHSW has as a strong multidisciplinary ethos and the role of the TASI Service is in promoting a trauma-informed response to NSSI. A social ecological perspective helps illustrate the different components of TASI across each layer of the system. Figure 9.1 depicts the range of contributions of the TASI Service, illustrating the influence of each part of the system, which all interact in a reciprocal way.

At the centre of the system is the patient, and the interventions that involve working directly with the patient. These interventions can be viewed in the context of the phased approach to trauma recovery (e.g., Herman, 1992/2015), which involves a safety and stabilisation phase, a processing phase, and a reintegration phase. Following admission to the service, an initial priority is to build an understanding of the patient's trauma history and trauma symptom profile. Patients are supported to complete a document that we refer to as a *Distress Signature* to help the development of a shared understanding of their experience of distress, ways of coping, and their preferences for how to be supported when in crisis. Patients are also supported to develop their own *Sensory Signature* document, which considers their sensory preferences, different ways of using their senses to modulate sensory input and arousal, and to develop sensory diets. A key aim for both the *Distress Signature* and *Sensory Signature* is to include patients' voice and choice to inform care planning, and promote trauma-informed sensory-supportive responses to distress and NSSI.

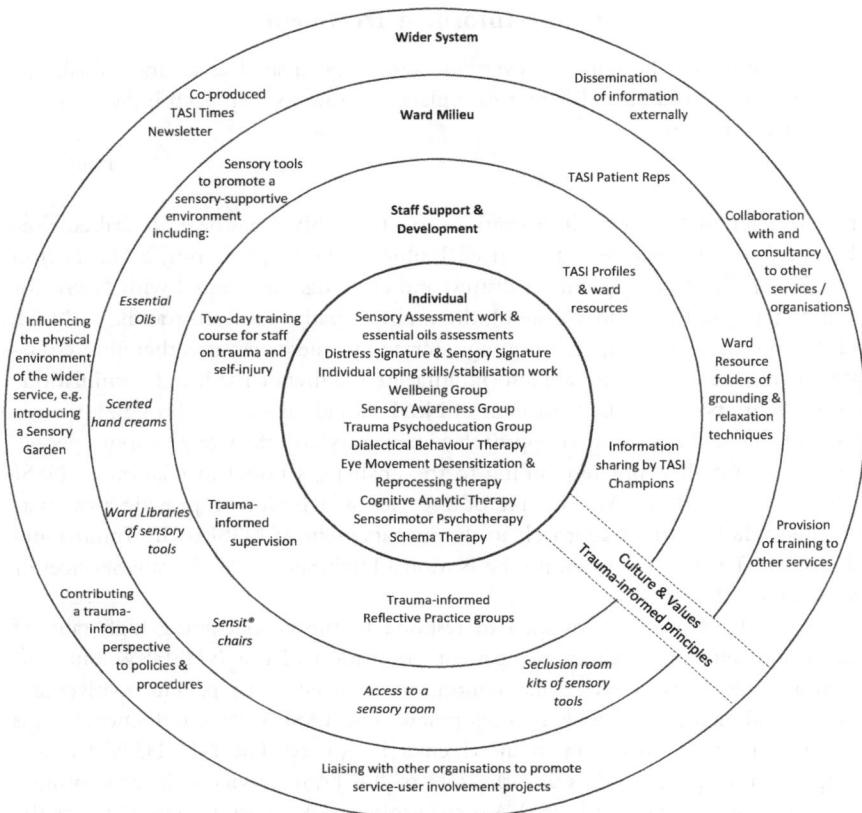

Figure 9.1   Elements of the TASI service

There are a range of therapeutic interventions within TASI that contribute heavily to the stabilisation phase of recovery, and to the pursuit of building emotional and bodily safety (Herman, 1992). These interventions are also focused on addressing the disconnect between cognition and affect, developing a greater understanding of, and language for, emotions, and learning skills to better regulate arousal/emotions and widen their window of tolerance. Three psychoeducational group interventions contribute to these aims: a Wellbeing Group, a Sensory Awareness Group, and a Trauma Psychoeducation Programme; additionally, Dialectical Behaviour Therapy also plays a key role in the provision of interventions to address NSSI. Whilst typically considered a key part of the *processing* phase of recovery, Eye Movement Desensitisation and Reprocessing (EMDR) can also be beneficial in the stabilisation phase, with the development of resources, and to specifically target NSSI (Annesley, Alabi, & Longdon, 2019).

The focus of psychoeducation, resource development, skills training and rehearsal within interventions contributes to addressing the difficulties highlighted within the regulatory and reactive pathways of Yates's model. The treatment needs associated with the representational pathway are typically addressed within the therapies that are offered as part of the *processing* and *reintegration* stages of recovery (see Figure 9.1). These trauma-focused interventions can also build on gains made in stabilisation therapies, to further develop the individual's understanding of their use of NSSI, target the underlying routes to these coping responses, and find new ways of managing distress and relating to others.

An essential component of trauma-informed care is the support and development of the staff team, which is necessary to enable the maintenance of compassionate care, and is highlighted as a priority in the long-term management of NSSI (National Institute for Health and Care Excellence, 2011). The staff support and development layer therefore focuses on interventions related to this, with a key part of this being the regular provision of trauma-informed supervision and reflective practice/case formulation sessions, as well as post-incident diffusion and debriefs; all of which are deemed essential to support staff with the emotional toll of engaging in this work (Beryl, Davies, & Völlm, 2016). A two-day training course on trauma and self-injury is central in efforts to increase knowledge about trauma and how it can affect people and groups; help staff to recognise the signs of trauma; explore power relations, ways of responding effectively, and resisting re-traumatisation. A key aim is to cultivate a compassionate understanding of NSSI and encourage therapeutic ways of responding to reduce harm, and the training has been found to increase staff confidence in working with trauma and self-injury and in asking for support (Robertson et al., 2013).

Supporting and encouraging trauma-informed principles within the ward milieu is another vital layer to foster an environment which can promote harm reduction. Central to this are the roles of the Ward TASI Champions and Ward TASI Patient Representatives. TASI Champions are members of the nursing team who contribute to the provision of TASI interventions and play a key role in promoting a trauma-informed perspective within the nursing team. The role of the TASI Patient Representative is to share information with, and from, the wider patient group, co-facilitate TASI groups and training, contribute to TASI Reference Group Meetings (where all TASI developments are initiated and reviewed), and to take part in the co-production of a quarterly *TASI Times* newsletters for the service. There is a strong emphasis on encouraging sensory approaches on the wards, with the aim of increasing sensory awareness and cultivating sensory-supportive environments. This includes promoting a range of sensory tools/equipment, as well as the use of essential oils, with assessments administered to identify a 'prescription' of oils to assist individuals with calming, activating, or grounding, as a means of helping navigate their window of tolerance.

The TASI Service also focuses on influencing the wider environment/system, for instance from co-producing projects to enhance the physical environment (such as the introduction of a sensory garden) to informing policies and procedures with the aim of promoting a trauma-informed perspective to service design and delivery. Running through each layer of the system, is the culture of the service, informed by its values and the principles of trauma-informed care: safety; trustworthiness and transparency; peer support; collaboration and mutuality; empowerment, voice, and choice; and cultural, historical, and gender issues (SAMHSA, 2014). The success of the TASI Service is in its multi-dimensional approach which keeps the patient at its centre, whilst recognising the need to influence all parts of the system in order to meet the needs of patients who engage in NSSI, and those staff who support them.

Conclusion

Unfortunately, there is no 'quick fix' to the challenges faced by forensic services when they try and support individuals who engage in NSSI. The complex, varied, and individualised reasons which lead to a person harming themselves makes it clear that no one treatment response is indicated. Traditional attempts by forensic services to 'manage and control' NSSI, often through restrictive interventions, can fail to address root causes, and may even negatively contribute to an individual's distress (both staff and patients). The TASI Service offers a way of approaching the challenge from a trauma-informed and multi-dimensional perspective, which involves encouraging an individualised understanding of distress and trauma, staff training to enhance skills and compassion, developing ward milieus which hold trauma in mind, and influencing the design of services and development of policy. The TASI Service is continually evolving, not least because of the central role of patient feedback and involvement. However, each incarnation holds the trauma-informed principles at its core, and strives to support each patient whilst they are on their therapeutic journey.

Note

1 Within this chapter, we use the term 'patient' to describe the women who reside in our service, as this is the terminology used within this setting.

Further Reading

Herman, J. (2015). *Trauma and recovery: The aftermath of violence from domestic abuse to political terror.* Basic Books.

Motz, A. (2009). *Managing self-harm: Psychological perspectives.* Routledge. This book offers a thought-provoking exploration self-harm, considering how it is understood, the wider context and systemic issues, as well as offering a focus on women and self-harm.

Nock, M. K. (Ed.) (2009). *Understanding nonsuicidal self-injury: Origins, assessment, and treatment.* American Psychological Association. This text provides a comprehensive overview of nonsuicidal self-injury, for readers who want to learn more about the origins, assessment, and treatment of NSSI.

References

Abrams, L. S., & Gordon, A. L. (2003). Self-harm narratives of urban and suburban young women. *Affilia, 18*(4), 429–444. doi:10.1177/0886109903257668

Aiyegbusi, A., & Kelly, D. (2015). 'This is the pain I feel!' Projection and emotional pain in the nurse–patient relationship with people diagnosed with personality disorders in forensic and specialist personality disorder services: Findings from a mixed methods study. *Psychoanalytic Psychotherapy, 29*(3), 276–294. doi:10.1080/02668734.2015.1025425

Annesley, P., Alabi, A., & Longdon, L. (2019). The EMDR DeTUR protocol for the treatment of self-injury in a patient with severe personality disorder: A case report. *Journal of Criminological Research, Policy and Practice, 5*(1), 27–38. doi:10.1108/JCRPP-11-2018-0034

Bennett, A. L., & Moss, M., 2013. Functions of deliberate self-injury of personality disordered prisoners: A small scale study. *Journal of Forensic Practice, 15*, 171–181. doi:10.1108/JFP-08-2012-0003

Beryl, R., Davies, J., & Völlm, B. (2016). Lived experience of working with female patients in a high-secure mental health setting. *International Journal of Mental Health Nursing, 27*(1), 82–91. doi:10.1111/inm.12297

Bhui, K., Stansfeld, S., Hull, S., Priebe, S., Mole, F. & Feder, G. (2003). Ethnic variations in pathways to and use of specialist mental health services in the UK. Systematic review. *British Journal of Psychiatry, 182*, 105–116. doi:10.1192/bjp.182.2.105

Boergers, J., Spirito, A., & Donaldson, D. (1998). Reasons for adolescent suicide attempts: Associations with psychological functioning. *Journal of the American Academy of Child & Adolescent Psychiatry, 37*(12), 1287–1293. doi:10.1097/00004583-199812000-00012

Carr, P. G. (2012). The use of mechanical restraint in mental health: A catalyst for change? *Journal of Psychiatric and Mental Health Nursing 19*, 657–664. doi:10.1111/j.1365-2850.2012.01912.x.

Chandler, A. (2014). *A sign that something is wrong: Young people talking about self-harm.* Centre for Research and Families and Relationships.

Cipriano, A., Cella, S., & Cotrufo, P. (2017). Non-suicidal self-injury: A systematic review. *Frontiers in Psychology, 8*, 1–14. doi:10.3389/fpsyg.2017.01946

Daffern, M., & Howells, K. (2009). Self-harm and aggression in dangerous and severely personality disordered patients of a high-security hospital. *Psychiatry, Psychology and Law, 16*(1), 150–154. doi:10.1080/13218710802471156De

De Genna, N. M., & Feske, U. (2013). Phenomenology of borderline personality disorder: The role of race and socioeconomic status. *Journal of Nervous and Mental Disease, 201*(12), 1027–1034. doi:10.1097/NMD.0000000000000053

DeHart, D. D., Smith, H. P., & Kaminski, R. J. (2009). Institutional responses to self-injurious behavior among inmates. *Journal of Correctional Health Care, 15*, 129–141. doi:10.1177/1078345809331444

Demming, V. A. (2008). *Women's reflections on their adolescent self-injury in relation to grief and loss* (Unpublished doctoral dissertation). Saybrook University.

Edmondson, A. J., Brennan, C. A., & House, A. O. (2016). Non-suicidal reasons for self-harm: A systematic review of self-reported accounts. *Journal of Affective Disorders, 191*, 109–117. doi:10.1016/j.jad.2015.11.043

Elcock, S., & Lewis, J. (2016). Mechanical restraint: Legal, ethical and clinical issues. In B. Völlm & N. Nedopil (Eds), *The use of coercive measures in forensic psychiatric care* (pp.315–331). Springer.

Favril, L., Yu, R., Hawton, K., & Fazel, S. (2020). Risk factors for self-harm in prison: A systematic review and meta-analysis. *Lancet Psychiatry, 7*, 682–691. doi:10.1016/S2215-0366(20)30190-5

Ford, J. D., & Gómez, J. M. (2015). The relationship of psychological trauma and dissociative and posttraumatic stress disorders to nonsuicidal self-injury and suicidality: A review. *Journal of Trauma and Dissociation, 16*(3), 232–271. doi:10.1080/15299732.2015.989563

Forkmann, T., Volz-Sidiropoulou, E., Helbing, T., Drüke, B., Mainz, V., Rath, D., ... & Teismann, T. (2019). Sense it and use it: Interoceptive accuracy and sensibility in suicide ideators. *BMC Psychiatry, 19*(1), 1–9. doi:10.1186/s12888-019-2322-1

Frueh, B. C., Knapp, R. G., Cusack, K. J., Grubaugh, A. L., Sauvageot, J. A., Cousins, V. C., ... & Hiers, T. G. (2005). Patients' reports of traumatic or harmful experiences within the psychiatric setting. *Psychiatric Services, 56*(9), 1123–1133. doi:10.1176/appi.ps.56.9.1123

Gallagher, J., & Sheldon, K. (2010). Assessing the functions of self-harm behaviours for dangerous and severely personality disordered males in a high secure hospital. *British Journal of Forensic Practice, 12*(1), 22–32. doi:10.5042/bjfp.2010.0035

Glassman, L. H., Weierich, M. R., Hooley, J. M., Deliberto, T. L., & Nock, M. K. (2007). Child maltreatment, non-suicidal self-injury, and the mediating role of self-criticism. *Behaviour Research and Therapy, 45*(10), 2483–2490. doi:10.1016/j.brat.2007.04.002

Gratz, K. L. (2003). Risk factors for and functions of deliberate self-harm: An empirical and conceptual review. *Clinical Psychology: Science and Practice, 10*(2), 192–205. doi:10.1093/clipsy/bpg022

Grocutt, E. (2009). 'Self-harm cessation in secure settings'. In A. Motz (Ed.), *Managing self-harm: Psychological perspectives* (pp.180–203). Routledge. doi:10.1093/clipsy.bpg022 | |

Gunter, T. D., Chibnall, J. T., Antoniak, S. K., Philibert, R. A., & Hollenbeck, N. (2011). Predictors of suicidal ideation, suicide attempts, and self-harm without lethal intent in a community corrections sample. *Journal of Criminal Justice, 39*(3), 238–245. doi:10.1016/j.jcrimjus.2011.02.005

Harris, J. (2000). Self-harm: Cutting the bad out of me. *Qualitative Health Research, 10*(2), 164–173. doi:10.1177/104973200129118345

Hawton, K., Linsell, L., Adeniji, T., Sariaslan, A., & Fazel, S. (2014). Self-harm in prisons in England and Wales: An epidemiological study of prevalence, risk factors, clustering and subsequent suicide. *Lancet, 383,* 1147–1154. doi:10.1016/S0140-6736(13)62118-2

Hawton, K., Witt, K. G., Salisbury, T. L. T., Arensman, E., Gunnell, D., Hazell, P., Townsend, E., & van Heeringen, K. (2016). Psychosocial interventions following self-harm in adults: A systematic review and meta-analysis. *The Lancet Psychiatry, 3*(8), 740–750. doi:10.1016/S2215-0366(16)30070-0

Hill, J., & Spreat, S. (1987). Staff injury rates associated with the implementation of contingent restraint. *Mental Retardation, 25*(3), 141–145.

Hetrick, S. E., Robinson, J., Spittal, M., & Carter, G. (2016). Effective psychological and psychosocial approaches to reduce repetition of deliberate self-harm: A systematic review and meta-regression. *BMJ Open, 6*(9), e011024. doi:10.1136/bmjopen-2016-011024

Herman, J. L. (1992). *Trauma and recovery.* Basic Books.

Himber, J. (1994). Blood rituals: Self-cutting in female psychiatric inpatients. *Psychotherapy, 31,* 620–631. doi:10.1037/0033-3204.31.4.620

Horne, O., & Csipke, E. (2009). From feeling too little and too much, to feeling more and less? A nonparadoxical theory of the functions of self-harm. *Qualitative Health Research, 19*(5), 655–667. doi:10.1177/1049732309334249

House, A. S., van Horn, E., Coppeans, C., & Stepleman, L. M. (2011). Interpersonal trauma and discriminatory events as predictors of suicidal and nonsuicidal self-injury in gay, lesbian, bisexual, and transgender persons. *Traumatology, 17*(2), 75–85. doi:10.1177/1534765610395621

Hui, A. (2016). Mental health workers' experiences of using coercive measures: "You can't tell people who don't understand". In B. Völlm & N. Nedopil (Eds), *The use of coercive measures in forensic psychiatric care* (pp.241–254). Springer.

Klonsky, E. D. (2007). The functions of deliberate self-injury: A review of the evidence. *Clinical Psychology Review, 27*(2), 226–239. doi:10.1016/j.cpr.2006.08.002

Klonsky, E. D., & Glenn, C. R. (2009). Assessing the functions of non-suicidal self-injury: Psychometric properties of the inventory of statements about self-injury (ISAS). *Journal of Psychopathology and Behavioral Assessment, 31*(3), 215–219. doi:10.1007/s10862-008-9107-z

Klonsky, E. D., & Muehlenkamp, J. J. (2007). Self-injury: A research review for the practitioner. *Journal of Clinical Psychology, 63*(11), 1045–1056. doi:10.1002/jclp.20412

Klonsky, E. D., Oltmanns, T. F., & Turkheimer, E. (2003). Deliberate self-harm in a nonclinical population: Prevalence and psychological correlates. *American Journal of Psychiatry, 160*(8), 1501–1508. doi:10.1176/appi.ajp.160.8.1501

Kontio, R., Antilla, M., Lantta, T., Kauppi, K., Joffe, G. & Valimaki, M. (2014). Towards a safer working environment on psychiatric wards: Service users' delayed perspectives of aggression and violence-related situations and development ideas. *Perspectives in Psychiatric Care, 50*(4), 271–279. doi:10.1111/ppc.12054 |

Lang, C. M., & Sharma-Patel, K. (2011). The relation between childhood maltreatment and self-injury: A review of the literature on conceptualization and intervention. *Trauma, Violence, & Abuse, 12*(1), 23–37. doi:10.1177/1524838010386975

Liu, R. T., Scopelliti, K. M., Pittman, S. K., & Zamora, A. S. (2018). Childhood maltreatment and non-suicidal self-injury: A systematic review and meta-analysis. *The Lancet Psychiatry, 5*(1), 51–64. doi:10.1016/S2215-0366(17)30469-8

Longdon, L., Beryl, R., & Siddall, Y. (2020). *An overview of trauma and trauma symptoms in the National High Secure Healthcare Service for Women*. Poster presented at Trauma in Forensic Settings Conference, 30–31 January. Nottinghamshire Healthcare, Nottingham.

Maniglio, R. (2011). The role of child sexual abuse in the etiology of suicide and non-suicidal self-injury. *Acta Psychiatrica Scandinavica, 124*(1), 30–41. doi:10.1111/j.1600-0447.2010.01612.x.

Messner, J. M., & Fremouw, W. J. (2008). A critical review of explanatory models for self-mutilating behaviors in adolescents. *Clinical Psychology Review, 28*, 162–178. doi:10.1016/j.cpr.2007.04.006

Ministry of Justice. (2021). *Safety in custody statistics, England and Wales: Deaths in prison custody to December 2020 assaults and self-harm to September 2020*. Ministry of Justice.

Motz, A. (2009). *Managing self-harm: Psychological perspectives*. Routledge.

National Institute for Health and Care Excellence. (2011). Self-harm in over 18s: long-term management (NICE Clinical Guideline CG133). Retrieved from www.nice.org.uk/guidance/cg133

Nock, M. K., & Cha, C. B. (2009). Psychological models of nonsuicidal self-injury. In M. K. Nock (Ed.), *Understanding nonsuicidal self-injury: Origins, assessment, and treatment* (pp. 65–77). American Psychological Association.

Ogden, P., Pain, C., & Fisher, J. (2006). A sensorimotor approach to the treatment of trauma and dissociation. *Psychiatric Clinics of North America, 29*(1), 263–279. doi:10.1016/j.psc.2005.10.012

Paivio, S. C., & McCulloch, C. R. (2004). Alexithymia as a mediator between childhood trauma and self-injurious behavior. *Child Abuse & Neglect, 28*(3), 339–354. doi:10.1016/j.chiabu.2003.11.018

Parfitt, A. (2005). On aggression turned against the self. *Psychoanalytic Psychotherapy, 19*, 160–173. doi:10.1080/02668730500115127

Robertson, K., Elcock, S., Milburn, C., Annesley, P., Jones, J., & Völlm, B. A. (2013). An evaluation of the staff training within the trauma and self-injury (TASI) programme in the National High Secure Healthcare Service for Women (NHSHSW). *Journal of Forensic Practice, 15*(2), 141–150. doi:10.1108/14636641311322322

SAMHSA. (2014). *SAMHSA's concept of trauma and guidance for a trauma-informed approach SAMHSA's trauma and justice strategic initiative*. Retrieved from http://store.samhsa.gov/product/SAMHSA-s-Concept-of-Trauma-and-Guidance-for-a-Trauma-Informed-Approach/SMA14-4884

Schaan, V. K., Schulz, A., Rubel, J. A., Bernstein, M., Domes, G., Schächinger, H., & Vögele, C. (2019). Childhood trauma affects stress-related interoceptive accuracy. *Frontiers in Psychiatry, 10*(October), 1–10. doi:10.3389/fpsyt.2019.00750

Serafini, G., Canepa, G., Adavastro, G., Nebbia, J., Murri, M. B., Erbuto, D., … & Amore, M. (2017). The relationship between childhood maltreatment and non-suicidal self-injury: A systematic review. *Frontiers in Psychiatry, 8*(August), 149. doi:10.3389/fpsyt.2017.00149

Shafti, M., Taylor, P. J., Forrester, A., & Pratt, D. (2021). The co-occurrence of self-harm and aggression: A cognitive-emotional model of dual-harm. *Frontiers in Psychology, 12*:586135. doi:10.3389/fpsyg.2021.586135

Siegel, D. J. (1999). *The developing mind*. Guilford.

Slade, K. (2019). Dual harm: The importance of recognising the duality of self-harm and violence in forensic populations. *Medicine, Science and the Law, 59*, 75–77. doi:10.1177%2F0025802419845161

Soininen, P., Konito, R., Joffe, G., & Putkonen, H. (2016). Patient experience of coercive measures. In B.Völlm & N. Nedopil (Eds), *The use of coercive measures in forensic psychiatric care* (pp.255–270). Springer.

Swannell, S., Martin, G., Page,A., Hasking, P., Hazell, P.,Taylor,A., & Protani, M. (2012). Child maltreatment, subsequent non-suicidal self-injury and the mediating roles of dissociation, alexithymia and self-blame. *Child Abuse and Neglect, 36*(7–8), 572–584. doi:10.1016/j.chiabu.2012.05.005

Swannell, S., Martin, G., Scott, J., Gibbons, M., & Gifford, S. (2008). Motivations for self-injury in an adolescent inpatient population: Development of a self-report measure. *Australasian Psychiatry, 16*, 98–103. doi:10.1080/10398560701636955

Uppal, G., & McMurran, M. (2009). Recorded incidents in a high-secure hospital:A descriptive analysis. *Criminal Behaviour and Mental Health, 19*, 265–276. doi:10.1002/cbm

van der Kolk, B. A. (1994). The body keeps the score: Memory and the evolving psycho-biology of posttraumatic stress. *Harvard Review of Psychiatry, 1*(5), 253–265. doi:10.3109/10673229409017088

van der Kolk, B. A., Perry, J. C., & Herman, J. L. (1991). Childhood origins of self-destructive behavior. *American Journal of Psychiatry, 148*(12), 1665–1671. doi:10.1176/ajp.148.12.1665

Völlm, B., & Nedopil, N. (Eds). (2016). *The use of coercive measures in forensic psychiatric care.* Springer.

Williams, M. T., Haeny,A. M., & Holmes, S. C. (2021). Posttraumatic stress disorder and racial trauma. *PTSD Research Quarterly, 32*(1), 1–3.

Yates, T. M. (2009). Developmental pathways from child maltreatment to non-suicidal self-injury. In M. Nock (Ed.), *Understanding non-suicidal self injury: Current science and practice* (pp.117–137).America Psychological Association.

Young, H. A., Davies, J., Freegard, G., & Benton, D. (2021). Nonsuicidal self-injury is associated with attenuated interoceptive responses to self-critical rumination. *Behavior Therapy, 52* (5), 1123–1136. doi:10.1016/j.beth.2021.02.010

Young, R.,Van Beinum, M., Sweeting, H., & West, P. (2007).Young people who self- harm. *British Journal of Psychiatry, 191*(1), 44–49. doi:10.1192/bjp.bp.106.034330

10

TRAUMA, SUBSTANCE USE, AND OFFENDING

John Farnsworth

A significant number of offenders who have survived childhood trauma go on to misuse drugs or alcohol. Relief from the psychological impact of these experiences is often sought through "self-medication" by legal or illicit means. Drugs are widely available in a number of forensic institutions and continue the cycle of offending as individuals seek substances to cope with re-traumatising experiences. This chapter will consider the routes to misuse and/or addiction, the consequences to social and psychological functioning, and the connections to crime, whether as a perpetrator or victim. It will look at treatment considerations when dealing with offenders who are survivors of trauma and who use substances.

Trauma, Substance Use, and Offending

The two most prevalent Axis 1 disorders in the prison population are substance use disorders and post-traumatic stress disorder (PTSD) (Butler et al., 2006; Butler & Kariminia, 2005; Sindicich et al., 2014). Substance use–related symptoms such as aggression, impulsivity, and reduced inhibitions, combined with PTSD symptoms including hypervigilance, anger, and irritability, may increase the likelihood that individuals will go on to perpetrate violence. These symptoms make individuals in prisons and hospitals difficult to manage and lead to poor staff morale. This translates into a group of individuals who are considered to be one of the most challenging groups in the criminal justice system (Chandler, Peters, Field, & Juliano-Bult, 2004).

It has been estimated that around one in ten children is neglected, or psychologically abused annually and that that between 4% and 16% are physically abused (Gilbert et al., 2009). Straus (1992) estimated that approximately ten million adolescents in the US are exposed to violence each year. Furthermore, reports of abuse and neglect are probably subject to underreporting because of embarrassment, shame, denial, or lack of insight (Widom, Ireland, & Glynn, 1995). One of the most widely cited

DOI: 10.4324/9781003120766-14

factors associated with juvenile delinquency is the use of illicit substances (Hawkins, Catalano, & Miller, 1992; Williams, Ayres, Abbott, Hawkins, & Catalano, 1999). The Adverse Childhood Experiences (ACEs) study concluded that the number of retrospectively reported ACEs experienced before the age of 18 was highly associated with addictive behaviours later in life (Felitti, et al., 1998). The prevalence of mental health conditions is also higher amongst substance using juvenile offenders (Montgomery, Vaughn, Thompson, & Howard, 2012). Substance use and mental health issues have been estimated to be roughly two to four times greater among those with histories of childhood trauma (Cusack, Herring, & Steadman, 2013).

Sommer et al. (2017) concluded that substance use prior to violence has been shown to make perpetrators feel more powerful, more aggressive, and less fearful in those who find aggression intrinsically rewarding (appetitive aggression). PTSD symptoms such as hyperarousal, hostility, and anger can be a behavioural precursor to aggression (Sommer et al.). When under the influence, substance use usually calms nerves and decreases inhibition, but this may also serve to increase the chances of becoming a victim of violence and thus increase the likelihood of being exposed to more traumatic experiences (Goldstein, Brownstein, Ryan, & Bellucci, 1989). Gang affiliation is often sought for protection from violence in disaffected youth. Gang affiliation is associated with drug abuse and violence which is reinforced by association with criminal peers and the desire to maintain status in the gang (Brunelle, Brochu, & Cousineau, 2000).

Exposure to violence significantly predicts substance use (Khoury, Tang, Bradley, Cubells, & Ressler, 2010), and exposure to traumatic events or dysfunctional childhood experiences are associated with a higher likelihood of depression, PTSD, substance use disorder, particularly intravenous drug use (Messina & Grella, 2006) and more sexual risk-taking behaviours (Davis, Combs-Lane, & Jackson, 2002). Poor social support and a high degree of family problems are related to higher levels of alcohol and marijuana use amongst teenagers (Rhodes & Jason, 1990). The converse was associated with less substance use among adolescents (Averna & Hesselbrock, 2001). Therefore, a positive supporting family network is a protective factor against adolescent substance misuse (Robertson, Xiaohe, & Stripling, 2010). Substance use can result in behavioural reactions such as impulsivity, reduced inhibitions, and aggression. These, coupled with PTSD symptoms such as hypervigilance, irritability, and anger, may serve to increase an individual's risk of violence (Barrett, Mills, & Teesson, 2011). Once comorbid substance use and PTSD have been established, they both act to maintain or exacerbate the other and this leads to significant harm (Sindicich et al., 2014).

Mechanisms that underlie the co-occurrence of substance use disorder and trauma are not yet fully understood. Biopsychosocial explanations have been suggested as including self-medication, heritability, social influence, and vulnerability factors such as poverty and a family history of mental illness. There is a substantial body of evidence that documents that PTSD occurs prior to the onset of substance use disorders, the suggestion being that substance use may be used to relieve the symptoms of PTSD. Green et al. (2016) studied the cumulative effective of multiple trauma types. They found a dose–response relationship between cumulative trauma exposure and the severity of mental disorders, including PTSD. Experiences of rape were associated with very high rates of PTSD in both men and women, whereas accidents and disasters were associated with a much lower rate. Ongoing sexual and/or physical abuse contributed significantly to lifetime PTSD, major depressive disorder, and substance abuse, compared with no trauma, traumatic bereavement, and single episode physical assault, suggesting the potency of repeated exposure to interpersonal violence. Briere, Kaltman, and Green (2008) found a linear relationship between a number of trauma types experienced by their participants before age 18 and trauma-related symptom complexity, suggesting a generalised effect of cumulative trauma.

The boundary between being a victim or a perpetrator is often blurred because of exposure to violence, trauma, and substance use (Sommer et al., 2017) and a reciprocal relationship also exists with being a victim and a perpetrator of violence. Howard, Karatzias, Power, and Mahony (2017) suggest the direction of causality in female offenders as the use of violence leading to PTSD and drug use. Those who are perpetrators of criminal acts are rarely thought of as being traumatised themselves (Butler & Kariminia, 2005), so PTSD often goes unrecognised. This is despite a substantial body of literature which documents the co-occurrence of past victimisation and psychological trauma amongst both male and female inmates (Gibson et al., 1999). Prisons can be toxic environments with a culture of violence. Therefore, individuals within prisons are often under threat of further re-traumatisation (Lovell, Johnson, Jemelka, Harris, & Allen, 2001). Up to 90% of prisoners of both sexes are exposed to traumatic events whilst incarcerated, with many having experienced multiple traumas (Indig et al., 2010). Does the system that includes intrusive searches, seclusions, limited privacy, and sanctions for misdemeanours constitute triggering re-traumatising events that lead to resurgence of PTSD symptoms and therefore substance misuse?

Substance Use and Trauma in Female Offenders

Incarcerated women often have extensive trauma histories. Cook, Smith, Tusher, and Raiford (2005) found that 81% had experienced five or more traumatic events in their lifetime. The rates of trauma amongst female prisoners have been reported at 94% for any trauma and 31% and 26% for childhood sexual and non-sexual abuse, respectively (Howard et al., 2017). Women are more likely to be diagnosed with PTSD and to use drugs more heavily than men prior to entering prison and have a higher rate of drug relapse (Kubiak, 2004). The prevalence of PTSD among female prisoners was found by Palmer, Jinks, and Hatcher (2010) to be 40%, compared with 12% of male prisoner. Drug abuse prevalence rates of 30–60% were reported among female prisoners and there were also indications that female prisoners report greater use of the most harmful and addictive drugs such as heroin, cocaine, ecstasy, and LSD than males (Komarovskaya, Booker-Loper, Warren, & Jackson, 2011).

The differences between female and male prisoners with substance use disorders and comorbid PTSD were predominantly in the types of trauma they experienced.

Female samples reported higher rates of sexual assault, which predominantly occurred in childhood (Salgado, Quinlan, & Zlotnick, 2007; Wolff & Shi, 2012), whereas male prisoners reported higher rates of physical assault which occurred in early adulthood. However, it was noteworthy that the prevalence of sexual assault amongst the sample of male prisoners was 47% (Sindicich et al., 2014). Fehrman (2019) reported that traumatic experience and subsequent PTSD are highly prevalent amongst female prisoners and that her findings support the view that this is related to their use of drugs. She stressed the importance of assessing differing needs for men and women who misuse substances, to ensure gender responsive treatment that is trauma informed.

Substance Use and Trauma in Black and Ethnic Minorities

In general, levels of substance use are lower in minority ethnic groups than among the white population. This is despite people of colour in the UK being disproportionately subject to "stop and search" (Beddoes, Sheikh, Khanna, & Francis, 2010). In the UK, the highest rates of substance use are by individuals from mixed ethnic backgrounds and the lowest levels from those from Asian backgrounds (Indian, Pakistani, or Bangladeshi). However, it is thought that substance use amongst minority ethnic communities is underreported due to the high levels of stigma associated with it in those communities. Furthermore, these communities may be at increased risk of drug use because they often live in disadvantaged and deprived areas where drug markets thrive (Beddoes et al.).

The Centre for Ethnicity and Health (2004) studied problematic drug use among asylum seekers and refugees. They reported that these groups experience considerable loneliness and isolation as they are often separated from their families and are living in a culture that is unfamiliar to them. Isolation and frustration also resulted from difficulties in accessing housing, health, and education. Ross Dawson (2003) reported that when accommodation was found it was often in areas where drug taking and dealing is problematic. Thus, substance misuse was not a problem generated by asylum seekers and refugees, rather it was one they had to face.

McCormack and Walker (2005) argue that the use of substances by asylum seekers and refugees is underreported, not only because not all institutions record refugee status, but also because most refugee and asylum seekers tend to hide any involvement in drugs for fear this may impact their status in the UK.

Personal Narratives

Over the course of a number of years I have spent documenting patients' narratives surrounding their substance use, there are a number of reoccurring themes associated with addiction. The most prominent one has been the experience of trauma. Patients speak of their use of drugs and alcohol as representing their failure to cope with life in general and their wish to escape from the realities associated with the painful memories that they have internalised with a sense of culpability. The shame they continue to experience is internalised as a sense of being fundamentally flawed.

Jay

Jay was one patient who told me of his traumatic experiences. He did so seemingly without an emotional connection to them. Jay told me he had learned to keep his emotions in check because he was scared if he began to "feel" he might not be able to control the outcome and that was a scary prospect. Jay told me that in his early years he had watched his father smoke cannabis and misuse prescription drugs to help with his own poor mental health. Jay was harshly punished on a regular basis when he misbehaved at school by getting into fights with others in his class. That was, he said, if he bothered to go to school at all. He told me that in retrospect, this behaviour started after he was sexually abused by one of his cousins. He said that he had told his mother about this. She dismissed what he had said as lies and an attempt to excuse his bad behaviour. He told me she was the only one who could stop what was happening, but she chose to ignore it. Jay said that this was the most difficult thing to cope with. He said he could "switch off" the pain of the abuse but could not come to terms with the feeling of not being believed and, worse still, not feeling protected. Jay tried to cope by using alcohol in the park with his friends, but he told me he would get aggressive when he drank, and his friends started to shun him as he directed his anger at them.

"Speed" (amphetamine) was a revelation to Jay the first time he took it. It made him feel invigorated, energetic, and superior to others. It gave him back the feeling that he was in control and that he was able to protect himself again. However, Jay's use of speed made him increasingly hypervigilant and paranoid. He said that although he did not recognise it at the time, his mental health was declining rapidly. He felt persecuted by everyone he encountered. He told me that his own sexual offence was committed because no one could be trusted and he wanted to humiliate someone else so they knew what it was like to feel the way he did.

Jay did not feel safe in prison, but he coped by using aggression as he had done in the community. In prison he found a drug that made him feel the same way as he did when he used speed, but it was better, a more intense feeling. Crack cocaine made him feel powerful against the harassment of others who persecuted him because of the nature of his offence. Jay fought back, but when restrained by prison officers it brought back the same feelings as those he had at the time of his own sexual abuse. He described these feelings to me as like a nightmare when he was awake. Crack was his medication; it numbed the painful emotions associated with the trauma such as guilt, shame, worthlessness, and anger at allowing himself to be a victim. Crack increased his sense of self-worth.

Ricky

Ricky grew up in a chaotic environment. He told me that he and his six siblings had to fend for themselves as their mother took prescribed benzodiazepines to escape from her own mental health problems and was "out of it" for most of the day. He told me that his stepfather was an alcoholic and violence was the norm at home. Other children at school would bully him because of the way he dressed in dirty clothing, and the fights he got into as a consequence of this resulted in multiple exclusions from school. Ricky struggled with his emotions. Rejection was particularly hard to manage. He could not deal with the emotional pain, but it hurt less if he turned some of it into physical pain. Ricky began cutting his forearms, which made him feel better for a fleeting moment but ended in feelings of shame. The trauma of previous neglect and violence was also relieved when he would sniff glue and butane in the park with some of the other children.

Ricky's safe base was at his grandmother's house where he would spend the weekends. When she died suddenly at the age of 55, he said that he felt alone as she was the only person who cared for him. He had been stealing his mother's benzodiazepine medication for some time. He took an overdose that almost killed him. Ricky told me how his mother was more upset that he had stolen her tablets than she was about the fact that he had almost died.

Ricky was moved into a children's home after that episode and had fond memories of being taken ice skating by the staff. He told me that he would go and visit his mother, who was now in psychiatric care and take her to McDonalds for lunch. He told me that he thought that they could live together, but the rejection continued, so this time he coped by drinking. He said that he was trying to prove that he could hurt himself more than anyone else could hurt him.

Ricky's life was chaotic – sofa surfing, drinking, and taking any substance he could get hold of. When he was ejected from a friend's house and faced the prospect of living on the streets, he set fire to the bins in the rubbish well of the block of flats he had been thrown out of.

Joe

Joe was considered a troubled child with disturbed behaviour that his foster family found difficult to cope with. They would lock him in a cupboard under the stairs in an attempt to address his unruly behaviour. He told me that it was frightening being in the dark, but he had experienced worse. Joe had been taken into care after he witnessed his mother being beaten by his alcoholic stepfather. He told me he was relieved at being taken away from the family home as he had suffered sexual abuse at the hands of his stepfather from the age of six. He told me he could not tell anyone about the abuse for fear of retribution, but he learned to live with the abuse by "taking my mind away to somewhere else" when it was taking place.

Joe's relationship with substances started when he began sniffing glue with a gang of older local "skinheads". Joe said that he felt a sense of belonging in their company, but they would "dare" him to drink the alcohol they gave him until he either passed out or was sick. By the age of 17 he said he would use anything he could get hold of to give himself "time away from bad thoughts". He told me he now knows he was self-medicating for the flashbacks to the abuse he had suffered as a child. Joe was a frequent patient in psychiatric units and said that when he was sectioned, he would constantly seek medication from the psychiatrist. Similarly, when he was on the streets, he said he would seek out his next "anaesthetic" from less legitimate drug suppliers.

Joe's substance use made him a victim of further trauma and abuse. He described a life where he was constantly trying to fit into a world where he felt isolated and alienated. He said that when he took cocaine or speed, he felt more confident. His said that his sexual promiscuity was also an attempt to manage his feelings of poor self-worth. Feelings of paranoia were dealt with by taking cocaine to make him more alert, and cannabis was smoked regularly to help him relax. His use of heroin gave him respite from the flashbacks of his sexual abuse, but anything else would do if he was offered it. Joe told me his substance use was his personality and that without it the traumatic memories would defeat him, so he would self-destruct with chemicals.

Joe had numerous convictions when I met him. He said that most were associated in some way with his substance use. He said that now he was "clean", he realised that the last 20 years of his life had been taken up by either being high on any substance he could get hold of, by trying to get hold of the means to get the drugs, or withdrawing from them. Even when Joe had managed to get hold of drugs or alcohol, he would be thinking about how he would get more when it ran out. He told me that, when sober, his mind would be constantly occupied with violent thoughts. He repeatedly told himself that he was to blame for the abuse he had suffered and that he could have stopped the violence his mother had endured.

Trauma, Substance Use, and Offending from a Treatment Perspective: What Might Work?

As we have seen, trauma and substance use frequently co-occur. This comorbidity makes both conditions harder to treat (Zlotnick et al., 2003) and patients with this clinical profile have poorer functioning, well-being, and treatment outcomes (Roberts, Roberts, Jones, & Bisson, 2016). Within the *risk needs responsivity model* (Bonta & Andrews, 2016), trauma may be considered as a responsivity factor that moderates the effectiveness of interventions that target the major risk factors for violence. A history of trauma has been linked to drop out from drug treatment programmes (Resko & Mendoza, 2012). Because patients with comorbid PTSD and substance use disorders are often excluded from clinical trials of psychological interventions, it can be difficult for clinicians to decide what treatment is best. Often this results in PTSD and substance use disorders being treated in a sequential fashion, leaving doubt as to whether this is the most effective approach, or whether an integrated treatment approach would be more effective (Roberts et al., 2016).

Pharmacological treatments can be used to block the effects of opioids, reduce cravings, or induce aversive sensations following consumption of, for example, alcohol. They have demonstrated mixed results (McHugh, Hearon, & Otto, 2010) and their use is usually accompanied by unwanted side effects.

The most common model of correctional addiction programme is Cognitive-Behavioural Treatment (CBT: Lipsey, Landenberger, & Wilson, 2007). CBT encourages patients to rethink their attitudes and modify their behaviours to remain abstinent. CBT relies heavily on self-control (Anthes, 2014). It teaches coping skills to deal with cravings and stress and teaches relapse prevention strategies. CBT incorporates homework tasks for patients to complete between sessions. However, trauma may interfere with participation in cognitive behavioural therapy (Miller & Najavits, 2012).

Eye movement desensitisation and reprocessing (EMDR: Shapiro, 2001) is often used to treat PTSD (Cusack et al., 2016) and has also been adapted to treat addiction (Markus & Hornsveld, 2017). The adaptive information processing model (AIP: Shapiro), theorises that dysfunctionally stored memories are accompanied with high levels of emotional arousal, which can be either positive or negative. In the case of substance use, these memories are thought to be weakened and modified using eye movements. Positive memories become less vivid and subsequently, less positive (Engelhard, van Uijen, & van den Hout, 2010; Hornsveld et al., 2011). EMDR does not rely as heavily on patients' self-control, as such it is thought it is better tolerated and accepted, with fewer retention and relapse problems than other therapies (Markus & Hornsveld, 2017). Roberts et al. (2016) reviewed the effectiveness of these combined treatments and concluded that trauma-focused therapy alongside substance use treatment had some effect, whereas stand-alone, non-trauma focused therapies had little or no effect.

Two treatment modalities that target the co-morbidity of substance use and personality disorder (the origins of which are understood to lie within early traumatic experience, see Chapter 4) are Dialectic Behaviour Therapy-Substance Abuse (DBT-S: Linehan, Schmidt, & Dimeff, 1999) and Dual Focus Schema Therapy (DFST: Ball, 1998). DBT-S was developed for patients with a diagnosis of borderline personality disorder and a history of substance abuse. Evidence suggests that this dual focus shows both decreased attrition rates and a reduction on substance use. DFST consists of a more individualised, formulation-based approach, built on a comprehensive assessment and conceptualisation of early maladaptive schemas and consequent maladaptive coping styles. The treatment consists of a cognitive-behavioural approach combined with experiential strategies (imagery and chair work) and has shown some promising findings in dissimilar populations of personality disordered and substance abusing individuals (Ball, 2007; Ball, Cobb-Richardson, Connolly, Bujosa, & O'Neil, 2005). However, in a review of all current dual focused treatments (including DFST) it was concluded that whilst it was more effective that regular mono-focused treatments, more valid and reliable research was needed before robust conclusions could be drawn (Shorey, Stuart, Anderson, & Strong, 2013).

Poor resilience has been associated with involvement in the development of PTSD (Fincham, Altes, Stein, & Seedat, 2009). Resilience has been defined as a dynamic or active factor that involves an interaction between risk and protective processes that reduces the effects of an adverse life event. It involves both internal and external factors that enable the individual to recover from crisis. Resilience has been found to moderate the relationship between risk factors and PTSD. Resilience is highlighted in *Seeking Safety* (Najavits, 2002), a treatment programme that focuses on both traumatic experiences and substance abuse. Navajits reported that those undergoing the programme showed more positive results on measures of substance abuse and PTSD than participants receiving treatment as usual. Lynch, Heath, Mathews, and Cepeda (2012) and Wolff, Frueh, Shi, and Schumann (2012) also demonstrated the feasibility and the effectiveness of a seeking safety intervention for PTSD and substance use disorders using the Seeking Safety programme with incarcerated women.

Whilst perceived coercion to enter treatment, such as pressure from family, criminal sanctions, loss of employment of financial concerns, can heighten psychological distress and may add additional pressure to seek treatment (Cimino, Mendoza, Nochajski, & Farrell, 2017), individuals who have been detained in hospital or prison are presented with an opportunity that they may not have in the community. Less chaotic living circumstances mean that access to treatment is more likely to address their complex needs (Butler et al., 2006). This in turn may also reduce their risk or relapse into substance misuse and criminal activity, particularly for those with comorbid substance use disorders and trauma. Integrated programmes address some of the reasons for substance abuse and criminal activity; they are more likely to influence future behaviour in order to break the cycle of violence (Greene, Haney, & Hurtado, 2000; Gunter, Chibnall, Antoniak, McCormick, & Black, 2012).

Treatment approaches that integrate treatments for trauma and substance abuse focus either on improving current coping skills or on exposure to past traumatic events. The review by Roberts et al. (2016) suggests that the latter are more effective.

Prison-based interventions targeting comorbid substance use and PTSD have been effective in reducing PTSD symptoms and substance use (Zlotnick, Johnson, & Najavits, 2009; Zlotnick, Najavits, Rohsenow, & Johnson, 2003). Brown, Perera, Masho, Mezuk, and Cohen (2015) advocate for an integrated treatment approach to intimate partner violence which includes intervention that addresses substance misuse and previous traumatic experience.

Murphy and Rosen (2014) suggest that promising data are emerging in support of combining trauma-informed therapeutic techniques with motivational enhancement techniques. Killian, Cimino, Mendoza, Shively, and Kunz (2018) suggest a possible link between positive outcomes from trauma treatment and subsequent readiness to change substance use disorders. However, the relationship between readiness to change behaviour and trauma history remains unclear.

Fehrman (2019) studied a female offender population and concluded that treating offending, substance use, and trauma needs in an integrated way would be hugely beneficial in reducing future violent offending. Wallace, Conner, and Dass-Brailsford (2011) reviewed integrated trauma interventions. They described a range of interventions that show promise in reducing trauma and mental health symptoms. Martin, Eljdupovic, McKenzie, and Colman (2015) highlight the multiple social, health and behavioural needs of prisoners who were at highest risk of violence, which should be considered as treatment targets. Wallace et al. stress the need for interventions for inmates with trauma histories to be integrated, that is to target multiple needs simultaneously, rather than sequentially in order to be effective.

Conclusions

There continues to be a need to clarify developmental pathways from traumatic experiences to criminal behaviour and substance use and to identify modifiable risk factors that can be targeted through treatment. There is also a need to disentangle causal relationships from associations. Offenders with substance use disorders and trauma are a vulnerable group with complex treatment needs. Yet despite their vulnerability and the complexity of their clinical profile, they receive little by way of treatment that would reduce recidivism whilst improving psychological well-being and further victimisation. Despite the lack of research into combining substance use and trauma treatment highlighted by Roberts et al. (2016), an integrated approach to treatment, formulating and targeting the interplay between trauma, substance use, and offending is indicated as being the most effective way forward.

Further Reading

Najavits, L. M. (2002). *Seeking safety: A treatment manual for PTSD and substance abuse*. Guilford Press. Whilst this manual was published in 2002 it represents the first, and most empirically supported, model to address the complex relationships between trauma and addiction.

Vujanovic, A. A., & Back, S. E. (Eds). (2019). *Posttraumatic stress and substance use disorders: A comprehensive clinical handbook*. Routledge. A summary of current evidence-based assessment and treatment of PTSD and substance abuse. The two areas are usually dealt with in isolation but this text combines clinical insight into both conditions.

Acknowledgements

Thanks to Naomi Thorpe, Nottinghamshire Healthcare NHS Foundation Trust, Library and Knowledge Services for additional evidence searches.

References

Anthes, E. (2014). Depression: A change of mind. *Nature, 515*(7526), 185–187. doi:10.1038/515185a

Averna, S., & Hesselbrock, V. (2001). The relationship of perceived social support to substance use in offspring of alcoholics. *Addictive Behaviors, 26(3)*, 363–374. doi:10.1016/S0306-4603(00)00112-X

Ball, S.A. (1998). Manualized treatment for substance abusers with personality disorders: Dual focus schema therapy. *Addictive Behaviours, 23*, 883–891. doi:10.1016/s0306-4603(98)00067-7

Ball, S. A. (2007). Comparing individual therapies for personality disordered opioid dependent patients. *Journal of Personality Disorders, 21(3)*, 305–321. doi:10.1159/000493644

Ball, S. A., Cobb-Richardson, P., Connolly, A. J., Bujosa, C. T., & O'Neil, T. W. (2005). Substance abuse and personality disorders in homeless drop-in centre clients: Symptom severity and psychotherapy retention in a randomized clinical trial. *Comprehensive Psychiatry, 46*, 317–379. doi:10.1016/j.comppsych.2004.11.003

Barrett, E. M., Mills, K. M., & Teesson, M. (2011). Hurt people who hurt people: Violence amongst individuals with comorbid substance use disorder and post-traumatic stress disorder. *Addictive Behaviors, 36*, 721–728. doi:10.1016/j.addbeh.2011.02.005

Beddoes, D., Sheikh, S., Khanna, M., & Francis, R. (2010). *The impact of drugs on different minority groups: A review of the UK literature*. The UK Drug Policy Commission (UKDPC).

Bonta, J., & Andrews, D. A. (2016). *The psychology of criminal conduct*. Routledge. doi:10.4324/9781315677187

Briere, J., Kaltman, S., & Green, B. L. (2008). Accumulated childhood trauma and symptom complexity. *Journal of Traumatic Stress, 21*, 223–226. doi:10.1002/jts.20317

Brown, M. J., Perera, R. A., Masho, S. W., Mezuk, B., & Cohen, S. A. (2015). Adverse childhood experiences and intimate partner aggression in the US: Sex differences and similarities in psychosocial mediation. *Social Science and Medicine, 131*, 48–57. doi:10.1016/j.socscimed.2015.02.044

Brunelle, N., Brochu, S., & Cousineau, M. M. (2000). Drug-crime relations among drug-consuming juvenile delinquents: A tripartite model and more. *Contemporary Drug Problems, 27*(4), 835–866. doi:10.1177/009145090002700406

Butler, T., Andrews, G., Allnutt, S., Sakashita, C., Smith, N., & Basson, J. (2006). Mental disorders in Australian prisoners: A comparison with a community sample. *Australian and New Zealand Journal of Psychiatry, 40,* 272–276. doi:10.1080/j.1440-1614.2006.01785.x

Butler, T., & Kariminia, A. (2005). Prison violence: Perspectives and epidemiology. *NSW Public Health Bulletin, 17,* 17–20. doi:10.1071/NB06005

Centre for Ethnicity and Health. (2004). *Young refugees and asylum seekers in Greater London: Vulnerability to problematic drug use.* Greater London Authority.

Chandler, R., Peters, R., Field, G., & Juliano-Bult, D. (2004). Challenges in implementing evidence-based treatment practices for co-occurring disorders in the criminal justice system. *Behavioral Sciences & the Law, 22,* 431–448. doi:10.1002/bsl.598

Cimino, A. N., Mendoza, N., Nochajski, T. H., & Farrell, M. G. (2017). Examining the relationship between psychological functioning, trauma history, and sources of perceived coercion among drug court enrollees. *Cogent Psychology, 4*(1), 1–8. doi:10.1080/23311908.2017.1320859

Cook, S. L., Smith, S. G., Tusher, C. P., & Raiford, J. (2005). Self-reports of traumatic events in a random sample of incarcerated women. *Women & Criminal Justice, 16*(1–2), 107–126. doi:10.1300/J012v16n01_05

Cusack, K. J., Herring, A. H., & Steadman, H. J. (2013). PTSD as a mediator between lifetime sexual abuse and substance use among jail diversion participants. *Psychiatric Services, 64,* 776–781. doi:10.1176/appi.ps.000052012

Cusack, K. J., Jonas, D. E., Forneris, C. A., Wines, C., Sonis, J., Middleton, J. C. Gaynes, B. N. (2016). Psychological treatments for adults with posttraumatic stress disorder: A systematic review and meta-analysis. *Clinical Psychology Review, 43,* 128–141. doi:10.1016/j.cpr.2015.10.003

Davis, J. L., Combs-Lane, A. M., & Jackson, T. L. (2002). Risky behaviors associated with interpersonal victimization: Comparisons based on type, number, and characteristics of assault incidents. *Journal of Interpersonal Violence, 17*(6), 611–629. doi:10.1177/0886260502017006002

Engelhard, I., van Uijen, S., & van den Hout, M. (2010). The impact of taxing working memory on negative and positive memories. *European Journal of Psychotraumatology, 1*(1), 5623. doi.org/10.3402/ejpt.v1i0.5623

Fehrman, E. (2019). *The relationship between trauma and substance misuse in high-risk mentally disordered offenders.* Trent Study Day: Substance Use and Forensic Mental Health. Nottingham. UK.

Felitti, V. J., Anda, R. F., Nordenburg, D., Williamson, D. F., Spitz, A. M., Edwards, V., & Marks, J. S. (1998). The relationship of adult health status to childhood abuse and household dysfunction. *American Journal of Preventative Medicine, 14 (4),* 245–258. doi:10.1016/s0749-3797(98)00017-8

Fincham, D. S., Altes, L. K., Stein, D. J., & Seedat, S. (2009). Posttraumatic stress disorder symptoms in adolescents: Risk factors versus resilience moderation. *Comprehensive Psychiatry, 50(3),* 193–199. doi:10.1016/j.comppsych.2008.09.001

Gibson, L., Holt, J., Fondacaro, K., Tang, T., Powell, T., & Turbitt, E. (1999). An examination of antecedent traumas and psychiatric comorbidity among male inmates with PTSD. *Journal of Traumatic Stress, 12,* 473–484. doi:10.1023/A:1024767020280

Gilbert, R., Widom, C. S., Browne, K., Fergusson, D., Webb, E., & Janson, S. (2009). Burden and consequences of child maltreatment in high-income countries. *Lancet, 373,* 68–81. doi:10.1016/S0140-6736(08)61706-7

Goldstein, P., Brownstein, H., Ryan, P., & Bellucci, P. (1989). Crack and homicide in New York: A conceptually based event analysis. *Contemporary Drug Problems, 16,* 651–687.

Green, L. G., Dass-Brailsford, P., Hurtado de Mendoza, A., Mete, M., Lynch, S. M., & DeHart, D. D. (2016). Trauma experiences and mental health among incarcerated women. *Psychological Trauma: Theory, Research, Practice and Policy, 8*(4): 455–463. doi:10.1037/tra0000113

Greene, S., Haney, C., & Hurtado, A. (2000). Cycles of pain: Risk factors in the lives of incarcerated mothers and their children. *The Prison Journal, 80,* 3–23. doi:10.1177/0032885500080001001

Gunter, T. D., Chibnall, J. T., Antoniak, S. K., McCormick, B., & Black, D. W. (2012). Relative contributions of gender and traumatic life experience to the prediction of mental disorders in a sample of incarcerated offenders. *Behavioral Sciences & the Law, 30,* 615–630. doi:10.1002/bsl.2037

Hawkins, J. D., Catalano, R. F., & Miller, J. Y. (1992). Risk and protective factors for alcohol and other drug problems in adolescence and early adulthood: Implications for substance abuse prevention. *Psychological Bulletin, 112,* 64–105. doi:10.1037/0033-2909.112.1.64

Hornsveld, H. K., Houtveen, J. H., Vroomen, M., Aalbers, I. K. D., Aalbers, D., & van den Hout, M. A. (2011). Evaluating the effect of eye movements on positive memories such as those used in resource development and installation. *Journal of EMDR Practice and Research, 5 (4),* 146–155. doi:10.1891/1933-3196.5.4.146

Howard, R., Karatzias, T., Power, K., & Mahony, A. (2017). Posttraumatic stress disorder (PTSD) symptoms mediate the relationship between substance misuse and violent offending among female prisoners. *Social Psychiatry & Psychiatric Epidemiology, 52 (1),* 21–25. doi:10.1007/s00127-016-1293-5

Indig, D., Topp, L., Ross, B., Mamoon, H., Kumar, S., & McNamara, M. (2010). *2009 NSW Inmate Health Survey: Key findings report.* Sydney: Justice Health.

Khoury, L., Tang, Y., Bradley, B., Cubells, J., & Ressler, K. (2010). Substance use, childhood traumatic experience and post-traumatic stress disorder in an urban civilian population. *Depression and Anxiety, 27,* 1077–1086. doi:10.1002/da.20751

Killian, M., Cimino, A. N., Mendoza, N. C., Shively, R., & Kunz, K. (2018). Examining trauma and readiness to change among women in a community re-entry program. *Substance Use & Misuse, 53(4),* 648–653. doi:10.1080/10826084.2017.1355387

Komarovskaya, I. A., Booker-Loper, A., Warren, J., & Jackson, S. (2011). Exploring gender differences in trauma exposure and the emergence of symptoms of PTSD among incarcerated men and women. *Journal of Forensic Psychiatry & Psychology, 22(3),* 395–410. doi:10.1080/14789949.2011.572989

Kubiak, S. P. (2004). The effects of PTSD on treatment adherence, drug relapse, and criminal recidivism in a sample of incarcerated men and women. *Research on Social Work Practice, 14(6),* 424–433. doi:10.1177/1049731504265837

Linehan, M. M., Schmidt, H., & Dimeff, L. A. (1999). Dialectical behavior therapy for patients with borderline personality disorder and drug dependence. *American Journal of Addictions, 8,* 279–292. doi:10.1080/105504999305686

Lipsey, M. W., Landenberger, N. A., & Wilson, S. J. (2007). Effects of cognitive-behavioral programs for criminal offenders. *Campbell Systematic Reviews, 6.* doi:10.4073/csr.2007.6

Lovell, D., Johnson, C., Jemelka, R., Harris, V., & Allen, D. (2001). Living in prison after residential mental health treatment: A program follow-up. *The Prison Journal, 81(4),* 473–490. doi:10.1177/0032885501081004004

Lynch, S. M., Heath, N. M., Mathews, K. C., & Cepeda, G. J. (2012). Seeking safety: An intervention for trauma-exposed incarcerated women? *Journal of Trauma & Dissociation, 13,* 88–101. doi:10.1080/15299732.2011.608780

Markus, W., & Hornsveld, H. K. (2017). EMDR interventions in addiction. *Journal of EMDR Practice and Research, 12,* 3–29. doi:10.1891/1933-3196.11.1.3

Martin, M. S., Eljdupovic, G., McKenzie, K., & Colman, I. (2015). Risk of violence by inmates with childhood trauma and mental health needs. *Law and Human Behavior, 39,* 614–623. doi:10.1037/lhb0000149

McCormack, M., & Walker, R. (2005). *Drug prevention for young asylum seekers and refugees: A review of current knowledge.* Mentor.

McHugh, R. K., Hearon, B. A., & Otto, M. W. (2010). Cognitive-behavioral therapy for substance use disorders. *Psychiatric Clinics of North America, 33(3),* 511–525. doi:10.1016/j.psc.2010.04.012

Messina, N., & Grella, C. (2006). Childhood trauma and women's health outcomes in a California prison population. *American Journal of Public Health, 96*(10), 1842–1848. doi:10.2105/AJPH.2005.082016

Miller, N. A., & Najavits, L. M. (2012). Creating trauma-informed correctional care: A balance of goals and environment. *European Journal of Psychotraumatology, 3,* 1–8. doi:10.3402/ejpt.v3i0.17246

Montgomery, K. L., Vaughn, M. G., Thompson, S. J., & Howard, M. O. (2012). Heterogeneity in drug abuse among juvenile offenders: Is mixture regression more informative than standard regression? *International Journal of Offender Therapy and Comparative Criminology, 57* (11), 1326–1346. doi:10.1177/0306624X12459185

Murphy, R. T., & Rosen, C. S. (2014). Addressing readiness to change PTSD with a brief intervention: A description of the PTSD motivation enhancement group. In J. Garrick & M. B. Williams (Eds), *Trauma treatment techniques: Innovative trends* (pp.7–28). New York, NY: Routledge.

Najavits, L. (2002). *Seeking safety: A treatment manual for PTSD and substance abuse.* Guilford Press. New York.

Palmer, E. J., Jinks, M., & Hatcher, R. M. (2010). Substance use, mental health, and relationships: A comparison of male and female offenders serving community sentences. *International Journal of Law and Psychiatry 33*(2), 89–93. doi:10.1016/j.ijlp.2009.12.007

Resko, S., & Mendoza, N. S. (2012). Early attrition from treatment among women with co-occurring substance use disorders and PTSD. *Journal of Social Work Practice in the Addictions, 12*(4), 348–369. doi:10.1080/1533256X.2012.728104

Rhodes, J. E., & Jason, L. A. (1990). A social stress model of substance abuse. *Journal of Consulting and Clinical Psychology, 58*(4), 395–401. doi:10.1037//0022-006x.58.4.395

Roberts, N. P., Roberts, P. A., Jones, N., & Bisson, J. I. (2016). Psychological therapies for post-traumatic stress disorder and comorbid substance use disorder. *Cochrane Database of Systematic Reviews, 4.* Art. No.: CD010204. doi:10.1002/14651858.CD010204.pub2

Robertson, A. A., Xiaohe, X., & Stripling, A. (2010). Adverse events and substance use among female adolescent offenders: Effects of coping and family support. *Substance Use & Misuse, 45,* 451–472. doi:10.3109/10826080903452512

Ross Dawson, C. (2003). *Drugs scoping study: Asylum seekers and refugee communities report.* Home Office.

Salgado, D., Quinlan, K., & Zlotnick, C. (2007). The relationship of lifetime polysubstance dependence to trauma exposure, symptomatology, and psychosocial functioning in incarcerated women with comorbid PTSD and substance use disorder. *Journal of Trauma & Dissociation, 8,* 9–26. doi:10.1300/J229v08n02_02

Shapiro, F. (2001). *Eye movement desensitization and reprocessing: Basic principles, protocols and procedures, 2nd Ed.* Guilford Press.

Shorey, R. C., Stuart, G. L., Anderson, S., & Strong, D. R. (2013). Changes in early maladaptive schemas after residential treatment for substance use. *Journal of Clinical Psychology, 69*(9), 912–922. doi:10.1002/jclp.21968

Sindicich, N., Mills, K. L., Barrett, E. L., Indig, D., Sunjic, S., Sannibale, C., … & Najavits, L. M. (2014). Offenders as victims: Post-traumatic stress disorder and substance use disorders among male prisoners, *The Journal of Forensic Psychiatry and Psychology, 25* (1), 44–60. doi:10.1080/14789949.2013.877516

Sommer, J., Hinsberger, M., Elbert, T., Holtzhausen, L., Kaminer, D., Seedat, S., Madikane, S., & Weierstall, R. (2017). The interplay between trauma, substance abuse and appetitive aggression and its relation to criminal activity among high-risk males in South Africa. *Addictive Behaviours, 64,* 29–34. doi:10.1016/j.addbeh.2016.08.008

Straus, M. A. (1992). *Children as witness to marital violence: A risk factor for lifelong problems among a nationally representative sample of American men and women* (Report of the Twenty-Third Ross Roundtable). Ross Laboratories.

Wallace, B. C., Conner, L. C., & Dass-Brailsford, P. (2011). Integrated trauma treatment in correctional health care and community-based treatment upon reentry. *Journal of Correctional Health Care, 17,* 329–343. doi:10.1177/1078345811413091

Widom, C. S., Ireland, T., Glynn, P. J. (1995). Alcohol abuse in abused and neglected children followed-up: Are they at increased risk? *Journal of Studies on Alcohol, 56(2),* 207–217. doi:10.15288/jsa.1995.56.207

Williams, J., Ayres, C., Abbott, R., Hawkins, J., & Catalano, R. (1999). Racial differences in risk factors for delinquency and substance use among adolescents. *Social Work Research, 23,* 241–256. doi:10.1093/swr/23.4.241

Wolff, N., Frueh, B. C., Shi, J., & Schumann, B. E. (2012). Effectiveness of cognitive–behavioral trauma treatment for incarcerated women with mental illnesses and substance abuse disorders. *Journal of Anxiety Disorders, 26,* 703–710. doi:10.1016/j.janxdis.2012.06.001

Wolff, N., & Shi, J. (2012). Childhood and adulthood trauma experiences of incarcerated persons and their relationship to adult behavioral health problems and treatment. *International Journal of Environmental Research and Public Health, 9,* 1908–1926. doi:10.3390/ijerph9051908

Zlotnick, C., Bruce, S. W., Weisberg, R. B., Shea, T., Machan, J. T., & Kelling, M. B. (2003). Social and health functioning in female primary care patients with post-traumatic stress disorders with or without comorbid substance abuse. *Comprehensive Psychiatry, 44,* 177–183. doi:10.1016/S0010-440X(03)00005-1

Zlotnick, C., Johnson, J., & Najavits, L. (2009). Randomized controlled pilot study of cognitive-behavioral therapy in a sample of incarcerated women with substance use disorder and PTSD. *Behavior Therapy, 40,* 325–336. doi:10.1016/j.beth.2008.09.004

Zlotnick, C., Najavits, L., Rohsenow, D., & Johnson, D. (2003). A cognitive-behavioral treatment for incarcerated women with substance abuse disorder and posttraumatic stress disorder: Findings from a pilot study. *Journal of Substance Abuse Treatment, 25,* 99–105. doi:10.1016/s0740-5472(03)00106-5

11

EARLY TRAUMA, PSYCHOSIS, AND VIOLENT OFFENDING

Claire Moore and Naomi Callender

though this is madness, yet there is a method in't

Shakespeare, Hamlet

Psychosis tends to be an experience that socially isolates the sufferer and generates fear and distance in others. This is likely intensified when this presentation is combined with offending. In this chapter, we aim to explore the role of trauma and the concept of *meaning* in these experiences. A brief review of relevant literature will be considered before sharing an insight into two patients' journey from trauma to psychosis and violent offending.

Several terms will be used interchangeably within this chapter to describe the same presenting problems. This reflects a split in the literature between the use of diagnostic and non-diagnostic descriptors. The word *psychosis* is used to define a range of symptoms. These are characterised by altered perceptual disturbance, such as delusional or overvalued beliefs; sensory experiences that others are not experiencing, often described as hallucinations; disorganised speech and a loss of characteristics, such as emotional connection either with oneself or others, lack of drive/motivation and social withdrawal. An aim in this chapter is to outline the importance of incorporating a psychological understanding of psychosis within the literature and clinical practice.

The Presence of Trauma in Psychosis

Until relatively recently, psychosis has been conceptualised through a medical lens as a neurodevelopmental disorder, historically described as a "brain disease". Therefore, pharmacological interventions have been viewed as the primary and most effective option. The relationship between childhood trauma and psychotic disorders has long been neglected (Read & Bentall, 2012), though there is a growing evidence for such a relationship. Additionally, research and clinical evidence highlight that those

DOI: 10.4324/9781003120766-15

suffering from psychotic experiences have an increased vulnerability for developing Post-Traumatic Stress Disorder (PTSD) from the psychotic experience and associated treatment such as involuntary detention, forced administration of medication, restraint and physical restrictions.

Green, Browne, and Chou (2017) conducted a systematic review and meta-analysis of the relationship between childhood abuse, psychosis, and violent offending. They concluded that individuals experiencing childhood adversity are more likely to develop psychosis in adulthood. Turner et al. (2020) explored the relationship between childhood adversity and psychosis, considering sexual, physical, emotional abuse, neglect, and inter-personal loss. Four in five of those individuals living with psychosis reported experiencing such an event. Bebbington and Freeman (2017) noted that disorders associated with delusional systems consistently occur in the context of a history of trauma. A Scottish census survey of forensic inpatients similarly supported this association (Karatzias et al., 2019). The majority (86%) of the patients included had been diagnosed with a psychotic disorder and childhood adversity was prevalent (79%), with physical abuse as the most reported experience (42%). McKenna, Jackson, and Browne (2019) explored the prevalence of childhood trauma in a UK high secure male forensic population. All 194 patients had been exposed to a traumatic event and 75% of these occurred in childhood, with 65% of individuals having experienced more than one type of trauma.

Within the Mental Health Service at Rampton, patients have attracted a range of psychiatric diagnoses, primarily paranoid schizophrenia (75%). Comorbid personality disorder is identified as present in 24%, 6% schizoaffective disorder, 2% delusional disorder, and 1% bipolar disorder. Only 2% have a diagnosis of PTSD or Complex PTSD (CPTSD). However, the prevalence of traumatic experience within this population is high. We found that, despite the low incidence of trauma-related diagnoses, 92% of our patients had experienced trauma throughout their lifetime, with 84% experiencing emotional, physical, and/or sexual abuse during childhood, 28% feeling traumatised by their offending, and 51% traumatised by the experience of psychosis itself and associated treatment.

Concerningly, only 4% had received treatment for trauma. The lack of acknowledgement regarding the experience of trauma in our patient group, and/or its relevance to diagnosis and treatment, could be partly explained, by an under-reporting of trauma. This is an essential component in the diagnostic criteria of PTSD. Therefore, mental images of sexual violence in an individual with disclosed sexual abuse might be conceptualised as flashbacks in an individual diagnosed with PTSD, but are more likely to be perceived as psychosis in an individual with an undisclosed sexual abuse history.

Another factor contributing to the lack of trauma treatment in this population may be the belief that psychotic and delusional experience do not inform or provide understanding of the internal world of the sufferer. That approach means that there is no relevance to their experience, thoughts, and/or feelings. We do not ask them what happened to them, we just accept that there is "something wrong with them". Nonetheless, there is growing evidence of the importance of understanding and formulating the function of psychosis (Andrew, Gray, & Snowden, 2008; British Psychological Society, 2013; Corstens, Longden, McCarty-Jones, Waddingham, & Thomas, 2014; Read & Bentall 2012).

Links Between Trauma, Psychosis, and Violent Offending?

It is widely accepted that the presence of "mental disorder" is a risk factor for violence and it is included as a relevant factor in structured risk assessment guides. Fazal, Gulati, Linsell, Geddes, and Grann (2009) completed a meta-analysis which suggested that men with schizophrenia are four times more likely to commit an act of violence compared to men in the general population. They also concluded that most of the excess risk was mediated by comorbid substance abuse, rather than directly the presence of psychotic symptoms. Similar assertions are made in relation to associations with schizophrenia and offences such as arson and murder (Anwar, Långström, Grann, & Fazal, 2011). However, the way in which psychosis and offending is linked continues to be debated.

Possible explanations for the association between mental illness and violence have highlighted the presence of positive symptoms of schizophrenia, in particular delusional beliefs and persecutory ideations. Swanson et al. (2006) suggested that the clusters and degree of prominence of these symptoms may also be important to consider, given the moderating effect of negative symptoms on the likelihood of committing serious violence. Skeem et al. (2006) highlighted the importance of looking beyond symptoms to understand violence in this group. An increase in symptoms may not necessarily equate to an imminent increase in risk and, conversely, an amelioration of symptoms may not equate to a reduction in risk. Again, this highlights the importance of understanding the presenting problem rather than grouping effect based on a broad diagnostic or categorical term.

The literature also highlights that the presence of childhood trauma, recent violent victimisation, previous conduct problems, co-morbidity, and specific delusions can be associated with an increased risk of violence to others, in individuals suffering from psychosis. Storvestre et al. (2020) suggest that childhood physical and emotional neglect may be of specific importance to later violent behaviour. They concluded that individuals with a diagnosis of schizophrenia and history of violence had higher exposure to childhood trauma compared to individuals with the same diagnosis and no history of violence. Buchanan, Sint, Swanson, and Rosenheck (2019) conducted a longitudinal multivariable analysis with 1,435 individuals, all with a diagnosis of schizophrenia. Follow-up after 18 month indicated that a history of previous injurious violence, recent violent victimisation, severity of drug use, childhood sexual abuse, and medication non-adherence were associated with future injurious violence. Buchanan et al. highlighted strong effects of previous injurious violence and recent violent victimisation on future violent behaviour. Green et al. (2017) concluded that individuals with psychosis who had also experienced childhood trauma were twice as likely to be violent as individuals with psychosis with no reported childhood trauma.

Understanding the Pathway to Psychosis

A comprehensive review of the literature and evolving chronology of the understanding of psychosis is outside the scope of this chapter; however, there are several emerging perspectives that have been useful in providing further understanding, and a review of relevant literature will be provided here.

Firstly, our understanding of the impact of early childhood trauma highlights biological changes in the brain which mirror those seen in individuals diagnosed with psychotic disorders. Fosse, Moskowitz, Shannon, and Mulholland (2019) outline how the structural changes in the brain, particularly to the hippocampus, amygdala, and prefrontal cortex, can be observed in individuals with psychotic disorders as well as those who have experienced early adversity. Interestingly, amongst other changes they note increased sensitivity to stress, deficits in episodic memory, and a prioritisation of biologically relevant information, thus leading to elevated levels of stress hormones. This is significant in considering that the causality of changes could equally, or alternatively, be explained by exposure to childhood trauma, rather than purely neurodevelopmental/genetic origins, often associated with psychotic disorders.

Consideration of the role of dissociation, attachment, and affect regulation are considered important in understanding the functional links between trauma and psychosis. Moskowitz, Heinmaa, and Van Der Hart (2019) describe psychosis as a form of dissociation – an attempt to cope with the experience of trauma by dividing the personality. This expands on the more common view of dissociation which can focus exclusively on depersonalisation and derealisation, and alternatively conceptualises it as a failure to integrate trauma experience. Individuals therefore become "stuck", with parts of them attempting to function as normal, and other parts "frozen" in the trauma experience. Moskowitz et al. hypothesise that, at some point in the individual's life, the ability to dissociate has been central to survival in an environment of adversity (physically and psychologically).

Integral to the extensive literature on trauma and attachment systems is an understanding of the need for processes like dissociation in children faced with early trauma, particularly when inflicted by a caregiver figure. Moskowitz and Montirosso (2019) describe a "relational trap" whereby the attachment system motivates the child to stay close to the caregiver who is responsible for keeping the child safe and nurtured, while the defence/threat system motivates them to flee from the person, who is also the source of emotional and physical harm.

Gumley and Liotti (2019) posit that disorganised attachment can lead to the increased likelihood that dissociation is implemented when faced with subsequent traumas. The process of dissociation, in this example, allows the child to feel safe, when unable to achieve physical safety, but keeps the adult stuck in a cycle where trauma is maintained and reinforced. The emotion regulation strategies, that an individual develops to "survive" their early attachment experiences, are the basis for the negative and positive symptoms identified within psychosis. As such, the individual with psychosis may be more likely to disconnect, focusing on threat rather than connection, leading to physical and social withdrawal and emotional inhibition, or to develop overvalued ideas or hallucinations which allow for symbolic expression.

Complementary to this explanation is the *double bind theory* and *communication deviance*, capturing the significance of developmental relational experiences. The double bind theory was proposed by Bateson, Jackson, Hayley, and Weakland (1956) and conceptualises trauma as a relational pattern rather than an event. Bateson et al. proposed that a child learns that what the caregiver *explicitly* and *implicitly* expresses are contradictory, and that this experience is forbidden to be acknowledged or discussed. A pattern then develops where the child is unable to trust their own perceptions and is required to suppress their own emotional responses, contributing to confusion about what is real and what is imagined, and what is an internal experience and what is another person's experience. Psychosis, particularly delusions, is therefore a means of avoiding the control of this double bind and expressing the emotion and behaviour that is forbidden. de Sousa, Varese, Sellwood, and Bentall (2014) explored this theory via meta-analysis, re-terming the concept communication deviance, finding that the prevalence was high in families of an individual who later developed psychosis.

Moskowitz and Montirosso (2019) highlight that although they would not, and could not insist, that all delusions must have their genesis in childhood experiences, they would suggest that many, if not most, delusions are explanations for powerful emotional experience, which may be memory-based. Hardy (2017) highlights the importance of memory processes in an individual's pathway from trauma to psychosis, drawing upon cognitive behavioural, attachment, and neuropsychological understanding of psychosis and PTSD. She proposes that vulnerability factors contribute to psychotic experience when combined with trauma. These are then reinforced and perpetuated by the coping responses of an individual. Vulnerability factors are identified as emotion regulation strategies, event memory processes, and personal semantic memories. Emotional regulation is considered in the context of trauma where there is repeated exposure to threat and the deprivation of core developmental needs. In the context of heightened emotional arousal of this kind, memory is affected. Hardy proposes that the perceptual and sensory information experienced tends to be enhanced, and episodic memory encoding inhibited. Therefore, intentional recall may be more difficult, whereas the associated sensory and perceptual stimuli are more intensely experienced and easily triggered. Implementation of emotion regulation may lead to increased fragmentation between the episodic memory and perceptual memories, leading to continued intrusions. The third vulnerability factor, personal semantic memory, holds an individual's core beliefs or appraisals of events where the meaning of experience is attributed. As this is also influenced by our internal working models and attachment systems, these filters are likely to be applied in understanding experiences, and in retrieving memories, therefore providing a reinforcing effect. In summary, Hardy posits that psychosis is associated with a weakened ability to integrate contextual information with trauma-based memory intrusion, occurring in the absence of any episodic context, so that they are experienced as occurring in the here and now, and as if the past is present.

Central therefore to the pathway to psychosis is the relevance of affect regulation in the experiencing of trauma, particularly when this is repetitive, complex, or chronic in nature. Porges (2004) explains the impact of psychological experience, such as trauma, on the body, allowing us to further understand the physiological and biological impact. Porges (2011) describes how we have evolved to cue and detect the affective states of others, and the environment, thus allowing us to safely engage, or to flee danger. This dialogue between social connection and threat response is key to us thriving as human beings.

Within Porges's *polyvagal theory*, physiological arousal is controlled by the autonomic nervous system (ANS) and made up of two main branches (sympathetic and parasympathetic), with the parasympathetic branch divided into two pathways (ventral-vagal and dorsal-vagal) (Porges, 1995; 2004; 2011). This gives the ANS three main states of responding: first, being safely engaged and socially connected (safe and engaged); second, being energised to move in response to danger (fight/flight); and third, shutting down or collapsing when escape is not possible (freeze/dissociate). Each state is associated with emotions, physical feelings, behaviour, styles of attachment and communication, and capacities for self-regulation through which we react to our environment (Dana, 2018; Gilbert, 2009).

Central to this is the concept of neuroception – the subconscious process of detecting threat. This involves scanning for sign of threat from the outside environment, within our own autonomic nervous system and between our own and other's systems (Dana, 2018). The ANS draws information from the current environment to ensure that we move between these states in an effective way, ensuring that we respond in a way that keeps us safe and socially connected. Trauma, particularly complex childhood trauma distorts the regulation of this system, resulting in overwhelming levels of physiological arousal characterised by chronic hypervigilance.

Of particular importance here is the freeze response (Levine & Frederick, 1997; Porges, 2011). When we are unable to escape or powerless to stop traumatic experience the ANS (mentally) shuts down, minimising the potential for psychological and physical damage. This state is controlled by the parasympathetic ANS (dorsal-vagal branch) and leads to adaptive survival responses overriding the other systems, particularly those linked to social engagement and connection. In this state of chronic hypervigilance, connection becomes at best deprioritised, at worst, unsafe and terrifying. Considering the relational trap described by Moskowitz and Montirosso (2019) we can see how such a physiological scar could lead an individual to neither feeling safe enough to stay, nor safe enough to leave.

Our current, and working, understanding draws from these emerging perspectives and is posited on several key principles.

- Psychosis symptomology has its base in a chronic hypervigilant state rooted in dissociation. This impacts on the individual's ability to filter and differentiate information from multiple systems and in turn leads to difficulty in deciphering what is past and present, theirs or mine, reality, or fantasy.
- Delusional and/or overvalued ideas are an individual's attempt to make sense of the body's heightened threat response, to facilitate disconnection and overcompensation, to achieve safety, and/or to promote action allowing expression of emotions, sensations, and actions suppressed through trauma (Moskowitz, Heinmaa, & Van Der Hart, 2019).
- The body's overriding focus on survival rather than connection exists as a wound between the person and the world (Van der Hart, Nijenhuis, & Steele, 2006).

This prevents re-connection and the potential for a corrective emotional experience. It maintains a disorganised attachment style, further damage to relationships, increased potential for victimisation, and emotional dysregulation (Levine & Frederick, 1997).

In this brief introduction, we have presented an overview of some of the important interrelated factors and systems we perceive are useful in understanding and formulating the experience of psychosis. These are developing ideas and require continued exploration, research, and clinical reflection. We hope to bring these to life in the following section through case examples, focusing on the importance of understanding risk and the role of psychosis in the use of violence.

Case Study 1: Nate

Nate is a 27-year-old male, who was admitted to our service after his mental health deteriorated in prison. He was at that time serving an Indeterminate sentence for Public Protection (IPP) following an assault and rape conviction, with a seven-year tariff, which expired four years ago. He had accessed mental health services since the age of 21, due to hearing voices, and had made numerous attempts to take his own life. Nate had spent little time in the community, moving between inpatient settings and prison. He was first convicted at the age of 13 and went onto amass over 40 convictions including violence, drug offences, and breaches of imposed orders.

Nate had also attracted labels of psychopathy, antisocial personality disorder, borderline personality disorder, and treatment-resistant paranoid schizophrenia.

On the ward, Nate would respond to unseen stimuli, was highly suspicious, and presented as aggressive, threatening, and intimidating. Meeting Nate for the first time was shocking, coloured by extreme distress and utter confusion (both his and mine); he could only tolerate sitting with me for ten minutes, before retreating to his room. Within that time, he shouted obscenities over his shoulder, poured water into his eyes, searched for cameras and recording equipment, showed me the "microbots" in his forearm and described small leprechaun-type creatures, which he perceived to be wreaking havoc.

Nate had experienced relational trauma. Given the evidence base that secure attachment is essential to recovery (Van der Hart et al., 2006) and the importance of understanding the function of psychotic symptomology, we focused on establishing a secure and consistent base, whilst acknowledging that this would not be an easy process for either of us. Over time, Nate spoke more openly about his range of experience, both in the past and present, but remained mistrusting. This was characterised by a disorganised attachment style, dismissal of the importance of the relationship – a push/pull approach where I was both desperately needed and feared as an attachment figure. At times, Nate would try to destroy the relationship, making threats to rape and harm me, but then frantically try to avoid abandonment.

In formulating his experience, we could see that he was haunted by several perceptual experiences which he found distressing and traumatising in nature. In addition to those already described, he believed that he was physically bent over – hunched in his appearance. He described the "aura" of a person changing into a "demon", which represented a sense that the person was evil and would ultimately harm him. Washing his eyes out with water would reset the image of that person. He also heard several voices, but the one which was most powerful, and distressing was the voice of a naked man, a ghost whom he described as cruel. This included telling Nate that he deserved to be abused, that he was disgusting, bent, defective, fat, ugly, violent, and a paedophile. Nate believed that this man kept him safe, by alerting him to those that he could not trust, that wanted to harm, abuse, and deceive him. Ultimately, the man told him that he could not and should not rely on anyone.

This voice also kept him disconnected; Nate believed that it had the power to inflict cancer and death on those that he cared about, those that cared for him, or that he was close to. Ultimately it was not safe for Nate, for those around him or for those forming a relationship with him. It was clear that his pushing and pulling in the therapeutic relationship was an attempt to both keep himself and me safe. In pushing people away and denying connection he was protecting others from the part of himself which he saw as bad – the part that raped and hurt others.

Nate's childhood history was characterised by experiences of mistreatment, abandonment, and neglect. He was unable to make sense of these early experiences or how he felt. This was particularly evident in his relationship with his main abuser, who inflicted horrific abuse, but who also provided Nate's only sense of attachment, belonging, and intimacy. It was unsafe to risk losing this attachment, but also risky to maintain it. Nate made sense of this dialectic by developing the belief that his abuse was a response to him being bad. It was punishment. However, his body's physical reactions to the abuse (i.e., sexual arousal and ejaculation) created further confusion and reinforced the sense that there was something wrong with him. Why would he enjoy this? Given the pleasure/comfort he felt, the only explanation he could find was that he was homosexual. This became enmeshed with the view of himself as bad and vulnerable, and a need to be punished.

Nate's inability to escape this situation, to have power over his abuser/s or his family meant that he was unable to mobilise, to fight back, or to flee. He used several regulation strategies to manage distress – abusing substances, inhibiting his emotions, and disengaging from others – but this did not alleviate his fear or make him feel safe. Even after the abuse had ended, his threat system remained hypervigilant and alarmed, altering his ability to accurately read the affect state and intent of others. He could not distinguish between past and present and began to misinterpret cues of social engagement as risky. This process maintained a cycle of threat and disconnection, preventing opportunities for connection that would help heal the wound with the world.

By the age of 14 Nate had started to hear the main voice. It initially provided him companionship and distance, through dissociation, by allowing him to separate from and dismiss the part of him that was a vulnerable child. It also provided a mechanism for managing anxiety; the voice was someone that would look after him and protect him, seek evidence for, and highlight risk of harm from others. Ultimately it allowed him to act violently in a "legitimate response" to threat. The voice encouraged him to remain disconnected, to rely solely on it. In this way it paralleled the relationship with his abuser, keeping Nate connected with the part of him that felt abused and alone. His sense of threat was reinforced by the belief that his vulnerability (which he linked to homosexuality) was physically manifested for all to see in that he was literally *bent over*. His use of intimidation and ultimately violence was a way of hiding that, to avoid feeling shameful and to regain control and power, when he felt controlled and powerless. His innate desire to connect, to feel love and/or kindness was thwarted by the belief that the voice had the power to kill those he cared about, or those that cared about him. This created another relational trap, where attachment was needed but feared. Ultimately this disconnect, hypervigilance, and misinterpretation of threat drove his violent behaviour. This in turn reinforced his feelings of defectiveness, shame, and a desire to be punished, perpetuating the cycle.

This process was also a critical factor in Nate's rape offence. He described the voice ridiculing him telling, him that he was ugly, fat, and gay, and that he needed to rape his victim to prove that he was heterosexual and therefore not vulnerable to further abuse. Nate described being desperate to escape his vulnerability; this, coupled with a desire to be attractive to his victim and to have connection and sexual contact, meant that he was able to dismiss her enough to force sexual contact/rape. However, this act also provided evidence that he was disgusting and worthy of punishment, thus keeping him trapped.

Case Study 2: Jason

Jason is a 34-year-old male, admitted whilst on remand for murder. His transfer from prison was due to a deterioration in his mental health. Jason had not engaged with mental health services before but had visited his doctor several times with concerns related to physical symptoms which did not appear to be organically caused. The GP on each occasion considered Jason's presentations as symptomatic of depression and anxiety, and prescribed pharmacological and psychological interventions, with which Jason did not engage. Prior to his admission Jason was diagnosed with delusional disorder.

Jason left school with qualifications and was in gainful employment prior to being arrested for the offence. He had no history of violence, no cautions, or convictions of any kind. He was a homeowner and had two stable relationships of note, one which had ended just prior to him offending. Jason is serving a life sentence, with a tariff of 27 years, after being found guilty of shooting a colleague.

On meeting Jason for the first time, I experienced him as shy and embarrassed. He was unwilling to make eye contact, placating and self-deprecating. He exhibited a great deal of shame for his offence, describing himself as a monster. Initially, we focused on establishing a therapeutic relationship. Jason was untrusting and suspicious, he struggled to talk about his life, the offence or his current situation.

Over time Jason described a long-standing sense of distrust for others, anxiety in social situations and a strong preference for isolation and small trusted groups of people. He used alcohol as a way of coping with day-to-day living because it allowed him to feel more confident around others. Just prior to the offence he had split with a long-term girlfriend with whom he lived and he had accepted a new job. This decision brought him back into contact with his father, from whom he was estranged.

Jason struggled to connect with his new colleagues and described how they bullied him. He believed that this was due to being brought into his father's business in a senior position. Jason reported that their behaviour escalated, he was assaulted, his car was tampered with and his house broken in to. One man in particular targeted Jason relentlessly and when he heard him talking about a contract killing, he became convinced that they were planning to kill him, or a member of his family. Jason became chronically hypervigilant, unable to leave his house, eat, or sleep. He stated that he could not run, due to the risk to his family, so borrowed a shot gun from a friend for protection. However, he was unable to tolerate the level of distress he was experiencing, and went to the victim's house, shooting him when he answered the door.

During the trial, and to date, Jason maintains that the threat of harm from the victim and his colleagues was real. Jason believed there was a failure by the court and his defence team, with a paucity of evidence presented to illustrate the harassment he had been exposed to.

So, what factors led to the deterioration of Jason's mental health to such an extent that he committed a fatal act of violence that appeared completely out of character? It emerged that Jason's history was peppered by physical abuse and emotional neglect; his father was a violent alcoholic who subjected the family to extreme levels of violence and control. At the age of three Jason was beaten for "noisily" eating an apple, resulting in him being hospitalised with a fractured skull and broken arm. Jason believes that neighbours and teachers knew what was happening but that his father was "untouchable"; people were too scared to stop or to even challenge him.

Jason felt that he needed to protect his mother and younger brother from this treatment and would try to direct his father's abuse away from them onto himself. He would often run away, to hide out, but he knew that his mother and brother would be punished for his "wrong doings". He was caught in a relational trap, unable to stay but unable to leave. Part of him remained frozen in that state, trying to become invisible, to remain below his father's radar whilst needing to be present to protect others.

His mother finally split from his father when Jason was 16, initially seeking refuge and then making the decision to move to another country to get away from her husband. Jason was left behind and spent time homeless and living in bedsit accommodation. He was subject to further abuse and intimidation in this environment and withdrew further. Despite these challenges he was able to secure an apprenticeship and achieved a period of stability, where he engaged in two long-term relationships. Often these relationships became stressful when Jason was unable to attend social or family events due to his high levels of mistrust and hypervigilance. The second of these relationships ended prior to his offence. He reported feeling ashamed that he was not and could not be "normal", and that this had resulted in the breakdown of a relationship with someone he cared deeply about. He felt defective and alone, paralleling his feelings as a child, and he started to rely on alcohol to help him manage his feelings of distress. He became dependant, and his employer arranged for him to have some time off and to complete a detox programme. This relationship was supportive and protective in nature, but Jason was ashamed, and struggled to return to work. It was at this point that his father offered him a job. Coming back into contact with his father was a difficult decision, but Jason hoped that his father could be the father he needed him to be.

Jason was exhibiting characteristics of undiagnosed PTSD/CPTSD for most of his life, and this had a significant impact on his ability to live adaptively and to connect with others. He suffered with chronic hypervigilance, flashbacks, nightmares, relationship difficulties, and used alcohol and social withdrawal to manage these symptoms, to no avail. It remains unclear whether Jason was subject to harassment in the build up to the offence, or whether his chronic hypervigilance, lack of support and exposure to stressful situations, distorted his reality. Either way his experience was real to him, and terrifying.

Regarding the pathway from trauma to psychosis, it is evident that as a child Jason was unable to mobilise, to fight or to flee. He remained traumatised throughout his adult life, unable to feel safe or secure. The breakdown of the relationships with his partner and at his previous workplace exacerbated a sense of shame and left him without the support that had previously been protective, allowing him to feel "safe enough" and to function, albeit, to a limited extent. His desire for his father to "be the dad I needed him to be", and for a new start, led to a recapitulation of neglect and abuse. His exposure to new social connections alongside his chronic hypervigilance led to an experiencing of others as unsafe and himself, as at risk. A further parallel to his childhood experience was a sense that he could not flee, once again feeling responsible for protecting his family from threat.

It is postulated that, given Jason's chronic arousal, he was unable to differentiate between past and present, leading to further traumatisation. This interpretation allowed him to make sense of the bodily fear that he was experiencing and prompted a symbolic enactment of events. Dissociation allowed him to express his anger, to act and to destroy the risk, eradicating it both from his childhood and adult experience, by ending the victim's life. Without the belief that he or a member of family would be killed, he would not have acted. In this way, "Psychosis" allowed him to react, to fight, and to ultimately be rid of the fear, in a way that he could not be as a child. Unfortunately, Jason's attempt to escape trauma in this way further traumatised him. He was unable to see the vulnerable traumatised boy, instead labelling himself as a monster who deserved to be punished and to never feel safe.

Whilst on remand, Jason's beliefs became more entrenched. He began to believe that his victim's associates had infiltrated the prison and poisoned his food. He described severe pain in his abdomen and a massive swelling on his jaw. He started to refuse food and water and his mental and physical health deteriorated further. Medical examination could find no reason for the physical ailments he described, which further added to his sense of distrust. This paralleled his first presentation at the GP where no organic cause could be found for physical ailments.

Jason still believes that he is at risk of being poisoned by his victim's associates. These beliefs keep him stuck in the trauma of the past, replicating the sense that he will never be free or safe. They have reinforced core beliefs which originated in childhood: that the world is not safe, that people will hurt him, and that he is defective. Killing his victim reinforced his sense of defectiveness and provided an explanation for his mistreatment. His punishment is now justified, in the way it felt justified as a child, but never was.

The child part of him, which remains frozen in trauma, continues to express and reach out for care. Its needs are dismissed and remain unheard. His somatisation of distress through physical ailments/pain, associated with poisoning and its residual effects, is postulated to be an attempt to gain care. This was the only way he could elicit care as a child and adolescent. Unfortunately, now, confirmation of a physical reason for the pain he feels reinforces his belief that he is not safe, while denial of a physical reason for his pain reinforces the sense that he will not be cared for and that he cannot trust others. Once again, this leads to a re-enactment of his trauma.

Conclusions

In this chapter we have discussed the pathway from trauma through psychosis to violence. We have embedded this within the current literature and highlighted relevant case examples. As illustrated, there is "method to madness", clear evidence for the need to understand and make sense of what is being communicated through delusional and/or psychotic experience. It is therefore vital to look beyond diagnostic frameworks and to ask, "what happened to you?" In doing so we can explore the function of hypervigilance, the parallels with childhood experience, and the efforts to avoid further victimisation. In these examples we can see that individual efforts to escape trauma led to re-enactment, keeping the victim trapped by their own means and creating other victims of trauma.

There are several barriers to working with this patient group, and we hope that those challenges are illustrated within the case examples. The development of a trusting relationship is clearly the biggest challenge, and the most important as a therapeutic factor. The relational impact of trauma and therefore the importance of connection within the therapeutic relationship has also been illustrated as key; trauma is fundamentally a chronic disruption of connection, and as such connection is essential to recovery. Given this the therapist may be pushed and pulled as a symbolic representation of the patient's experience of disorganised attachments in the past. Learning to sit with them in the chaos, uncertainty and fear is key to this process.

The exact mechanism that links trauma to psychosis needs further exploration. However, several key characteristics are emerging:

- Firstly, the child experiences trauma where they are unable to mobilise, either related to the relational trap, or Porges's (2011) "Freeze" state.
- Secondly, there remains an inability to accurately detect affective states of others, and the environment, or to integrate contextual information and/or an overreliance or prioritisation of feedback from the threat system or parasympathetic ANS (dorsal-vagal branch) (Hardy, 2017; Porges, 2011).
- Thirdly, the adaptive survival responses override the other systems in response to this threat, particularly linked to social engagement and connection (Dana, 2018; Gilbert, 2009). The interpretation of information is distorted in a way that the individual experiences the past, and therefore the threat, as present.

We posit that this process of paranoid overcontrol is an effort to avoid fear which focuses attention and recall on fear. In trying to understand their bodily reactions to this threat, they focus on the need to survive rather than to thrive. Connection, which would be the antidote to their experience, is dismissed. This process keeps the person frozen in a reality which is based in past trauma and drives future trauma. For the men in our service, the use of violence is a defence against fear, one which does not allow them to escape from the original trauma, and one that reinforces their sense of defectiveness and lack of connectedness. Levine and Frederick (1997) comment that much of the violence that plagues humanity is the result of unresolved trauma and attempts to establish empowerment. Psychosis or delusional belief systems can facilitate the use of violence, providing justification and thereby making the act more tolerable. The urge to solve trauma through re-enactment can be severe and compulsive; we are inexorably drawn into situations that repeat the original trauma in both obvious and subtle ways.

This working model of psychosis is useful in facilitating understanding, connection, and healing. It allows us, and the patient, to better understand the function of their psychotic experience and related beliefs and enables multidisciplinary teams to respond to underlying drivers of presenting behaviours, rather than reacting to the behaviour. It limits re-traumatisation and re-enactment, further facilitating the ability to separate the past from the present, through a reduction in chronic levels of arousal and greater ability to integrate contextual information when faced with trauma-based memory retrieval. The focus can therefore shift back to social connection, away from threat, thus allowing corrective emotional experience, and a healing of the "wound with the world" that Van der Hart et al. (2006) so powerfully describes.

Given the functional nature of delusions and perceptual disturbance described, we have also seen a reduction in the most disturbing symptoms (i.e., derogatory and abusive voices); there is greater integration of parts and a reduced need to make sense of the body's heightened threat response, to facilitate disconnection or overcompensation. Targeting trauma as a treatment for psychosis in our service has also contributed to reductions in risk-related ratings as measured by structured assessment measures, as well as local system clinical observation measures and progression to lower security placements.

We continue to explore this working model; early findings are promising and although the sample size is small, there is a growing number of case examples, such as those presented here, which further strengthen the hypothesis presented within this chapter. We hope that this approach will contribute to the steadily improving understanding of the trajectory of psychosis.

Further Reading

Levine, P.A., & Frederick, A. (1997). *Waking the tiger; healing trauma.* North Atlantic Books.

Moskowitz, A., Dorahy, M.J., & Schafer, I. (2019). *Psychosis, trauma and dissociation, evolving perspectives on severe psychopathology second edition,* Wiley Blackwell. For an overview of the developing understanding of psychosis and the emerging consideration of the role of trauma within this.

Porges, S.W. (2011). *The polyvagal theory: Neurophysiological foundations of emotions, attachment, communication, and self-regulation.* W. W. Norton.

References

Andrew, E.M., Gray, N.S., & Snowden, R.J. (2008).The relationship between trauma and beliefs about hearing voices: A study of psychiatric and non-psychiatric voice hearers. *Psychological Medicine, 38*(10), 1409–1717. doi:10.1017/S003329170700253X

Anwar, S., Långström, N., Grann, M., & Fazal, S. (2011). Is arson the crime most strongly associated with Psychosis? A national case-control study of arson risk in schizophrenia and other psychoses. *Schizophrenia Bulletin, 37*(3), 580–586. doi:10.1093/schbul/sbp098

Bateson, G., Jackson, D.D., Hayley, J., & Weakland, J.H. (1956).Toward a theory of Schizophrenia. *Behavioural Science, 1*, 251–264. doi:10.1002/bs.3830010402

Bebbington, P., & Freeman, D. (2017). Transdiagnostic extension of delusions: Schizophrenia and Beyond. *Schizophrenia Bulletin, 43*, 273–282. doi:10.1093/schbul/sbw191

British Psychological Society. (2013). *Classification of behaviour and experience in relation to functional psychiatric diagnosis: Time for a paradigm shift. DCP Position Statement.* BPS.

Buchanan, A., Sint, K., Swanson, J., & Rosenheck, R. (2019). Correlates of future violence in people being treated for schizophrenia. *American Journal of Psychiatry, 176*(9), 694–701. doi:10.1176/appi.ajp.2019.18080909

Corstens, D., Longden, E., McCarty-Jones, S., Waddingham, R., & Thomas, N. (2014). Emerging perspectives form the hearing voices movement: Implications for research and practice. *Schizophrenia Bulletin, 40*(S4), S285–294. doi:10.1093/schbul/sbu007

Dana, D.A. (2018). *The polyvagal theory in therapy: Engaging the rhythm of regulation.* W.W. Norton and Company.

de Sousa, P., Varese, F., Sellwood, W., & Bentall, R. (2014). Parental communication and psychosis: A meta-analysis. *Schizophrenia Bulletin, 40*, 756–768. doi:10.1093/schbul/sbt088

Fazal, S., Gulati, G., Linsell, L., Geddes, J.R., & Grann, M. (2009). Schizophrenia and violence: Systematic review and meta-analysis. *PLoS Medicine, 6*(8), e1000120. doi:10.1371/journal.pmed.1000120.

Fosse, R., Moskowitz, A., Shannon, C., & Mulholland, C. (2019). Structural brain changes in psychotic disorders, dissociative disorders, and after childhood adversity: Similarities and differences. In A. Moskowitz, M.J. Dorahy & I. Shafer (Eds), *Psychosis trauma and dissociation: Evolving perspectives on severe psychopathology* (pp.159–178). John Wiley and Sons. doi:10.1002/9781118585948.ch10

Gilbert, P. (2009). *The compassionate mind: A new approach to life's challenges.* Constable and Robinson.

Green, K., Browne, K., & Chou, S. (2017). The relationship between childhood maltreatment and violence to others in individuals with psychosis: A systematic review and meta-analysis. *Trauma, Violence and Abuse, 20*(3), 358–373. doi:10.1177/1524838017708786.

Gumley, A., & Liotti, G. (2019). An attachment perspective on schizophrenia, the role of disorganised attachment, dissociation and mentalisation. In A. Moskowitz, M.J. Dorahy & I. Shafer (Eds), *Psychosis trauma and dissociation: Evolving perspectives on severe psychopathology* (pp.97–116). John Wiley & Sons Ltd.

Hardy, A. (2017). Pathways from trauma to psychotic experience. A theoretically informed model of posttraumatic stress in psychosis. *Frontiers in Psychology, 8*, 697. doi:10.3389?fp syg.2017.00697

Karatzias, T., Shevlin, M., Pitcairn, J., Thomson, L., Mahoney, A., & Hyland, P. (2019). Childhood adversity and psychosis in detained inpatients from medium to high secured units: Results from the Scottish census survey. *Child Abuse and Neglect, 96*, 104094. doi:10.1016/j.chiabu.2019.104094

Levine, P.A., & Frederick, A. (1997). *Waking the tiger; healing trauma.* North Atlantic Books.

McKenna, G., Jackson, N., & Browne, C. (2019).Trauma history in a high secure male forensic inpatient population. *International Journal of Law and Psychiatry, 66*, 101475. doi:10.1016/j.ijlp.2019.101475

Moskowitz, A., Heinmaa, M., & Van Der Hart, O. (2019). Defining psychosis, trauma and dissociation; historical and contemporary conceptions. In A. Moskowitz, M.J. Dorahy & I.

Shafer (Eds), *Psychosis trauma and dissociation: Evolving perspectives on severe psychopathology* (pp.7–27). John Wiley & Sons Ltd.

Moskowitz, A. & Montirosso, R. (2019). Childhood experiences and delusions: Trauma, memory and the double bind, A. In A. Moskowitz, M.J. Dorahy & I. Shafer (Eds), *Psychosis trauma and dissociation: Evolving perspectives on severe psychopathology* (pp.117–140). John Wiley & Sons Ltd.

Porges, S.W. (1995). Orienting in a defensive world: Mammalian modifications of our evolutionary heritage: A polyvagal theory. *Psychophysiology, 32,*301–318. doi:10.1111/j.1469-8986.1995.tb01213.x

Porges, S.W. (2004). Neuroception: A subconscious system for detecting threats and safety. *Zero to Three, 24*(5), 19–24.

Porges, S.W. (2011). *The polyvagal theory: Neurophysiological foundations of emotions, attachment, communication, and self-regulation.* W.W. Norton.

Read, J., & Bentall, R.P. (2012). Negative childhood experiences and mental health: Theoretical, clinical and primary prevention implications. *British Journal of Psychiatry, 200*(2), 89–91. doi:10.11.92/bjp.bp.111.096727

Skeem, J.L., Schubert, C., Odgers, C., Mulvey, E.P., Gardner, W., & Lidz, C. (2006). Psychiatric symptoms and community violence among high-risk patients: A test of the relationship at the weekly level. *Journal of Consulting and Clinical Psychology, 74*(5), 967–979. doi:10.1037/0022-006X.74.5.967

Storvestre, G.B., Jensen, A., Bjerke, E., Tesli, N., Rosaeg, C., Friestad, C., ... & Haukvik, U.K. (2020). Childhood trauma in persons with schizophrenia and a history of interpersonal violence. *Frontiers in Psychiatry, 11*, 383. doi:10.3389/fpsyt.2020.00383

Swanson, J.W., Swartz, M.S., Van Dorn, R.A., Elbogen, E.B., Wagner, H.R., Rosenheck, R.A., & Lieberman, J.A. (2006). A national study of violent behaviour in persons with schizophrenia. *Archives of General Psychiatry, 63*(5), 490–499. doi:10.1001/archpsyc.63.5.490

Turner, S., Harvey, C., Hayes, L., Castle, D., Galletly, C., Sweeney, S., ... & Spittal, M.J. (2020). Childhood adversity and clinical and psychosocial outcomes in psychosis. *Epidemiology and Psychiatric Sciences, 29*, e78, 1–10. doi:10.1017/S2045796019000684.

Van der Hart, O., Nijenhuis, E.R.S., & Steele, K. (2006). *The haunted self: Structural dissociation and the treatment of chronic traumatisation.* W.W. Norton &Co.

12

TRAUMA AND SEXUAL OFFENDING

Causal Mechanisms and Change Processes

Lawrence Jones

In this chapter the links between different kinds of trauma and sexual offending, in men, will be explored. Heffernen and Ward (2020), bemoaning the lack of theoretical literacy in forensic psychology, have argued that it is important to identify theoretically plausible psychological processes driving dynamic risk factors in order to make them clinically meaningful and useful. It is increasingly evident from the literature that men who offend sexually often have a range of different kinds of trauma in their histories. As with other kinds of offending, trauma in the backgrounds of people who offend sexually is often complex and pervasive. Some of these processes will be generic processes and others will be more specific to sexual offending of different kinds. Biological, psychological, and social mechanisms underpinning these links will be outlined and strategies for bringing about change based on these mechanisms will be briefly highlighted.

The processes outlined in this chapter are aimed at helping the practitioner to think about the kinds of resource loss processes (see Chapter 3) that are derived from trauma and adverse experiences that might be linked with sexual offending. Figure 12.1 offers an overview of some of the ways in which these processes contribute to offending processes.

Evidence of Links Between Trauma and Sexual Offending

Much of the evidence suggests that a combination of different kinds of abuse, the severity of abuse, and the degree of family dysfunction are associated with sexual offending (e.g., DeLisi & Beauregard, 2018; Leach, Stewart, & Smallbone, 2016; Levenson & Socia, 2016). Jespersen, Lalumière, and Seto (2009) found that sexual abuse was a significant factor in the background of those who offend sexually and that this was also linked with atypical sexual interests.

DOI: 10.4324/9781003120766-16

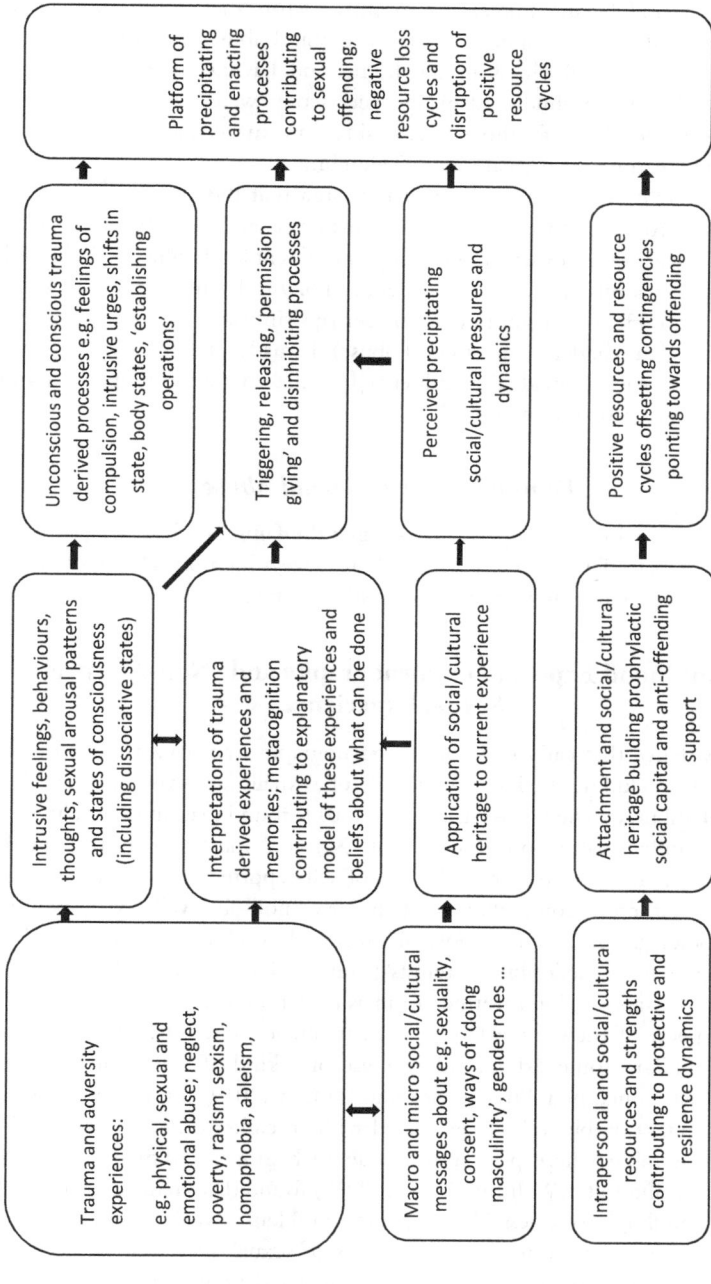

Figure 12.1 Diagrammatic illustration of ways in which trauma-derived processes can contribute to sexual offending processes

Levenson and Grady (2016) found, for male "sex offenders", factors that significantly predicted sexual deviance included histories of childhood sexual abuse, emotional neglect, and having unmarried parents. Factors that significantly predicted violent sexual offending included childhood physical abuse, substance abuse in the childhood home, mental illness in the home, and having an incarcerated family member. ACE (adverse childhood experience) scores were significantly higher for "generalist offenders" than for those "specialising" in sexual crime, suggesting different developmental pathways for each kind of offending.

Lamade (2020), in a narrative review, indicated that the overall adversity of the childhood environment should be a significant consideration, as well as looking at specifics, in the aetiology of sexual offending of different kinds. She also indicated that offenders against adults had a higher incidence of physical abuse in their backgrounds than those who offended against children (perhaps similar to violent offenders who also have a higher incidence of physical abuse). Lamade highlights that the impact of the abuse for each individual is influenced by the context it happens in and the meaning given to it by the individual.

Family History of Sexual Abuse

McCuish, Cale, and Corrado (2017) found that the families of adolescents who had committed sexual offences were more likely to have a high prevalence of abuse and sexual abuse experiences in particular, suggesting an intergenerational process.

Childhood Exposure to Pornography and "Non-Abusive" Sexual Experiences

There is evidence that early exposure to pornography can have a range of adverse consequences including an increase in risk of sexually abusive behaviour. Ybarra, Mitchell, Hamburger, Diener-West, and Leaf (2011) found that, amongst children and adolescents, intentional exposure to violent "X-rated" material over time predicted an almost six-fold increase in the chances of self-reported sexually abusive behaviour. Similarly, there is some evidence that early "non-abusive" sexual experiences such as "doctor games", seen as "normal" in sexual development, can contribute to the development of paedophilic interests (Breiling, Rettenberger, & Turner, 2020). I have put "non-abusive" in inverted commas to denote the fact that being exposed to some aspects of these experiences (e.g., frequency, intensity, and ages of those involved) could, to some extent, reflect abuse or a kind of neglect in parenting of the individuals concerned. Puszkiewicz and Stinson (2019) found that exposure to "sexual boundary problems" was associated with an earlier onset of sexually abusive behaviour. Defining where play ends and abuse begins is a difficult issue. Dillard, Maguire-Jack, Showalter, Wolf, and Letson (2019) found that victims disclosing abuse involving "fondling" were less likely to show problem sexualised behaviour (PSB) than those who had experienced other kinds of sexual abuse. However, exposure to pornography and to physical abuse was associated with PSB and suggested, in addition to power differences, exposure to coercion and objectification as a factor.

Simons, Wurtele, and Durham (2008) found that people who had offended against children reported more experiences of early exposure to pornography, sexual activities with animals, and an earlier onset of masturbation and child sexual abuse – all contexts where the individual is prematurely exposed to learning about sexual behaviour, particularly of a coercive kind.

Male Caregiver Abuse

Davis and Knight (2019) found that psychological abuse by a male caregiver may be a particularly salient factor in the development of problematic sexual interests and behaviours. Kingston, Graham, and Knight (2017) found that male caregiver psychological abuse was the most prominent correlate of hypersexual thoughts (a common risk factor linked with offending) and behaviours in adulthood, above and beyond the effects of other abuse types, such as physical abuse and sexual abuse. Together these studies suggest male caregiver abuse can have a significant impact. Clearly it is the meaning of the experience in each individual case that determines how it impacts.

Abuse by Women

Harris and Mayba (2017) found that 20.3% of a sample of 71 adult men incarcerated for serious sexual offences reported experiencing physical or sexual abuse by one or more women. Little work has been done exploring this link. Some individuals do not recognise such sexual abuse as abuse, seeing it as a desirable early sexual experience. Clinically this is an area that is often avoided due to the difficulty people have accepting that this can happen (Murphy & McVey, 2010).

Biological Processes

Trauma Causing an Alternative Development of the Brain

Sometimes conceptualised as damage to the brain, the impact of trauma on the brain can result in an, sometimes state-dependent, altered capacity to problem solve and think. Yoder, Grady, and Precht (2019) found that young people who had offended sexually had impairments in working memory, planning, and organising, and suggested that this was linked with a history of sexual abuse and with their sexual offending behaviour. Others (e.g., Creeden, 2004) have argued that one of the main links between trauma of different kinds and sexual offending is the impact of trauma on the brain. There is little literature on the interaction between unusual neuropsychological presentations and the process of meaning making in relation to traumatic experiences. It is the interaction between these very different kinds of process that we need to look to clinically.

Schmidt and Imhoff (2021) propose a difficulty in people committing child sexual offences linked with lack of skill in responding to bodily signs of adulthood, – hypothesised to be caused by "neurodevelopmental perturbations", but acknowledged to be unclear in origin, which means that they only respond to bodily signs of youth.

Whatever the source, it is not difficult to see how this kind of difficulty can result in a cascade of adverse consequences in an individual's life.

Several aspects of the neuropsychological presentation of people who have offended sexually could be attributed to sequelae of sexual or other kinds of trauma (Turner & Rettenberger, 2020). The finding that some dissociative states are linked with diminished frontal lobe activation suggests that this may be a contributory factor. Few studies look at dynamic shifts in neuropsychological functioning linked with offending (see Chapter 3).

Jones (2020a) describes the approach used in the UK prison service that explicitly targets thinking skills amongst people who offend sexually. The evidence supporting this kind of intervention comes from Travers, Mann, and Hollin (2014), who found that people who had offended sexually who had engaged in the Enhanced Thinking Skills programme were less likely to re-offend.

Each Evolved "Interpersonal System" Can Be Shaped by Adversity and Trauma

Jones (e.g., 2016, 2020b) proposed that an evolutionary approach should incorporate several biological systems (fear, dominance, sexual, attachment, and violence). Each one of these "hard wired" systems can be impacted significantly by early experiences in ways that can contribute to offending behaviour.

Early Experiences of Sexual Abuse Impacting on the Sexual System

Jones (2016, 2020b) based on work by Pfaus et al. (2012) and Miccio-Fonseca (2014) indicated that early sexual experiences can have an impact on an individual's sexual development and shape their ways of relating as well as what kinds of activity are sexually arousing for them. He highlighted the role that harmful experiences can have on sexual systems and sexual development and the link that this can have to some risk process. It is not clear to what extent this process is a longstanding learning experience. However, the findings of Ricci and Clayton (2016) that, following EMDR focusing on early traumatic sexual experiences, perpetrators no longer evidenced the same degree of offence-related sexual arousal when assessed using penile plethysmography, suggest that these kinds of apparently powerful early learning experiences can be changed.

Sexualisation

Vizard (2013) reports that inappropriate sexual knowledge, sexual interest, and sexual acting out appear to be the strongest indicators of past abuse in children. An early age of onset of being sexually abused has been shown to predict hypersexual, exposing, and victimising sexual behaviours (Vizard, 2013). This is a reaction in young people experiencing sexual arousal at an early age and then becoming sexually preoccupied and acting out with peers. It is probable that this kind of reaction is linked with premature activation of the sexual system as well as the kinds of meaning that people attribute to their experience of arousal.

Being sexually pre-occupied and repeatedly re-enacting of one's own victimisation history are not uncommon amongst children who have been sexually traumatised (e.g., Burton, 2003; Veneziano, Veneziano, & LeGrande, 2000). The question here is: what is "re-enacting" and why do children do this? Hunter (2010) suggests that this may be a process reflecting a "re-experiencing phenomenon (i.e., intrusive sexual cognitions and affects)" associated with PTSD (p.369). The child re-experiences aspects of the abuse, such as sexual feelings and thoughts, that they do not understand and cannot make sense of. This conceptualisation is Van der Kolk's (2014) formulation, whereby it is the body that experiences and replays much of what is experienced in trauma, not some intellectual cognitive process. Here it is not only fear-based experiences that return intrusively, but also sexual experiences in the context of abuse that return. This can then be an antecedent process to later sexual acting out and sexual preoccupation or compulsivity (Katehakis, 2016).

One implication of this is a "knight's move" causal process whereby a child is exposed to sexual abuse from an adult and then, in engaging in sexualised behaviour with other children, exposes other children to inappropriate sexual experiences thereby potentially impacting on their sexual development. This process can be further complicated by the active collusion, incitement, or coercion of children into engaging in sexual behaviour with other children in the context of abuse.

Erectile Dysfunction

There is evidence that for some people who have experienced sexual abuse, one reaction is problems with sexual arousal, either erectile dysfunction or a range of affective reactions linked with sexual arousal deriving from the traumatic experiences of sexual abuse. Laumann, Paik, and Rosen (1999) found that male victims of adult-child contact are three times as likely as non-victims, to experience erectile dysfunction and men who have sexually assaulted women were 3.5 times as likely to report erectile dysfunction. Erectile problems linked with diabetes or physical deformity can also be intrinsically traumatising. Whatever the origin this needs to be addressed (see Chapter 3 on interpretations of abuse-related arousal).

Clinical experience suggests that this can lead to a range of downstream consequences; some individuals describe becoming sexually frustrated and going through periods of sexual abstinence followed by periods acting out. Others describe seeking out contexts in which they can feel aroused, perhaps where feelings of fear and threat are not evident, i.e., contexts in which they are in control or where the victim is vulnerable and consequently are not experienced as posing a threat, maybe because they are using a weapon or violence of some kind, or because the victim is younger or vulnerable in some way (emotionally or cognitively). Another pathway is for the individual to seek out increasingly "extreme" sexual material to become sexually aroused, resulting in offending behaviour.

Psychological Processes

Meaning Ascribed to Sexual Arousal in the Context of Abuse

Bullock and Beckson (2011) describe how male victims of sexual assault can experience sexual arousal and ejaculation in the context of the abuse. In their review of the literature on the impact of sexual abuse on male victims, King and Woollett (1997) found that just under 20% of the men were stimulated by their assailant until they ejaculated. Bullock and Beckson also provide evidence to support sexual arousal during anal sex resulting in ejaculation in the victim. This kind of experience of arousal in the context of abuse can then lead the individual to believe that they are somehow complicit in the abuse, triggering a cascade of emotions and inferences based on this. The confusion is worsened by social narratives, including, sadly, ones used in legal contexts on occasion, where becoming aroused and ejaculation can be construed as a form of consent. Bullock and Benson also highlight that in some victims, sexual arousal is evoked by anxiety or fear. They describe evidence for a range of emotions often associated with abuse – anger, fright, and pain – being associated with sexual arousal.

Clinically helping people to understand and make sense of these processes is critical. Clinically it is important to:

- Recognise that some aspects of the self-experience during abuse are involuntary and do not represent an act of agency. Arousal, erection, and ejaculation are not acts that indicate consent on the part of the individual. Some individuals who have experienced abuse as children, often in the context of grooming, believe that what happened to them was not abusive, or that it was enjoyable. They may also believe that maintaining relationships with caregivers can justify "turning a blind eye" to abuse. This perception is then used to justify their own offending, which is construed as being enjoyable for the victims.
- Acknowledge the fact that sexual arousal, in this involuntary scenario, has been paired with feelings of rage, anxiety, or pain that may have had a significant impact on the individual's later experiences (based on the principle that early sexual experiences can become the template for later ones, e.g., Pfaus et al., 2012). They may find themselves experiencing sexual arousal later in life, primarily in contexts where these emotions are elicited.
- Look out for the mistaken inference that because they have "consented-through-arousal" therefore victims are also "consenting through their arousal". Similarly, look out for the inference, explicit or implicit, that their victim's experiences of arousal are going to be "enhanced" by experiences of pain, anxiety, or anger is mistaken.

Perpetrator Beliefs about Their Own Sexual Abuse Not Being Harmful

In order to get to a position where they are able to recognise that they have harmed the victim, perpetrators must first acknowledge that they themselves have been harmed by the experience. This work is done by exploring the consequences of the abuse on their own lives. Shifting this belief involves psychoeducation about sexual arousal and recognition that sexual arousal is not necessarily *intentional*. Attribution of intent is a significant problem in the way that people make sense of unsolicited reactions. Helping the individual to see that they did not intend to become aroused is useful in helping them recognise that they were being exploited in the act of abuse. Other attributions of intent also need to be addressed. For example, having intrusive thoughts about sexual abuse does not mean that the individual *wants* to have these thoughts.

Another approach is to look at the power difference between their perpetrator and them. Ask questions like "if an adult were to give a child heroin and they claimed to enjoy it would it be OK?". If the answer to this is "no" then using Socratic questions to elicit the reasons the individual would consider it not to be OK. Exploring the morality of having power, different kinds of privilege, the nature of innocence, powerlessness, and harm linked with trauma in the self and the victim is an important therapeutic task.

Re-enactment

Veneziano et al. (2000) found a significant correlation between the ways in which adolescent individuals offended – their age, gender, relationship with the person who offended as well as specific arousal behaviour – and what the behaviours were that they had been subjected to in the context of their own abusive experiences. For example, people who had been sexually abused before the age of five were much more likely to have abused somebody under the age of five themselves.

Shaughnessy-Mogil (2014) argues that a number of variables including age of sexual victimisation, severity of the victimisation, use of force, gender of the perpetrator, duration and frequency of abuse, and number of perpetrators differentiate those victims of sexual abuse who go on to abuse from those who do not. Burton (2000) suggests a proportional relationship between high levels of ongoing, prolonged trauma (including sexual and emotional abuse and other traumas) and possible sexual offending behaviour. In a review by Plummer (2019), older abuse onset age, over 10 years, for males, is reported to be predictive of subsequent offending and a greater chance of developing sexually intrusive behaviour before the age of 14.

Intervention with this aspect of abuse in an individual's history involves trying to develop ways of being sexual that are not paired with a need for threat or control. Part of this is working on the trauma of the abuse itself and helping the individual to process this. Another aspect is to help the individual to develop sexual interests and fantasies that do not involve coercive or violent ways of managing threat, for example, involving activating attachment experiences that also have the impact of downregulating fear or threat responses. Psychoeducation is also useful in helping the individual to understand why their sexuality has developed in the way it has.

Unprocessed Traumatic Memories

Another aspect of the link between trauma and sexual offending is the idea that some kinds of traumatic experiences are linked with a process of blocking or, at least, atypical processing of memories. This model proposes that individuals in unusually heightened states of fear arousal do not establish memories in the same way as people in everyday states of arousal. Whilst memories are formed, they are not integrated into memory in the same way. As a consequence, the memories can be triggered and played out in relatively unprocessed ways. Typically, unprocessed memories are experienced as intrusive when triggered by trauma reminders. Memories are typically conceptualised as being in the form of experiences in the body, images, smells, thoughts, states of dissociation, and interpersonal patterns of relating. These are usually unsolicited memories and experienced as intrusive, sometimes to the extent of the individual actually reliving the traumatic experience.

Prospective studies in the United States with victims brought as children to hospital after sexual abuse showed that, when interviewed, 17 and 20 years later, 38% to 40% *did not recall the abuse* that they had suffered as children and that had been reported and documented by the hospital (Widom & Shepard, 1996; Williams, 1994). Amnesia is a key element of dissociation, so this lack of recollection suggests that a dissociative process may have been in play whereby experiences are compartmentalised, unprocessed, and apparently forgotten.

In the psychodynamic literature on sexual offending, some theorists suggest that some behaviour can be the result of an intrusive memory. The behaviour itself is an intrusive phenomenon, recapitulating aspect of the individual's own traumatic experience. Examples of this might be committing an identical offence to the one that was perpetrated against them or playing out in the offence some aspects of the traumatic experience, for instance people who had experienced a lot of corporal punishment as children developing a sexual preoccupation with spanking and playing this out in the context of the offence (without necessarily making the link between the two).

Social Learning

Perhaps the most frequently used model for explaining the links between trauma and offending is social learning theory. Essentially, this model proposes that sexual offending is driven by learning experiences that result in the child learning vicariously from witnessing others' behaviour. This model is based on the assumption that witnessing another individual experiencing reward or punishment results in the individual learning about reward and punishment themselves.

Social learning can be changed by further social learning and can be reinforced by exposure to social behaviour that is similar to that which generated the problematic behaviour in the first place. There are a number of ways in which social learning can lead to both change and reinstatement of offence-related beliefs and ways of behaving outlined below.

The Role of Attachment

Barra, Bessler, Landolt, and Aebi (2018) found that juveniles who had experienced neglect and had offended sexually had anxious attachment styles that made it difficult for them to meet intimacy needs. It was hypothesised that they sexually abused children out of fear of being refused by peers. Juveniles abused by a family member were hypothesised to develop avoidant attachment styles which predicted elevated severity of sexual coercion. Peer attachment problems were hypothesised to be linked with being less popular with peers, consequently experiencing low self-esteem and turning to children with whom they could experience power and control. Grady, Looman, and Abracen (2019) found an association between childhood abuse of any kind, amongst people who had offended sexually and fearful attachment. Secure attachment was found to be a protective factor from offending.

Wyre (2000) argues that the relational characteristics of the abuse, including the nature of controlling behaviour, contribute to the chances of the victim going on to victimise others, more than the nature of the abuse itself. Social learning from caregivers is forming an internal working model in attachment terms, one which is both a source – or not as the case may be – of safety and a model for how to be an adult.

Cicchetti and Lynch (1995) reported that a range of childhood adversities may result in the failure to establish secure attachment bonds to parents, and this then leads to a range of developmental impacts. Grady et al. (2019) found in a sample of men, who had committed sexual offences, that those who had experienced childhood abuse of any kind were more likely to demonstrate a fearful or preoccupied attachment style. Those who were securely attached were less likely to engage in antisocial behaviour, and those who were more anxiously attached were less arrogant and deceptive in interpersonal relationships. Neglect is also evidenced as impacting on attachment and offending. Burton (2008) and Leibowitz, Laser, and Burton (2011) found higher levels of physical and emotional neglect amongst juvenile "sex offenders" compared to generally delinquent male adolescents. Grady, Yoder, and Brown (2018) found that sexual abuse predicted the later commission of sexual crimes with no influence from attachment style. So there is also some evidence of a possible independent pathway from sexual abuse to offending.

Jones (2020a) highlighted the way that many psychodynamic formulations of sexual offending hypothesise early (prior to the age of five) terrifying experiences of abandonment or feeling overwhelmed by the caregiver, resulting in problematic attachment. These result in unprocessed experiences of "nameless dread" and/or fear of psychological annihilation that are then played out in the offence through a process whereby the perpetrator (often unconsciously) makes the victim experience the trauma that they themselves fear, i.e., getting the victim to experience some form of nameless dread.

Therapy, in psychodynamic approaches, aims to offer a healthier attachment experience to the client which undermines the harmful version of attachment learned previously. In addition, helping the individual to understand the patterns of relating they have evolved is thought to equip the individual with the ability to prevent the patterns from being repeated.

Attachment is generally discussed in a broader way in the literature however (Jones 2020a). A common formulation for its role in the genesis of sexual offending is that it is caused by the impact of lack of secure attachment on the individual's development and the consequent lack of capacity to (a) understand their own psychological experience and those of others; (b) develop the capacity for self and emotional regulation or compassion and emotional understanding due to emotional abuse; (c) protect themselves, through an internalised secure attachment experience, from the impact of other traumatic experiences, particularly sexual abuse; and (d) develop intimacy skills and therefore turn to children out of fear of rejection from similar aged peers. Attachment difficulties can also be played out in relationships generally, resulting in problematic relationships with a greater chance of deteriorating thereby precipitating a crisis that increases the chances of offending behaviour.

There seems to be a consensus that forming a strong attachment as part of the therapy and as a way of addressing attachment traumas is a critical component of therapy with this group. This offers a reparative experience or reparenting, thereby helping the individual to develop a safe base and a healthier internal working model of relationships.

Family Secrets

Jones (2016) argued that there were a range of other trauma-related pathways for the development of sexual offending. For example, if an individual's mother believed that the individual was the product of abusive relationship with their father, then not only is the quality of attachment impacted, but also the relationship contaminated in a very specific way; the individual is a trauma trigger for the parent, and may be perceived as being like or the same as the perpetrator and responded to correspondingly.

Family secrets around parentage, where an individual is either not the child of the "father" or the result of an incestuous relationship or was conceived when the mother was underage, can impact in complex ways on narrative identity and core beliefs about self and others. Individuals may grow up with knowledge about their parentage that is unspoken or discovered at some point. They may then implicitly take up some aspects of the narrative and see themselves as being *like the perpetrator* against their mother.

Parents with difficulties in particular areas may play this out with their children. For example, wishing that they had a female child when they had a male child and dressing them up as a girl in reaction to this, and this then resulting in difficulties deriving from internalised messages about gender that then impact on later navigation towards a working sexual identity later in life.

Dissociation

Trauma-related dissociated, or partly dissociated, parts of the self can also be offence-related (Schwartz, 2016). The individual might fragment into parts that, in some way, identify with the perpetrator at the time of the offence. The dissociation might be linked with not being aware of themselves when they are in offending states. This kind of trauma experience – trauma-related beliefs and trauma-related fragmentation in the experience of self – can be addressed using standard trauma therapies that look at the origins and impacts of traumatic experience on the individual (e.g., Schwartz, 2016).

Socio-Cultural Processes

Patriarchal and Misogynistic Attitudes to Women, Sexuality, and Power as a Socially Constructed Response to the Experience of Trauma

McKibbin, Humphreys, and Hamilton (2016) describe a contrasting stance in relation to causal processes that critiques the notion of the individual being "a receptacle of biological process or as an ecologically nested identity" (p.663), preferring to construe the individual as "a socially constructed subject". Messerschmidt's (2000) life history analysis of boys who had sexually abused children theorises this offending as "performance of hegemonic masculinity", a dominant culture of masculinity that defines status in terms of activities involving dominating women and other men. This is seen as the most powerful position within the configuration of masculine subjectivities (i.e., way of experiencing masculinity in this social culture). Messerschmitt suggested that the boys abused children in order to achieve a movement from a subordinate subject position to a dominant masculine subject position.

Sexual Activity as Being Linked with Power Associated with Masculine Status

Multiple ACEs were hypothesised by Barra et al. (2018) as being linked with generalised feelings of powerlessness and loss of control – the desire to regain power being hypothesised to be amplified in poly-victims. This goal is hypothesised to be easier to attain by offending against children than against adults.

Plummer (2019), highlighting social construction of masculinities and sexualities, questions simple social learning theory models and Ward's pathways models (e.g., Ward & Siegert, 2002), arguing that people who had experienced sexual abuse and gone on to commit sexual offences differed from those who did not go on to commit sexual offences in the extent to which they saw sexual abuse as being linked with masculine identity.

Arguing that the process linking trauma to perpetration was primarily evident in males and not evident in female victims of abuse, Plummer (2019) proposed that the key link between victimisation and offending was the victim's perception that sexual activity affirmed power and masculine identity. Individuals who did not perceive their own victim experiences as being sexual were less likely to offend sexually. Sexual offending was seen as *a way of doing masculinity* linked with patriarchal attitudes. Plummer found that people who offended against children, when contrasted with people who had been sexually abused who did not offend, were more likely to interpret their abuse experience as sexual and that they identified sexuality as an area of their lives where they were more reliably to experience power. Plummer found that they were more likely to describe CSA (child sexual abuse) involving less severity, shorter duration, and less frequency and suggested this made it easier for putative offenders to deny or minimise harm. Plummer argued that the results suggest that the different interpretations of CSA experiences for offenders and non-offenders resulted in different constructions of sexuality, with offenders constructing their sexualities around control and power ... the transition from victim to offender is impacted by experiences of abuse that result in victims understanding the abuse to be sexual in nature, and that allow the victim to minimise his experience of abuse (to himself and/or to others) such that he may not self-define as a 'victim' of CSA.

pp.244–245

Plummer argues that "findings may be better explained by the Power/ Powerlessness theory, which suggests that the experience of powerlessness as an abuse victim, together with subsequent experiences of powerlessness in relationships ... may impact the transition from victim to offender" (p.267). Offenders were described as being more likely to have worries in relation to their sexual identities following sexual abuse, whereas non-offenders were more confused about the experience generally. Denial of abuse was also linked by Plummer with the victim's experience of the abuse as something they were complicit with and were aroused by and also as a strategic way of protecting their masculine status. All of these cultural perspectives can be seen as learned through a process of social learning.

This approach suggests multiple layers (e.g., in the family, in school, in care, in prison) of social denial of trauma and lack of action to protect the individual from traumatic harms – particularly as the individual becomes stigmatised with labels like conduct disordered or delinquent. Masculinity is conveyed as being:

• Achieved through the use and misuse of power and dominance;
• Treated as being about power and dominance misuse which is, moreover, 'above the law' and validated through a culture of denial and impunity;
• Achieved through internalising oppressive attitudes and habits of crushing and objectifying vulnerability and avoiding emotional awareness.

Any recurrence of a lack of responsiveness to this kind of issue in the custodial context replays this social learning. Misuse of power amongst prison officers, police, therapists, or probation officers corroborates this learning.

Whilst it is clear that this describes a cultural process linked with a predominating patriarchal set of beliefs, at its heart is the notion of the desirability and rewarding capacity of experiences of status, power, and dominance. The tension between constructivist formulations and biological formulations must, in the end, resolve around the construction an individual develops in relation to their lived embodied experiences of emotions, pleasure, consciousness, and pain. The proper domain for trauma-based formulations must be the culturally influenced meanings that people attribute to their social emotions (particularly those involving power/powerlessness, sex, fear, and attachment), feelings, and non-intentional altered states of consciousness such as dissociation, in the context of actions (seen here as fundamentally social in all aspects). A less Eurocentric formulation might involve exploring the meanings given to these experiences outside an evolutionary framework and informed by religious and cultural explanatory frameworks unique to each individual.

Intervention for this process involves using narrative strategies, to find alternative less harmful and more rewarding ways of construing masculinity, responding to powerlessness, and nurturing a more mature version of sexuality that isn't about power and control. Revisiting and re-construing early traumatic experiences of powerlessness is critical to this task.

Briere (2019) describes the importance of offering *relational disparity*, i.e., systemically and systematically endeavouring not to behave in ways that trauma has led people to expect. This dissonance then brings about change. Relational disparity involves not letting people down by being inconsistent, attending to their state and inner worlds, not behaving in ways that corroborate toxic messages about how to "do masculinity" and not playing out privilege. With time this can undermine lack of epistemic and emotional trust.

Risk Processes

Link Between Risk Factors Identified in the Literature and Sexual Offending

Chapter 1 highlights the links between trauma and generic risk. In this section more specific sexual offending risk processes are considered. Table 12.1 illustrates some examples of links between risk factors identified by Mann, Hanson, and Thornton (2010) and trauma histories. Links should be used to hypothesise about the psychological mechanisms behind dynamic risk (e.g., Heffernan & Ward, 2020) in the process of case formulation. Ricci and Clayton (2016) have also explored this approach looking at the drivers behind risk factors for sexual offending.

Table 12.1 Examples of trauma "risk" propensity processes linked with sexual offending risk factors identified by Mann, Hanson, and Thornton (2010); adapted from Jones (2016)

Risk propensity from Mann, Hanson, Thornton (2010)	*Attachment and trauma processes*	*Trauma-related sexualisation and hyper-sexuality*
Sexual pre-occupation	Sexualisation developed in context of abuse (e.g., Vizard, 2013)	Sexual thoughts intruding with high level of intensity and frequency (Katehakis, 2016)
Sexual preference for pubescent or pre-pubescent children	Abuse involved sexual contact with other children, abuse modelled by perpetrator, believed it did no harm	Hypersexuality fixated on specific trigger (Pfaus et al., 2012)
Sexualised violence	Arousal linked with anger through conditioning (e.g., Bullock & Beckson, 2011)	Sexual arousal generalised to wide range of triggers (e.g., Bullock & Beckson, 2011)

(continued)

Table 12.1 Cont.

Risk propensity from Mann, Hanson, Thornton (2010)	Attachment and trauma processes	Trauma-related sexualisation and hyper-sexuality
Paraphilic interest	Sexual behaviour shaped by unusual early sexual experiences (e.g., Pfaus et al., 2012)	Hypersexuality fixated on specific trigger (Pfaus et al., 2012)
Offence supportive attitudes	Believe it did no harm, think all people are sexual offenders, believe own arousal indicated complicity (e.g., Jones, 2016)	Sexual arousal linked with sexualised thoughts and sense of entitlement; countervailing thoughts crowded out (e.g., Jones, 2016)
Lack of emotionally intimate relationships with adults	Fear or dislike adults as they are associated with abuse, attachment trauma – betrayal trauma (i.e., by cared for caregiver) (e.g., Jones, 2016)	Acting on hypersexual impulses has lead to lack of intimate relationships (e.g., Katehakis, 2016)
Lifestyle impulsiveness	Impulsive behaviour used to avoid or distract from trauma intrusions (e.g., Jones, 2016)	Sexual impulsivity linked with sexualisation in childhood (e.g., Katehakis, 2016)
Poor problem solving	Trauma-related states impede capacity to think (Jones, 2016)	Sexual arousal inhibits capacity or willingness to think (Katehakis, 2016)
Resistance to rules and supervision	Dislike of people in authority due to abuse by adults in context of care/school	Taking a dismissive stance towards sexual boundaries
Grievance/hostility	Anger and vengeful thinking about people who have abused them or about others for not protecting them (Levenson & Grady, 2016)	Feeling persecuted by people who react to hypersexualised acting out
Negative social influences	Turn to delinquent peer group due to neglect or disaffiliation from families where abuse is taking place	Socialisation limited to others with similar hypersexual interests
Hostile beliefs about women	Witnessing sexual assaults on caregivers, hostility linked with not being believed or protected	Experiences of rejection linked with sexual acting out drive hostility towards women
Lack of concern for others/callousness	Emotional numbing, acquired callousness (Kerig & Becker, 2010)	Overwhelming states linked with arousal impede capacity to empathise or mentalise (Katehakis, 2016)

Table 12.1 Cont.

Risk propensity from Mann, Hanson, Thornton (2010)	Attachment and trauma processes	Trauma-related sexualisation and hyper-sexuality
Lack of empathy	As above	As above
Sexualised coping	Sexual abuse linked with precocious sexualisation and beliefs about sex as a way of coping (e.g., Levenson & Grady, 2016)	Stress linked with exacerbation of hyper-sexualisation

Conclusion

This chapter has explored the links between trauma and sexual offending. It has not, however, explored the other factors that contribute towards the development of sexual offending. Whilst a significant proportion of the antecedent drivers for sexual offending are trauma-linked, there are some that are not, for example, neurodiversity of different kinds. Often however these also have trauma and adversity consequences that cascade forwards and contribute to the platform of contributory factors to offending. Space does not permit an exploration of these processes. A genetic perspective needs to have a trajectory of developmental events that explains the links between the genetic disposition and the epigenetic outcome. It is likely that this trajectory has a significant element of trauma and ACE components in it.

Hopefully, this chapter has encouraged readers to explore and think about the heterogeneous trauma- and adversity-related factors linked with sexual offending and consider approaches to addressing some of these.

Further Reading

Jones L. F. (2020a). Treatment approaches to trauma for those convicted of sexual crime: Interventions globally. In H. Swaby, B. Winder, R. Lievesley, K. Hocken, N. Blagden, & P. Banyard (Eds), *Sexual crime and trauma* (pp.1–32). Palgrave.

Levenson, J. S., & Grady, M. D. (2016). The influence of childhood trauma on sexual violence and sexual deviance in adulthood. *Traumatology, 22*(2), 94–103.

References

Barra, S., Bessler, C., Landolt, M. A., & Aebi, M. (2018). Patterns of adverse childhood experiences in juveniles who sexually offended. *Sexual Abuse, 30*(7), 803–827. doi:10.1177/1079063217697135

Breiling, L., Rettenberger, M., & Turner, D. (2020). The relevance of sexual biographies in individuals convicted of child sexual abuse offenses for the development of pedosexual interests and sexual recidivism. *Sexual Offending: Theory, Research, and Prevention, 15*(1), 1–26. doi:10.5964/sotrap.3711

Briere, J. (2019). *Treating risky and compulsive behavior in trauma survivors*. Guilford.

Bullock, C., & Beckson, M. (2011). Male victims of sexual assault: Phenomenology, psychology, physiology. *Journal of the American Academy of Psychiatry and the Law, 39*(2), 195–205.

Burton, D. L. (2000). Were adolescent sexual offenders children with sexual behavior problems? *Sex Abuse: Journal of Research and Treatment, 12*(1), 37–48. doi:10.1023/A:1009511804302

Burton, D. L. (2003). Male adolescents: Sexual victimization and subsequent sexual abuse. Child and Adolescent *Social Work Journal, 20*(4), 277–296. doi:10.1023/A:1024556909087

Burton, D. L. (2008). An exploratory evaluation of the contribution of personality and childhood sexual victimization to the development of sexually abusive behavior. *Sexual Abuse: A Journal of Research and Treatment, 20*(1), 102–115. doi:10.1177/1079063208315352

Cicchetti, D., & Lynch, M. (1995). Failures in the expectable environment and their impact on individual development: The case of child maltreatment. In D. Cichetti & D. J. Cohen (Eds), *Developmental psychopathology* (Vol. 2, pp. 32–71). Wiley.

Creeden, K. (2004). Integrating trauma and attachment research into the treatment of sexually abusive youth. In M. C. Calder (Ed.), *Children and young people who sexually abuse: New theory and practice developments* (pp. 202–216). Russell House Publishing.

Davis, K. A., & Knight, R. A. (2019). Childhood maltreatment experiences and problematic sexual outcomes in adult males who have sexually offended: Further evidence of the potency of male caregiver psychological abuse. *Child Abuse & Neglect, 96,* 104097. doi:10.1016/j.chiabu.2019.104097

DeLisi, M., & Beauregard, E. (2018). Adverse childhood experiences and criminal extremity: New evidence for sexual homicide. *Journal of Forensic Sciences, 63*(2), 484–489. doi:10.1111/1556-4029.13584

Dillard, R., Maguire-Jack, K., Showalter, K., Wolf, K. G., & Letson, M. M. (2019). Abuse disclosures of youth with problem sexualized behaviors and trauma symptomology. *Child Abuse & Neglect, 88,* 201–211. doi:10.1016/j.chiabu.2018.11.019

Grady, M. D., Looman, J., & Abracen, J. (2019). Childhood abuse, attachment, and psychopathy among individuals who commit sexual offenses. *Sexual Addiction & Compulsivity, 26*(1-2), 77–102. doi:10.1080/10720162.2019.1620660

Grady, M. D., Yoder, J., & Brown, A. (2018). Childhood maltreatment experiences, attachment, sexual offending: Testing a theory. *Journal of Interpersonal Violence, 36*(11-12), NP6183–NP6217. doi:10.1177/0886260518814262

Harris, D. A., & Mayba, Y. (2017). An exploratory study of spontaneous recollections of female-perpetrated childhood abuse by men convicted of sexual offenses. *Journal of Child & Adolescent Trauma, 10*(2), 109–120. doi:10.1007/s40653-017-0134-3

Heffernan, R., & Ward, T. (2020). *Dynamic risk factors for sexual offending.* Springer.

Hunter, J. A. (2010). Prolonged exposure treatment of chronic PTSD in juvenile sex offenders: Promising results from two case studies. *Child Youth Care Forum, 39*(5), 367–384. doi:10.1007/s10566-010-9108-4

Jespersen, A. F., Lalumière, M. L., & Seto, M. C. (2009). Sexual abuse history among adult sex offenders and non-sex offenders: A meta-analysis. *Child Abuse & Neglect, 33*(3), 179–192. doi:10.1016/j.chiabu.2008.07.004

Jones, L. (2016). *Trauma and sexual offending from a developmental perspective.* Paper presented at HMP Whatton conference on sexual offending.

Jones L. F. (2020a). Treatment approaches to trauma for those convicted of sexual crime: Interventions globally. In H. Swaby, B. Winder, R. Lievesley, K. Hocken, N. Blagden, & P. Banyard (Eds), *Sexual crime and trauma* (pp. 1–32). Palgrave.

Jones, L. F. (2020b). Trauma, adverse experiences, and offence-paralleling behaviour in the assessment and management of sexual interest. In G. Akerman, D. Perkins, & R. M. Bartels (Eds), *Assessing and managing problematic sexual interests: A practitioner's guide* (pp. 251–274). Routledge. doi:10.4324/9780429287695

Katehakis, A. (2016). *Sex addiction as affect dysregulation: A neurobiologically informed holistic treatment.* Norton.

Kerig, P. K., & Becker, S. P. (2010). From internalizing to externalizing: Theoretical models of the processes linking PTSD to juvenile delinquency. In S. J. Egan (Ed.), *Posttraumatic stress disorder (PTSD): Causes, symptoms and treatment* (pp.33–78). Nova Science Publishers.

King, M., & Woollett, E. (1997). Sexually assaulted males: 115 men consulting a counselling service. *Archives of Sexual Behavior, 26*, 579–585. doi10.1023/A:1024520225196

Kingston, D. A., Graham, F. J., & Knight, R. A. (2017). Relations between self-reported adverse events in childhood and hypersexuality in adult male sexual offenders. *Archives of Sexual Behavior, 46*(3), 707–720. doi:10.1007/s10508-016-0873-5

Lamade, R. V. (2020). Trauma, assessment and management in sex offender contexts. In R. A. Javier, E. A. Owen, & J. A. Maddux (Eds), *Assessing trauma in forensic contexts* (pp.379–414). Springer.

Laumann, E. O., Paik, A., & Rosen, R. C. (1999). Sexual dysfunction in the United States: Prevalence and predictors. *JAMA, 281*(6), 537–544. doi:10.1001/jama.281.6.537

Leach, C., Stewart, A., & Smallbone, S. (2016). Testing the sexually abused-sexual abuser hypothesis: A prospective longitudinal birth cohort study. *Child Abuse & Neglect, 51*, 144–153. doi:10.1016/j.chiabu.2015.10.024

Leibowitz, G. S., Laser, J. A., & Burton, D. L. (2011). Exploring the relationships between dissociation, victimization, and juvenile sexual offending. *Journal of Trauma and Dissociation, 12*(1), 38–52. doi:10.1080/15299732.2010.496143

Levenson, J. S., & Grady, M. D. (2016). The influence of childhood trauma on sexual violence and sexual deviance in adulthood. *Traumatology, 22*(2), 94–103. doi:10.1037/trm0000067

Levenson, J. S., & Socia, K. M. (2016). Adverse childhood experiences and arrest patterns in a sample of sexual offenders. *Journal of Interpersonal Violence, 31*(10), 1883–1911. doi.org/10.1177/0886260515570751

Mann, R. E., Hanson, R. K., & Thornton, D. (2010). Assessing risk for sexual recidivism: Some proposals on the nature of psychologically meaningful risk factors. *Sexual Abuse: A Journal of Research and Treatment, 22*, 191–217. doi:10.1177/1079063210366039

McCuish, E. C., Cale, J., & Corrado, R. R. (2017). Abuse experiences of family members, child maltreatment, and the development of sex offending among incarcerated adolescent males: Differences between adolescent sex offenders and adolescent non-sex offenders. *International Journal of Offender Therapy & Comparative Criminology, 61*(2), 127–149. doi:10.1177/0306624X15597492

McKibbin, G., Humphreys, C., & Hamilton, B. (2016). Prevention-enhancing interactions: A critical interpretive synthesis of the evidence about children who sexually abuse other children. *Health & Social Care in the Community, 24*(6), 657–671. doi:10.1111/hsc.12260

Messerschmidt, J. W. (2000). Becoming "real men" adolescent masculinity challenges and sexual violence. *Men and Masculinities, 2*(3), 286–307. doi:10.1177/1097184X00002003003

Miccio-Fonseca, L. C. (2014). Family lovemap, eroticized children, and a constellation of sexually related risk variables. *Journal of Forensic Practice, 16*(1), 3–17. doi:10.1108/JFP-03-2013-0019

Murphy, M., & McVey, D. (2010). Fundamental treatment strategies for optimising interventions with people with personality disorder. In M. Murphy & D. McVey (Eds), *Treating personality disorder: Creating robust services for people with complex mental health needs* (pp.89–132). Routledge.

Pfaus, J. G., Kippin, T. E., Coria-Avila, G. A., Gelez, H., Afonso, V. M., Ismail, N., & Parada, M. (2012). Who, what, where, when (and maybe even why)? How the experience of sexual reward connects sexual desire, preference, and performance. *Archives of Sexual Behavior, 41*, 31–62. doi:10.1007/s10508-012-9935-5

Plummer, M. (2019). *Explaining the transition from victim to offender among men who experienced child sexual abuse* (Unpublished doctoral thesis). University of New South Wales School of Law.

Puszkiewicz, K. L., & Stinson, J. D. (2019). Pathways to delinquent and sex offending behavior: The role of childhood adversity and environmental context in a treatment sample of male adolescents. *Child Abuse & Neglect, 98*, 104184. doi:10.1016/j.chiabu.2019.104184

Ricci, R. J., & Clayton C. A. (2016). EMDR with sex offenders: Using offense drivers to guide conceptualization and treatment. *Journal of EMDR Practice and Research, 10*(2), 104–118. doi:10.1891/1933-3196.10.2.104

Schmidt, A. F., & Imhoff, R. (2021). Towards a theory of chronophilic sexual orientation in heterosexual men. In L. A. Craig & R. M. Bartels (Eds), *Sexual deviance: Understanding and managing deviant sexual interest and paraphilic disorders* (pp. 41–52). Wiley-Blackwell.

Schwartz, R. C. (2016). Perpetrator parts. In M. Sweezy & E. L. Ziskind (Eds), *Innovations and elaborations in internal family systems therapy* (109–123). Routledge

Shaughnessy-Mogil, M. E. (2014). *Trauma, criminalization, and movements for healing justice: A theoretical study of relational theory and transformative interventions in the treatment of juvenile sexual offending* (Unpublished Masters thesis). Smith College.

Simons, D. A., Wurtele, S. K., & Durham, R. L. (2008). Developmental experiences of child sexual abusers and rapists. *Child Abuse & Neglect, 32*, 549–560. doi:10.1016/j.chiabu.2007.03.027

Travers, R., Mann, R. E., & Hollin, C. R. (2014). Who benefits from cognitive skills programmes? Differential impact by risk and offence type. *Criminal Justice and Behavior, 41*, 1103–1129. doi:10.1177/0093854814543826

Turner, D., & Rettenberger, M. (2020). Neuropsychological functioning in child sexual abusers: A systematic review. *Aggression & Violent Behavior, 54*, 101405. doi:10.1016/j.avb.2020.101405

Van der Kolk, B. (2014). *The body keeps the score: Mind, brain and body in the transformation of trauma.* Penguin.

Veneziano, C., Veneziano, L., & LeGrande, S. (2000). The relationship between adolescent sex offender behaviors and victim characteristics with prior victimization. *Journal of Interpersonal Violence 15*(4), 363–374. Org:10.1177/088626000015004002

Vizard, E. (2013). Practitioner review: The victims and juvenile perpetrators of child sexual abuse – assessment and intervention. *Journal of Child Psychology and Psychiatry, 54*(5), 503–515. doi:10.1111/jcpp.12047

Ward, T., & Siegert, R. J. (2002). Toward a comprehensive theory of child sexual abuse: A theory knitting perspective. *Psychology, Crime and Law, 8*(4), 319–351. doi:10.1080/10683160208401823

Widom, C. S., & Shepard, R. L. (1996). Accuracy of adult recollections of childhood victimization: Part 1. *Childhood physical abuse. Psychological Assessment, 8*(4), 412–421. doi:10.1037/1040-3590.8.4.412

Williams, L. M. (1994). Recall of childhood trauma: A prospective study of women's memory of child sexual abuse. *Journal of Consulting and Clinical psychology, 62*(6) 1167–1176. doi:10.1037/0022-006X.62.6.1167

Wyre, R. (2000). Paedophile characteristics and patterns of behaviour: Developing and using a typology. In C. Itzin (Ed.), *Home truths about child sexual abuse: Influencing policy and practice, a reader* (pp. 49–69). Routledge.

Ybarra, M. L., Mitchell, K. J., Hamburger, M., Diener-West, M., & Leaf, P. J. (2011). X-rated material and perpetration of sexually aggressive behavior among children and adolescents: Is there a link? *Aggressive Behavior, 37*(1), 1–18. doi:10.1002/ab.20367

Yoder, J., Grady, M. D., & Precht, M. (2019). Relationships between early life victimization, antisocial traits, and sexual violence: Executive functioning as a mediator. *Journal of Child Sexual Abuse, 28*(6), 667–689. doi:10.1080/10538712.2019.1588819

13

THE TRAUMATIC IMPACT OF VIOLENT CRIME ON OFFENDERS

Jennifer Pink and Nicola S. Gray

Introduction

The development and emergence of post-traumatic stress disorder (PTSD) are most commonly associated with being a victim of a traumatic event. However, it is increasingly acknowledged through research and practice that, in addition to the victims of violent and sexual crimes, those who commit the offences can also develop PTSD as a result of their own actions (Gray et al., 2003). In committing offences of this nature, perpetrators witness the serious injury, sexual assault, or death involved or caused by their own offences. Offence-related trauma can lead to a full range of PTSD symptoms that can endure over time, impact longer-term mental health, and increase the risk of violence and aggression (Ternes, Cooper, & Griesel, 2020). This chapter discusses the prevalence of offence-related trauma in offending populations and illustrates through a series of case studies the survival response that some offenders may use in response to their trauma and the complexity in identifying and working with such cases. The case studies are all based on real cases, but with all identifying features changed to protect the anonymity of those involved. It concludes with a practical framework for identifying those with offence-related PTSD and working with them.

The Prevalence of Offence-Related Trauma

While the extent to which offence-related trauma is present in offending populations has not been extensively explored, several studies have identified prevalence rates ranging from around 33% to over 50% in samples of adult offenders with convictions of serious interpersonal violence. Within a group of mentally disordered adult offenders with violent and sexual index offences (n = 37), one third met the criteria for PTSD as a consequence of their offending behaviour, while over half reported symptoms of intrusion, avoidance, and hyperarousal (Gray et al., 2003). Similarly, Crisford, Dare, and Evangeli (2008) identified a prevalence rate of 40% for offence-related PTSD in

DOI: 10.4324/9781003120766-17

their mainly male sample of 45 mentally disordered violent and sexual offenders. In studies with samples of only homicide perpetrators, prevalence rates of offence-related PTSD exceeding 50% have emerged (Papanastassiou, Waldron, Boyle, & Chesterman, 2004; Pollock, 1999). Of the 80 offenders in Pollock's (1999) study, 42 met the criteria for current PTSD, with 82% of these reporting their offence as traumatic. In Papanastassiou et al.'s (2004) study, 58% of the participants had full PTSD since the index offence, and an additional 21% displayed one or more of DSM-IV's B, C, or D criteria. However, high prevalence rates of this type of trauma have not emerged in all studies in this area. Only 9% (n = 5) of a sample of adult forensic inpatients (n = 53), all with convictions for violence ranging from arson through to homicide, reported that their own offence had led to symptoms of PTSD (Spitzer et al., 2001). Interestingly, these five inpatients with offence-related trauma included all three of the sample who had committed a murder, and the remaining two were violent and sexual offenders. Therefore, while it is challenging to determine any general prevalence rates for offence-related PTSD, it appears that offence-related trauma is most prevalent in those who have offended violently but is also present in lower levels for sexual offenders.

Of further interest is a possible distinction in trauma symptomatology between violent and sexual offenders: higher levels of PTSD symptoms have been identified in violent offenders compared to levels of symptomatology in those with sexual index offences (Gray et al., 2003). This difference in prevalence and symptomology may be largely driven by the nature of the trauma caused by the offence. However, the deliberateness of the offence may also play a role in this differentiation. Violent interpersonal offences can sometimes be committed "in hot blood" when a person is angered or frightened and does not consider the possible consequences of their actions. This is often the case in forensic psychiatric populations, where the offender may be acting violently when experiencing severe mental health issues, causing them to be fearful or paranoid. Contrastingly, sexual offences are often planned, intentional, and desired (Gray et al., 2003). Thus, the traumatic reaction to committing different types of offence may be driven by both what is witnessed and experienced during the offence, and its intentionality.

In younger forensic populations, evidence suggests comparable prevalence rates to those found in adult populations. Evans, Ehlers, Mezey, and Clark (2007) conducted research with young male offenders (n = 105) with convictions for serious violent crime. Similarly high levels of offence-related PTSD symptomatology emerged to those found in the adult samples previously discussed, with 46% of the participants reporting intrusive memories related to their offence. Comparable levels of trauma symptoms emerged in another sample of young male offenders (n = 34) with convictions for serious violence or murder (Welfare & Hollin, 2015). While many of these participants reported symptoms related to their own experiences of trauma as well as their index offence, all of the offenders with an index offence of murder (n = 8) reported ruminations relating to the offence, and six reported intrusions, both experiences thought to exacerbate symptoms of PTSD and maintain the disorder (Arendt, Riisager, Larsen, Christiansen, & Moeller, 2021). Of the 26 serious violent offenders who did not have a murder conviction, only 9 reported intrusions and 6 reported ruminations related to their index offence. Thus, the type of offence committed appears to be important in the mediation of offence-related PTSD.

In addition to differing levels of prevalence and symptoms emerging for those with murder, serious violence, and sexual offence convictions, research indicates that symptoms and instances of offence-related trauma may vary depending on the nature of the relationship between victim and offender. In a large sample of male violent offenders (n = 150), Ternes et al. (2020) found that those whose victims were friends or family members experienced greater trauma symptoms than those where there was no relationship with the victim. Consistent with this, Papanastassiou et al. (2004) identified that homicide perpetrators were more likely to develop PTSD when the victim was a family member: of the 12 participants in their sample where there was a victim-offender relationship, eight had developed full PTSD, while the remaining four had developed partial PTSD. Interestingly, the victim relationship was not found to be important in Gray et al.'s (2003) sample: there was no difference in symptoms of intrusion or avoidance between offenders who had a close relationship to their victim and those offenders where the victim was previously unknown. Therefore, while not definitive, the relationship with victims may be a factor to consider when identifying instances of offence-related trauma in forensic populations.

It is important to note that prevalence rates of offence-related trauma may differ across different types of forensic population. Aside from the Ternes et al. (2020) study, many of the studies published have featured relatively small samples and focused on, or included, offender groups with high levels of mental health difficulties and per-sonality disorders (Gray et al., 2003; Papanastassiou et al., 2004; Pollock, 1999; Spitzer et al., 2001). The relatively small sample sizes are understandable given the specialist nature of the populations being studied and the difficulties in conducting this type of research, which can cause emotional dysregulation and distress in the service-users and offenders. This can raise important ethical issues in balancing the risks of com-pleting the research with the benefits of knowledge acquisition. Due to the high levels of mental disorder in the offender samples that have been investigated to date, the emerging prevalence rates of offence-related PTSD may not generalise within main-stream prison populations. Further, the prevalence of offence-related trauma may differ in female offenders as while the majority of the research has been completed with mixed-gender samples, these have mostly consisted of male offenders (Gray et al., 2003; Papanastassiou et al., 2004; Spitzer et al., 2001).

Another demographic factor largely overlooked in the literature to date is whether differences emerge in the prevalence of offence-related trauma or symptomatology between those from different racial/ethnic minority groups. Of the studies discussed here, only Evans et al. (2007) explored ethnicity and its relation to symptoms of offence-related PTSD. In their sample of young male offenders with serious violent criminal convictions, a correlation emerged between being of non-white ethnicity and reporting higher levels of PTSD symptom severity. This is an important area requiring further research and investigatory focus, particularly given a recent review (Asnaani & Hall-Clark, 2017) which suggested elevated rates of PTSD in some non-white groups. While Asnaani and Hall-Clark's review focused upon rates within the general population, it is possible that particular racial/ethnic minority groups may experience greater levels of offence-related trauma and its sequelae. This would have important treatment implications for these service-users. Furthermore, the existing data on prevalence of trauma and its sequelae may conceal the true level of those experiencing offence-related trauma, as those with trauma may be more reticent to participate in such research studies and may engage in avoidance behaviours (Spitzer et al., 2001). Therefore, it is essential to extend the research in this area to quantify the incidence of offence-related trauma across different racial/ethnic minority groups, genders, and forensic environments.

Identifying and Working with Cases of Offence-Related Trauma

Together, the research on the prevalence and the factors associated with the development of offence-related trauma provides a useful starting point for clinicians when thinking about and identifying those service users who may be experiencing offence-related trauma. Firstly, the nature of the offence should be considered, as evidence suggests that the development of offence-related PTSD is greatest in those who have committed a serious violent offence or murder. This is particularly the case if the violent act was conducted in the context of strong emotion (e.g., fear or anger). However, this does not preclude those with sexual offending or other offending histories from developing the disorder, with the likelihood of the development of symptoms of PTSD arising in violent interpersonal offenders. Secondly, the impulsivity of the offence appears to be important. Those who did not plan their offence or committed it impulsively out of rage or fear may be more likely to develop PTSD symptoms as a consequence of their offence. Thirdly, the relationship between the offender and their victim should be examined, as greater levels of symptoms have emerged in those whose victims were friends or family members. The relevance of these issues is illuminated in a case study set out below, which Gray and colleagues describe in detail in Rogers, Gray, Williams, and Kitchiner (2000).

Case Study 1: Offence-Related Trauma in the Absence of Any Pre-Existing Traumatic History

CH (Rogers et al., 2000), a 51-year-old white British woman, was convicted of manslaughter on the grounds of diminished responsibility after stabbing one of her employers in the back with a knife over 40 times. Following her conviction, CH was admitted as a mentally disordered inpatient in a medium secure unit. At the time of the offence, she was suffering from major depression, which gave grounds for the findings of diminished responsibility.

CH had been employed as a chef within a hotel for two years, and over time had built a good working relationship with both her employers, who were a married couple. However, the relationship with her female employer began to deteriorate in the three months leading up to the offence. CH perceived that her employer became increasingly critical of her, both professionally and personally (although it is possible that this perceived criticism may have been due to CH's symptoms of major depression). On the day of the offence, CH believed that her employer was critical and insulting about CH's failed marriage. This resulted in an outburst of rage and anger whereby CH stabbed her employer repeatedly, resulting in the woman's death.

Following conviction, CH was admitted to a medium secure psychiatric service. In the secure unit, CH continued to suffer from periods of severe depression over four years. Once the depression had been treated successfully, efforts were made to prepare her for community discharge and rehabilitation. As part of the preparatory work for discharge, CH came into increased contact with knives as her rehabilitation programme required her to demonstrate cooking skills. As she was encouraged to engage with knives, CH became increasingly avoidant of them, even refusing to use a knife when eating. Her avoidance of knives impacted her daily functioning, affecting her day-to-day living and future prospects for work upon release from the unit. She felt that she could not be trusted with knives and that the responsibility for the safety of others was beyond herself. She reported being "frightened by them in case they make me kill again" (Rogers et al., 2000), and she started to experience offence-related nightmares and intrusive thoughts and memories. Thus, the requirement to use a knife, a significant offence-related stimulus, as part of her rehabilitation programme triggered the acute onset of symptoms of offence-related PTSD. She began to avoid not only physical knives in her presence, but other stimuli related to knives, such as reading about or watching films about assaults using a knife, as well as talking about the offence itself and saying the victim's name. Therefore, for CH, a strong association had developed between knives and the intrusive thoughts, feelings of fear, and flashbacks to the offence.

A treatment programme was established looking at exposure to triggers to the symptoms of PTSD related to the offence. Through imaginal and live graded exposure, CH was successfully treated and later successfully discharged into the community without any further offending behaviour.

The details of CH's offence illustrate all of the earlier factors identified as placing her at greater risk for developing offence-related trauma. She had committed a violent interpersonal offence that resulted in the death of another, the attack was impulsive and unplanned, was committed in the context of extreme emotion, and CH knew the victim through working together. However, her case is also an example of offence-related trauma being triggered years after the offence itself, following a change in circumstances. The onset of offence-related trauma differs between individuals. As such, it is important to be aware that while for some it may emerge almost immediately after committing a crime, for others there may be a substantial time delay before the onset of symptoms. The onset of symptoms may correspond to the person coming into contact with stimuli that are potent triggers to traumatic symptomatology (in this case, the use of knives and cooking as part of a rehabilitative process). Prior to this, CH had been protected from these triggers due to her residence within medium secure psychiatric provision (where knives were carefully restricted, for obvious reasons).

The Association Between Pre-Existing Trauma and Offence-Related Trauma

While CH's risk factors are present in the next case study, this client (DB) had a pre-existing trauma that presented different therapeutic challenges. DB had experienced a preceding violent and sexual trauma that led to him committing a violent offence, which subsequently triggered offence-related PTSD. However, as the case study demonstrates, the initial trauma and the offence-related trauma became intertwined in terms of triggers and symptoms of trauma, requiring an integrated treatment approach. DB's case highlights the importance of identifying any prior traumatic events when working with offence-related trauma, and of carefully considering this in conjunction with what may initially appear to be triggers that are unrelated to the offence itself.

Case Study 2: Pre-Existing Single Trauma with Offence-Related Trauma

DB was a 22-year-old Afro-Caribbean British male. He arrived at a low secure forensic psychiatric unit after a court diversion process identified that he was suffering from severe PTSD. At the time of the mental health evaluation DB was on remand, having hit a woman around the head in her home with a bottle of vodka.

The year before the offence, DB had shared a cell with another prisoner while he was serving a short prison sentence for burglary. He had no previous offences for violence. One evening DB's cellmate tied him up as he told him he was planning to escape and had informed DB that it would look better for him if it appeared that he had been overpowered and was not part of the escape plan. However, once DB had been tied up, he was sexually assaulted and raped. His cellmate had then strangled him and left him for dead. DB was found by prison staff the following morning when the cells were unlocked. He was severely injured and unconscious and rushed to the hospital for emergency medical assistance. When he awoke in the hospital DB had extensive physical injuries and severe bruising to his face and neck. DB reported experiencing severe PTSD, beginning a few days after he regained consciousness in hospital. He endured multiple daily flashbacks and intrusive memories of the sexual assault and strangulation and displayed high levels of hypervigilance, fear, and anger. After DB's physical recovery, he was returned to prison to complete his sentence, but was extremely anxious and fearful, and became acutely suicidal. DB was therefore transferred to the healthcare wing of the prison. A few weeks later, at the completion of his sentence, DB was discharged into the community. Soon after release from prison, DB began to heavily abuse alcohol to try to cope with his symptoms of trauma, reportedly drinking up to 30 pints of lager each day.

Two months later, DB met a young woman in a local pub. They connected, and she invited him back to her house for a few more drinks. Unfortunately, as they began to kiss at her home, the young woman touched DB's neck. DB reported that her touch triggered a sudden feeling of terror associated with vivid memories and flashbacks of being strangled and raped flooding back to him, leading to an impulsive anger outburst. He grabbed the nearest thing in reach, which was a vodka bottle, hitting her around the head. DB stated that he was not aware of what he was doing until after the incident. DB was horrified by his actions and immediately telephoned the police. The young woman survived the attack but suffered a significant head injury. DB was convicted of attempted murder.

When he arrived at the low secure psychiatric unit, DB was experiencing frequent flashbacks and nightmares of the attack upon the young woman and was severely depressed. He could not bear anyone or anything to touch his neck. If anything did so, he became very frightened and was immediately explosively violent, often leading to self-harming behaviour, such as headbutting walls, punching doors, and throwing furniture. DB's sensitivity to his neck being touched even extended to the sensation of clothing against his neck. The severity of these episodes of extreme emotional dysregulation and anger outbursts delayed any opportunities for rehabilitation and discharge as his trigger point was almost unavoidable daily.

In order to treat his PTSD, its source and meaning needed to be understood. The inability to cope with being touched on the neck was clearly related to the initial trauma but was disconnected from the offence-related trauma. However, DB reported that the sensation of being touched on his neck not only triggered memories and feelings associated with him being a victim of assault, but also now images and flashbacks of his offence of violence. Somehow the two traumatic events had become intertwined. DB also reported strong feelings of guilt and remorse for the offence, especially since his victim had been nothing but kind and attentive to him. These feelings of offence-related guilt became intertwined and associated with strong feelings of embarrassment and shame for the rape he had suffered, with one emotion immediately triggering the other. DB reported that he would repeatedly ruminate about how he could have been "so stupid" to willingly allow his cellmate to tie him up prior to the rape and strangulation, thereby placing himself in such a vulnerable position. Through exploring his personal history, the clinician was able to understand the meaning of the touch to DB, how it related to his unresolved trauma from being raped, strangled, and left for dead, and how it then acted as the precipitating factor to his violent offence.

Importantly, the original trauma as a victim had become interwoven and associated with the offence-related trauma, something which DB stated he was unaware of prior to cognitive behavioural therapy. Through discussions with DB, it was clear that his self-view had completely changed and that he struggled to understand his actions in light of his personal experience of being a victim. He said, "I never thought of myself as violent, then I did this terrible thing" and "my cellmate raped and strangled me even though I had done nothing to deserve this. I then did exactly the same to Alice (the victim's name). I am just as bad as him". DB also stated that "I can understand I am vulnerable after what happened to me, but then I went and done it to someone else. I am just as bad as my attacker, if not worse, as she was just a young girl".

DB's treatment required careful exploration of the meaning of both the pre-existing trauma and the offence-related trauma, exploring the themes that connected these two traumatic experiences and their shared trigger factors. Exposure therapy and desensitisation to key triggers was completed, initially via imaginal exposure and then building to in vivo exposure. DB was provided with exposure therapy and eye movement desensitisation reprocessing (EMDR) to attempt to treat his symptoms of PTSD. Exposure therapy with DB was challenging due to his tendency to explosive violence and self-harm, often with little insight, prior warning, or control of these violent outbursts in response to strong feelings of fear and anger and symptoms of excessive arousal. Much of the therapy was conducted in the presence of two staff nurses, who were present solely to ensure the safety of the therapist and DB himself. However, the presence of other people within the therapy session caused DB to feel greater shame and reinforced his belief of being a bad person who could not be trusted. Treatment progress accelerated once it was felt that therapy was safe to progress on a one-to-one basis, with the trust placed in DB by the therapist supporting his ability to begin to challenge his own negative beliefs about himself. The therapeutic process was a difficult and lengthy process, taking almost two years of weekly therapy. The final stages of therapy involved DB allowing the therapist to touch, and then hold, his neck while he focussed on remaining calm and regulating his emotions. The establishment of mutual trust between DB and the therapist was essential for the success of this therapeutic process. It was felt that this treatment stage was important for DB's rehabilitation as, without this, he could not be considered safe to rehabilitate to the community. After completion of cognitive behavioural therapy and EMDR, DB reported few symptoms of trauma to either the pre-existing traumatic event or the offence-related trauma and was no longer explosively violent, indicating broad treatment success. However, the changes to his negative sense of self, including feelings of shame and guilt, and to his beliefs about the wider community and his own safety, did not undergo significant change.

Complex Trauma and Offence-Related Trauma

The experience of DB relates to the literature on PTSD and cognitive perspectives following personal trauma. After a personal trauma, there is thought to be a shift in previously held belief structures and life goals, which contribute to an individual's belief system and personal meanings that give direction to day-to-day living (Park, Mills, & Edmondson, 2012). Before a trauma, a person may feel safe and in control. Yet, following a traumatic experience, these belief systems and feelings of personal safety, or trust in oneself to make good decisions, may be violated. For DB, his traumatic experience of being assaulted and raped led him to feel unsafe and extremely fearful, as well as to feelings of self-blame and shame. These feelings of shame and self-blame are a common consequence of interpersonal assault and trauma (Bhuptani & Messman, 2021). Such a meaning system violation can give rise to negative appraisals of global beliefs and personal goals and may sensitise individuals to developing PTSD symptoms.

Park et al. (2012) found that, in a sample of people who had experienced a DSM-IV criterion trauma (n = 130), cognitive appraisals of goal and belief violation predicted PTSD symptoms. This is nothing new to those of us that work in trauma-informed clinical practice. However, what is important to consider here is the association between the pre-existing trauma and the offence-related trauma, and how the beliefs and meaning violations of the pre-existing traumatic incident became intertwined and associated with the beliefs and meanings of the offence-related trauma. For DB, this meant that the consequences of the pre-existing trauma could not be successfully treated without taking a simultaneous therapeutic approach to the offence-related trauma, and vice versa. It is well known that it is frequently the case that people who have committed serious offences against the person (both violent and sexually violent offences) have complex and severe pre-existing trauma histories, often stemming from interpersonal violence experienced in childhood (Fox, Perez, Cass, Baglivio, & Epps, 2015; Ternes et al., 2020; Levenson, Willis, & Prescott, 2016). This suggests that successful treatment of these pre-existing complex traumas is only possible if clinicians also address offence-related trauma and explore therapeutically how the person has connected and associated these disparate traumatic incidents. If we consider this in light of DB's case, his preceding trauma violated his meaning system, giving rise to negative appraisals of global beliefs and goals, which in combination with excessive arousal and anger outbursts led to his serious violent offence. This, in turn, sensitised him to developing PTSD symptoms as a consequence of his own offending behaviour.

More clinically complex than cases of simple PTSD (where there is a single, albeit severe, traumatic event, as with DB) are cases of offence-related PTSD where there is a history of repeated trauma or abuse during childhood and adolescence. At the time of trauma, a range of emotional reactions can arise, including fear, horror, and helplessness (Brewin & Holmes, 2003). Beyond the trauma, other emotions can develop, including anger, guilt, and shame. These are thought to result from cognitive appraisals of the trauma and its causes, and to misplaced beliefs about blame and responsibility and its longer-term implications (Brewin & Holmes, 2003). Such longstanding negative cognitive appraisals of this nature significantly impact upon later life experiences, as illustrated in research by Andrews, Brewin, Rose, and Kirk (2000). These authors found that experiencing childhood abuse, and symptoms of shame and anger towards the self and others, led to the prediction of PTSD following a violent crime in adulthood. Thus, pre-existing shame or anger arising from experiences of childhood abuse can be re-triggered when being a victim of crime within adulthood, leading to the development of crime-related PTSD. While this research explores these relationships between pre-existing trauma and the development of PTSD in *victims of crime*, it seems reasonable to consider that a similar process may apply in the development of offence-related PTSD. Shame and anger arising from complex trauma in childhood and adolescence may trigger violent offending, reinforcing pervasive feelings of shame and anger, and sensitising the individual to develop offence-related PTSD. Such an association between traumatic personal histories and elevated levels of offence-related trauma has emerged in one study: offenders who reported the greatest exposure to previous traumas, including those early in life, reported the highest level of offence-related PTSD symptoms (Payne, Watt, Rogers, & McMurran, 2008). However, as Ternes et al. (2020) notes, the exploration of this association has been limited thus far, and findings have been inconsistent (see Papanastassiou et al., 2004; Pollock, 1999).

This link between being a victim of early repeated trauma, offending in adulthood, and sensitisation to offence-related PTSD is illustrated in the case study below. These issues are more challenging to resolve therapeutically, as the different traumas constituting the repeated and complex trauma in early life become intertwined and highly associated both with each other and with the offence-related trauma. As with DB, the case set out below highlights the need for clinicians to explore the associations between prior victim experiences and the nature of a person's offending behaviour. As outlined below, there can be parallels between personal experiences of unresolved early trauma and subsequent offence-related trauma, which are important to understand within the psychological formulation and therapeutic approach. However, as AL's case below demonstrates, cases of offence-related trauma where there is pre-existing complex trauma can be challenging to treat.

Case Study 3: Pre-Existing Complex Trauma and Offence-Related Trauma

"AL" was a 20-year-old white British woman. Throughout her life, as far back as she could remember, she witnessed domestic violence in the family home. Her father would regularly come home late from work drunk, shout at and threaten her and her siblings, and physically assault her mother. On occasions, AL witnessed her older sisters being beaten and, as she grew older, her father began to periodically physically assault and hit her. As he hit her, her father would tell AL, "you're a bad person", "this is all your fault", "you deserve this", and tell her that she was "not good enough" as a daughter and as a person more generally. She described feeling useless and stupid, and struggled to make friends.

AL reported that in secondary school these issues of emotional and verbal abuse within the home by her father were replicated within school. She stated that a group of girls and boys in school would taunt and bully her, telling her that she was fat, ugly, and stupid. This led AL to isolate herself from people within school and she reported internalising the negative comments of her peers and believing that she was deserving of the emotional and physical abuse sustained by her father, and the bullying experienced at school. AL stated that she had never reported any form of abuse to a safe adult (e.g., teacher) as she felt that help would not be provided, believing that she was deserving of such treatment.

When she was 19, AL gave birth to a baby boy. The pregnancy was unplanned and was the result of a brief relationship with a neighbour who was significantly older than she was. At the time, AL was still living at home with her parents, but she decided to move out into a flat for the child's safety as her father was continuing to be abusive and violent. She tried to bring the child up alone due to the informal nature of her relationship with the child's father who, she later discovered, was already in a committed relationship with another woman. Once moving to her own accommodation, AL became isolated: she had few, if any, friends and could not rely on her mother to help her with caring for the baby as her father would not let her mother visit the flat. AL's sleep became very disrupted, and she quickly became extremely stressed and anxious, reporting that she felt that she was "not good enough" to care for the baby and was "a bad mother". When the baby was around one month old, AL began hearing derogatory voices telling her that she "was a bad person" and that her "baby hated her". AL's mental state and level of functioning deteriorated rapidly, and she struggled to cope. She reported that she prioritised feeding and changing the baby, but neglected all other aspects of her own self-care or care of the home. AL stated that her typical day involved getting up in the morning to feed the baby, but that after this she would return to bed and lie in bed all day next to the baby with the curtains drawn. She reported that she would attempt to drown out the voices by turning up the television very loudly, but that this sometimes distressed the child, reinforcing her sense of guilt and self-blame. AL subsequently stated that she felt worthless and not deserving of help or support, with the voices reinforcing her sense of worthlessness. AL became totally isolated, not leaving the home for a period of 10 days prior to the offence.

On the day of the offence, AL reported that the baby was crying, and she was unable to soothe him. She reported that the voices were telling her that she was "a terrible mother", that she was "not good enough", and "did not deserve to live". She picked up a pillow next to her, placed it over the baby's face, and smothered her baby. Shortly afterwards, AL took a large overdose of paracetamol and telephoned her mother. AL's mother arrived to find the baby was not breathing and lifeless, and her daughter unconscious. AL subsequently reported that neither the murder nor her attempted suicide was planned and that she felt that she acted on "auto-pilot" and as if she were watching someone else perform these actions from a distance.

AL was charged with infanticide and was later convicted of manslaughter due to diminished responsibility on the basis of a postpartum psychosis. She was admitted to a medium secure psychiatric facility for assessment and treatment. She was displaying symptoms of offence-related PTSD, along with complex trauma associated with the physical and emotional abuse she had suffered throughout childhood and beyond. AL's traumatic symptoms from childhood had become associated with the traumatic memories and flashbacks related to the offence, with each symptom becoming interwoven and connected. Triggers to traumatic memories from childhood would then trigger offence-related traumatic memories, and vice versa: each symptom cluster from each trauma (the childhood abuse, and the infanticide) becoming connected and acting as a potent trigger for the other.

During therapeutic sessions, attempts to work with AL on resolving her offence-related trauma would trigger thoughts and intrusive memories of childhood trauma, and vice versa. She described frequent memories of the sounds she heard while she smothered her baby, flashbacks to the face of her child after she lifted the pillow from its face, alongside experiencing nightmares of her childhood traumatic experiences and her diminished and negative sense of self. AL's arrest and police interviews following the offence, which she interpreted as highly punitive and intimidatory, became strongly associated in her mind with the abuse she had experienced at the hands of her father. Of note, there was no evidence that the police had treated AL negatively and these attributions were thought to be false and associated with a persecutory frame of self-reference. Importantly, however, AL did not attribute blame to either the police (for what she believed was punitive treatment of her) or her father for his past abusive actions towards her. Rather, she turned these attributions of blame inwards and firmly believed that she was a "terrible person" who deserved such treatment. These negative self-beliefs formed the genesis of AL's suicidal ideation and intent, and for a number of months following the infanticide AL had to be managed via close observations to ensure her continued safety and to manage a number of incidents of attempted suicide. However, due to the many instances of early trauma, which each became enmeshed with the offence-related trauma, treatment attempts were largely unsuccessful.

In EMDR sessions, AL reported being unable to focus on one traumatic event and stated that as soon as she attempted to focus on one aspect of a single trauma, many other associated traumatic memories would pop into consciousness, with all the associated emotions of fear, anxiety, guilt, and shame. This made AL feel overwhelmed emotionally and she was often unable to tolerate therapeutic sessions, becoming highly emotionally dysregulated (mainly displayed via excessive anxiety, feelings of panic, or distress and tearfulness). As such, AL would typically attempt to avoid therapeutic work and used numerous strategies of avoidance, both explicit (such as refusing to attend therapy sessions) and implicit (such as chanting silently in her head, rather than focussing on traumatic events and their meaning to her). Identifying such avoidant strategies proved difficult therapeutically and AL would often appear outwardly to be engaging, but with no sign of therapeutic progress.

AL also struggled to form therapeutic rapport and was unable to learn to trust the therapist, firmly believing that the therapist thought negatively about her and was "lying" when anything positive was said to her. This placed the therapist in a difficult situation, acting as a double-bind and an inherent dilemma: positive comments were met with strong negative affect by AL, due to her firm belief that the therapist was lying to her about this and was being disingenuous. However, neutral comments were also always interpreted negatively by AL and as "punishment" for being a bad person. Thus, much therapeutic effort was spent on attempting to address issues of interpersonal trust with the therapist, to develop therapeutic rapport, and to resolve breaches in the therapeutic relationship (such as AL's distress if the therapeutic paid her a compliment, and her belief that this was a lie). These interpersonal difficulties and AL's continued avoidant behaviour meant that little progress was made therapeutically, despite extensive and intensive engagement in psychological therapy within medium secure psychiatric services over a period of five years.

We believe that AL's case illustrates the difficulties of working with people who have experienced both complex trauma and offence-related trauma. There is also a dearth of research in this area with which to guide clinicians in the assessment and formulation process, or how they may address the many hurdles that arise when engaging these individuals in psychological therapy as part of a rehabilitative process. We would encourage researchers and scientist-practitioners to begin research into this important area of clinical practice.

A Clinical Framework for Offence-Related Trauma

Bringing together clinical experience and research in the field, we have attempted to put together a framework which we hope will be helpful to assist clinicians in identifying key issues when assessing possible cases of offence-related trauma, and when working therapeutically with those experiencing this form of trauma and its repercussions. Fundamental to both assessment and treatment is the importance of asking the right questions, as the answers given by our service users will fundamentally depend on the questions asked.

Identifying Key Issues in Cases of Offence-Related PTSD

- Was the index offence violent?
- Was the crime reactive or impulsive as opposed to planned?
- Did the offence result in death or serious injury?

- Was there a personal relationship with the victim?
- Is there an experience of pre-existing trauma in the past?
- Were previous traumatic incidents interpersonal in nature?
- If yes, was this a single (or simple) trauma or did it represent multiple and complex trauma?

Considerations When Working Therapeutically with Those Who Have Offence-Related PTSD

- How does offence-related trauma impact on rehabilitation potential and future risk of offending?
- Is there previous unresolved trauma that may as yet be unexplored or unidentified?
- Are there issues of re-enactment of trauma in sexual or aggressive acts? If so, what function does the re-enactment have for the person (e.g., in reestablishing a sense of power or control)?
- In what ways are pre-existing trauma associated with offence-related trauma in personal meaning, or similarities of events or actions of the person?
- Are the offence-related PTSD triggers associated with the triggers to pre-existing trauma and have these issues become intertwined and associated each with the other? This may make so-called simple trauma, complex.
- Do treatment strategies need to integrate consideration of both pre-existing trauma and offence-related trauma simultaneously? If so, how should this be organised and prioritised within the therapeutic framework?
- Does offence-related trauma lead to excessive arousal and affect dysregulation which increases the risk of violence to self or others? If so, this needs to be a key treatment target in terms of rehabilitation and safety planning.
- Are there core issues of guilt and shame arising from offence-related PTSD that keep the person within a negative self-view and that serve as barriers to therapeutic progress and rehabilitation?
- Are there avoidant strategies being utilised by the person that act to ensure actual or emotional disengagement in therapy? These avoidant strategies may be overt and explicit (e.g., refusing to engage in therapy or refusing to talk about the offence-related trauma) or implicit and secretive avoidance strategies (e.g., internal chanting or silent singing to avoid engagement with thoughts and memories of traumatic symptoms, or substance abuse and/or medication-seeking as attempts to numb emotional engagement). It should be remembered that severe restriction of eating can serve as an emotional avoidance strategy, effectively numbing the person's emotions and serving to distract all thoughts from everything but food and sustenance.
- Do offence-related traumatic symptoms trigger issues of dissociation or a sense of disconnection from themselves and the people around them? Can this keep the person distanced in interpersonal relationships and affective connection with others, preventing rehabilitative potential?
- Have there been elemental changes in the person's core beliefs or values, or sense of self and the future (e.g., hopelessness and helplessness) that act to prevent therapeutic progress or rehabilitation potential?

- Are there fundamental issues of interpersonal trust and suspiciousness that need to be addressed as a preliminary to trauma-focused work? If so, how are these associated with offence-related PTSD or pre-existing trauma, or both?

Further Reading

Fleurkens, P., Hendriks, L., & Minnen, A. v. (2018). Eye movement desensitization and reprocessing (EMDR) in a forensic patient with posttraumatic stress disorder (PTSD) resulting from homicide: A case study. *The Journal of Forensic Psychiatry & Psychology, 29*(6), 901–913. doi.org/10.1080/14789949.2018.1459786. For clinicians who wish to read further on the use of EMDR in offence-related trauma, this paper describes its successful use in a case of PTSD following perpetration.

Harry, B., & Resnick, P. J. (1986). Posttraumatic stress disorder in murderers. *Journal of Forensic Sciences, 31*(2), 609–613. This paper provides a further three offence-related trauma case studies which may be of interest to clinicians in the field.

References

Andrews, B., Brewin, C. R., Rose, S., & Kirk, M. (2000). Predicting PTSD symptoms in victims of violent crime: The role of shame, anger, and childhood abuse. *Journal of Abnormal Psychology, 109*(1), 69. doi:10.1037//0021-843x.109.1.69

Arendt, I., Riisager, L., Larsen, J., Christiansen, T., & Moeller, S. (2021). Distinguishing between rumination and intrusive memories in PTSD using a wearable self-tracking instrument: A proof-of-concept case study. *The Cognitive Behaviour Therapist, 14*, E15. doi:10.1017/S1754470X2100012X

Asnaani, A., & Hall-Clark, B. (2017). Recent developments in understanding ethnocultural and race differences in trauma exposure and PTSD. *Current Opinion in Psychology, 14*, 96–101. doi:10.1016/j.copsyc.2016.12.005

Bhuptani, P. H., & Messman, T. L. (2021). Self-compassion and shame among rape survivors. *Journal of Interpersonal Violence.* doi:10.1177/08862605211021994

Brewin, C. R., & Holmes, E. A. (2003). Psychological theories of posttraumatic stress disorder. *Clinical Psychology Review, 23*(3), 339–376. doi:10.1016/S0272-7358(03)00033-3

Crisford, H., Dare, H., & Evangeli, M. (2008). Offence-related posttraumatic stress disorder (PTSD) symptomatology and guilt in mentally disordered violent and sexual offenders. *Journal of Forensic Psychiatry & Psychology, 19*(1), 86–107. doi:10.1080/14789940701596673

Evans, C., Ehlers, A., Mezey, G., & Clark, D. M. (2007). Intrusive memories and ruminations related to violent crime among young offenders: Phenomenological characteristics. *Journal of Traumatic Stress, 20*(2), 183–196. doi:10.1002/jts.20204

Fox, B. H., Perez, N., Cass, E., Baglivio, M. T., & Epps, N. (2015). Trauma changes everything: Examining the relationship between adverse childhood experiences and serious, violent and chronic juvenile offenders. *Child Abuse & Neglect, 46*, 163–173. doi:10.1016/j.chiabu.2015.01.011

Gray, N. S., Carman, N. G., Rogers, P., MacCulloch, M. J., Hayward, P., & Snowden, R. J. (2003). Post-traumatic stress disorder caused in mentally ill offenders by the committing of a serious violent or sexual offence. *Journal of Forensic Psychiatry & Psychology, 14*(1), 27–43. doi:10.1080/1478994031000074289

Levenson, J. S., Willis, G. M., & Prescott, D. S. (2016). Adverse childhood experiences in the lives of male sex offenders: Implications for trauma-informed care. *Sexual Abuse, 28*(4), 340–359. doi:10.1177/1079063214535819

Papanastassiou, M., Waldron, G., Boyle, J., & Chesterman, L. P. (2004). Post-traumatic stress disorder in mentally ill perpetrators of homicide. *Journal of Forensic Psychiatry & Psychology, 15*(1), 66–75. doi:10.1080/14789940310001630419

Park, C. L., Mills, M. A., & Edmondson, D. (2012). PTSD as meaning violation: Testing a cognitive worldview perspective. *Psychological Trauma: Theory, Research, Practice, and Policy, 4*(1), 66–73. doi:10.1037/a0018792

Payne, E., Watt, A., Rogers, P., & McMurran, M. (2008). Offence characteristics, trauma histories and post-traumatic stress disorder symptoms in life sentenced prisoners. *British Journal of Forensic Practice, 10*(1), 17–25. doi:10.1108/14636646200800004

Pollock, P. H. (1999). When the killer suffers: Post-traumatic stress reactions following homicide. *Legal and Criminological Psychology, 4*, 185–202. doi:10.1348/135532599167842

Rogers, P., Gray, N. S., Williams, T., & Kitchiner, N. (2000). Behavioral treatment of PTSD in a perpetrator of manslaughter: A single case study. *Journal of Traumatic Stress, 13*(3), 511–519. doi:10.1023/A:1007793510239

Spitzer, C., Dudeck, M., Liss, H., Orlob, S., Gillner, M., & Freyberger, H. J. (2001). Post-traumatic stress disorder in forensic inpatients. *Journal of Forensic Psychiatry, 12*(1), 63–77. doi:10.1080/09585180121757

Ternes, M., Cooper, B. S., & Griesel, D. (2020). The perpetration of violence and the experience of trauma: Exploring predictors of PTSD symptoms in male violent offenders. *International Journal of Forensic Mental Health, 19*(1), 68–83. doi:0.1080/14999013.2019.1643428

Welfare, H. R., & Hollin, C. R. (2015). Childhood and offense-related trauma in young people imprisoned in England and Wales for murder and other acts of serious violence: A descriptive study. *Journal of Aggression, Maltreatment & Trauma, 24*(8), 955–969. doi:10.1080/10926771.2015.1070230

PART IV

Trauma-Responsive Treatment

14

A THERAPEUTIC COMMUNITY APPROACH TO ADDRESS HARMFUL SEXUAL BEHAVIOUR IN OLDER TEENAGERS

Karen Parish and Peter Clarke

Introduction

Glebe House is a specialist residential therapeutic community for adolescent males who display harmful sexual behaviour. This chapter provides an overview of the history and theoretical underpinnings of therapeutic communities, focusing on the Glebe House model. It then explores the impact of trauma and disrupted attachment on the development of harmful sexual behaviour. The therapeutic community model can be a useful approach to respond to complex trauma and associated behaviours. This chapter explores some of the key ways in which Glebe House addresses these issues, considering relationships, emotional regulation, power and control, learning normative social behaviour and considering development into adulthood and transition into the wider community. The chapter concludes by exploring the effectiveness of the Therapeutic Community approach.

Therapeutic Community Approach

Main (1946) coined the term *therapeutic community*, describing therapeutic communities as structured, psychologically informed environments where the social relationships, structure of the day, and activities are designed to help promote health and well-being. This approach is designed to provide a safe and containing environment where trauma can be explored and responded to.

For an organisation to move from a community that includes therapy to a therapeutic community, Main argued, requires a questioning approach which he identified

DOI: 10.4324/9781003120766-19

as a *culture of enquiry*. A culture of enquiry encourages the questioning of fundamental beliefs and practices held by professionals, questioning the roles professionals
play and the impact of their experiences on the work. Psychoanalysis supports the
development of democratic therapeutic regimes as it offers ways of understanding
and making sense of apparently irrational thoughts and behaviours. Three aspects of
psychoanalytical thinking are particularly present in therapeutic communities: the use
of psychoanalytic approaches to understand group dynamics; the use of theoretical
structures to promote reflection and thinking; and the use of psychoanalytic thinking
to understand relationship dynamics especially transference (directing feelings on to
therapist), counter-transference (therapist directing feelings onto patient), projection
(attributing undesired feelings onto others), and scapegoating (blaming others for
own difficulties).

During the Second World War the therapeutic intervention at the Northfield
Military Hospital led to a sophisticated model for understanding group dynamics.
Bion (1961) identified that working collectively with war veterans now understood
to be experiencing PTSD was beneficial. He identified that using the power and
strength of the patients as *experts by experience* can drive treatment, and that the sharing
of individuals' lived experiences can help them and the group to understand the
effects of trauma and can aid patient recovery. It was in the publication of *Experiences
in Groups* in 1961 that the ideas came together and reached prominence.

In the late 1960s, Glebe House was established as a therapeutic community by
three Quakers: Geoffrey Brogden, a probation officer; David Clark, a psychiatrist;
and David Wills, an educationalist. The therapeutic community approach adopted at
Glebe House is based on Rapoport's *Four Cornerstones*. Rapoport (1960) published
Community as Doctor which detailed his experiences and observations at the Social
Rehabilitation Unit at Belmont Hospital. Rapoport identified four characteristics
(or cornerstones) that he felt distinguished the unit as a therapeutic community and
provided a structure to assist the individual and the group to make sense of their
experiences:

- **Democracy:** the concept that each member of the community should share
  decision-making. At Glebe House the model is one of consensus which reflects
  both Quaker values and the decision-making described by Jones (1968). This gives
  opportunity to prolong discussion and increase reflection. There is a Director's
  veto to prevent unsafe or illegal decision, which is rarely used.
- **Permissiveness:** renamed *Tolerance* due to the cultural meaning of permissiveness
  changing after Rapoport's work was published, tolerance is the idea that community members might bring distressing behaviours into the community and these
  should be understood and tolerated as much as possible – with a feedback loop
  regarding the effect of behaviour on others.
- **Communalism:** the idea that the process of living together, solving the problems
  that this generates is itself a healing medium.
- **Reality-Confrontation:** this refers to the practice where the "patients" are continuously presented with interpretations of their behaviour to counteract processes of
  denial, distortion, or withdrawal. This encourages the verbalisation of thinking. It is

possible for different and apparently mutually exclusive interpretations to both be valid – in the way that at times any individual may hold conscious or unconscious core beliefs that are themselves mutually exclusive.

Kennard (1998) identifies two key principles of social psychiatry that can be applied to understand therapeutic communities: firstly, that an organisation fosters therapeutic relationships where safety, collaboration, and open communication are engrained in its structures to enhance recovery; and secondly, that treatment is more effective in organisations where genuine and appropriate responsibility and ownership for personal recovery is given to the patient. The terms *Planned Environment Therapy* and *Living/Learning Environments* have been coined to describe this structured therapeutic approach. The principles of therapeutic communities are echoed in the current thinking and principles of trauma-informed care, reaffirming the importance of the therapeutically informed environment and the need for safety, choice, collaboration, trustworthiness, and empowerment.

Although a snapshot of a therapeutic community can sometimes give the impression of a place with a degree of chaos and lack of boundaries, the framework requires a thinking approach that offers containment to those whose experience of persistent trauma has led to a world view where others cannot be trusted and emotions cannot be contained (Bath, 2008). The intervention to interrupt that process and "reset" the pattern requires persistent experiences of containment (the holding of anxiety) and reflection (the processing of thoughts and feelings). The striving to get to that functionality offers a sense of hope and improvement. The use of self and the concept of *experts by experience* provide a context that makes change achievable. Bloom (2010) highlights how the presence of trauma can impact on an organisation's ability to create a healthy culture, with the staff group experiencing the impact of transferential trauma. Bion (1961) suggests that groups that experience high levels of anxiety caused by unprocessed trauma can oscillate between three different emotional states: dependency, pairing, and fight or flight. In order to work with trauma in such an intensive environment there need to be structures in place to allow all community members, staff, and young people, the space to reflect, to process what they are experiencing, and to recognise the emotional impact this can have. This links to the culture of enquiry referenced previously. It is important that behaviour is not just experienced but time is dedicated to exploring and understanding the meaning of behaviour through a nuanced theoretically informed lens.

It is helpful to understand behaviour through the lens of misdirected communication. The attempt to reflect and think about trauma and distress in the here and now can often be met with resistance and self-protective defences, such as challenging behaviour. "The children we work with will also attack our attempts to think about and understand them. This is linked to their overwhelming sense of mistrust" (Tominson, 2004; p.112).

The fundamental principles of the therapeutic community model encourage behaviour to be understood as a means of communication and help individuals to feel respected and valued through both positive and negative experiences. These are necessary for healthy development of the individual, the group, and the wider community. This is achieved by providing healthy attachments and interdependence between people, recognising the importance of mutual need, and an understanding of wider social relationships. This helps create a safe, supportive, and containing environment that allows the individual to develop, grow, and change by actively being involved in decision-making, sharing responsibility, and ownership.

Trauma and Harmful Sexual Behaviour

Attachment theory (Bowlby, 1969) highlights the importance of the relationship between an infant and their primary caregiver. A secure attachment allows the infant the safety to explore the world knowing there is a secure base to which they can return. This learning process offers opportunity to develop emotional well-being and self-regulation, adaptability and resilience, and to form and maintain healthy relationships with others. Marshall (1993) highlights how those who offend sexually often do not form secure attachments in childhood. Marshall suggests that these attachment insecurities can result in young people experiencing developmental deficits in relation to interpersonal skills, self-esteem, and empathy. Zaniewski, Dallos, Stedmon, and Welbourne (2019) explored attachment strategies among young people who engage in harmful sexual behaviour, concluding that young people who display harmful sexual behaviour often hold complex insecure attachment strategies that have the intrusion of trauma and loss. They also found that there were intergenerational patterns of avoidant attachment with unresolved trauma and loss for these young people.

It is important to consider the impact of adverse childhood experiences on the development of harmful sexual behaviour. Felitti et al. (1998) highlight seven adverse childhood experiences (ACEs): psychological, physical, and sexual abuse; family members with mental illness or substance abuse problems; exposure to domestic violence; and a family member in prison. Felitti et al. highlight how these experiences increase the likelihood of young people experiencing difficulties in later life. Shonkoff et al. (2012) suggest that, if ACEs are continuous and unresolved, young people's bodies can produce too much cortisol, affecting the nervous and immune systems. Longo (2008) further suggests that traumatic histories can cause neurological and developmental deficits, and that adolescents who display inappropriate and harmful sexual behaviours must be viewed holistically because of these developmental factors.

McMackin, Leisen, Cusack, LaFratta, and Litwin (2002) highlight how trauma-associated feelings can be triggers for harmful sexual behaviours in adolescents. They found that 95% of the adolescents who displayed harmful sexual behaviour in their study had experienced a traumatic event and 65% were assessed as meeting the criteria for PTSD. Braga, Goncalves, Basto-Pereira, and Maia (2016) highlight a link between experiencing trauma and ACEs and increased rates of antisocial behaviour and a strong link between childhood experiences of physical and sexual abuse and adolescent aggression.

The impact of ACEs is magnified during adolescence; adolescence is a time when independence and responsibility are striven for. However, young people may not have the skills or emotional capacity to manage the change in responsibility and independence (Crittenden & Ainsworth, 1989). Ward and Siegert's (2002) Pathways Model posits that harmful sexual behaviours develop from difficulties with intimacy and social skills deficits, emotional dysregulation, distorted sexual scripts, antisocial cognition, or a combination of these factors that may affect the development of independence and responsibility. These deficits appear to originate from early ACEs and attachment difficulties. If left unresolved they can affect the individual's ability to regulate their emotions, manage relationships and trust, leading to maladaptive behaviours.

Gil and Cavanagh-Johnson (1993) highlight how adolescent sexual behaviour should be understood as a continuum between consensual behaviour at one end and sexual abuse at the other. The difficulty for professionals assessing harmful sexual behaviour is that once there has been an incident of sexual abuse, being able to distinguish between behaviours that are concerning and part of an abusive pattern and behaviours that are part of normal development can be extremely difficult. Many adolescents experiment with drugs and alcohol, risk taking behaviour, and egocentric behaviour. Often, however, these behaviours are viewed as factors that increase risk when seen through the lens of harmful sexual behaviour. If these behaviours in adolescence are considered a "normal" part of development, it could be argued that rather than being considered a risk factor they should be considered as a vulnerability that needs addressing.

Asmumssen, Fischer, Drayton, and McBride (2020) highlight how trauma-informed care can reduce the impact of ACEs if a young person is placed in an environment where there is safety, personal choice, and a degree of control, coupled with positive and trusting relationships. Elliot, Bjelajac, and Fallot (2005) highlight how recovery from trauma must be a primary goal and that this is best achieved through empowerment, personal control, and positive relationships. The therapeutic community approach provides a wide range of potential healing relationships and, as such, is an effective structure for responding to young people who have displayed harmful sexual behaviours and have a history of ACEs. The structure and containment of the therapeutic environment allows for some of the effects of these developmental deficits and childhood adversities to be addressed and responded to.

Therapeutic Community and the Importance of Relationship

Within psychotherapy there is clear reference to the importance of the therapeutic relationship/working alliance between professional and young person. It is considered to be one of the most significant factors in changing behaviour, even more important than the type of intervention model used. It is believed that a positive relationship is essential to achieve desired outcomes in treatment (Mallinckrodt, 2000). The importance of the therapeutic relationship for promoting positive outcomes is also highlighted by Horvath, Del Re, Fluckiger, and Symonds (2011). Rogers (1957) identifies conditions that are necessary for therapeutic change in clients; these are that the counsellor has congruence/genuineness in the therapeutic relationship, unconditional positive regard (warmth), and the ability to empathise and communicate empathy. Relational factors and the importance of family, peers, and intimate relationships are highlighted within the literature in relation to harmful sexual behaviour (Smallbone, 2006; Altschuler & Brash, 2004).

Young people who display harmful sexual behaviour, who have experienced ACEs and insecure attachment relationships, need to be placed within therapeutic settings that can focus on providing specially adapted environments that offer nurturance, security, and safety so that recovery can take place. Young people who have experienced ACEs will often display psychological (heightened emotional arousal or controlling behaviour) and physical (fight or flight) defences, perceiving the environment and people around them as frightening, hostile, and unsafe. The lived therapeutic experience that a therapeutic community provides can aid a young person to build the confidence to try to form relationships (Lanyado, 2001). Whilst outpatient therapeutic support can also aid these developments, some young people with significant ACEs need their primary lived experience to be therapeutic (Dockar-Drysdale, 1990).

The primary lived experience needs to contain the young person both emotionally and physically. Within a therapeutic residential setting this occurs in a variety of ways. Young people can seek and be willing to receive positive physical contact in the form of hugs, but this can also be through the young person creating situations to have physical containment through restraint and physical intervention. Within therapeutic communities the meaning of behaviour is considered and reflected on, this allows there to be a thoughtful approach to responses, early intervention to redirect behaviour and the young people having consistency and containment in the responses they receive. It offers a platform for a young person to develop alternative working models concerning their identity, relationships, and behaviour options. In considering relationships one Glebe House young person stated:

> Relationships are not easy for me; they always end up going wrong. Glebe has taught me that I don't need to use sex as a way to make friends.
>
> *Young Person DK*

Within the therapeutic community model there is a focus on the relationship between the staff and young people; these relationships are based in psychodynamic principles that highlight a two-way process, with both parties bringing conscious and unconscious dynamics. There will be expectations, assumptions, and agendas for those involved that need to be acknowledged and understood. This mutuality in the relationship is a strength of the therapeutic community model and aids the development of perspective taking and empathy.

In a therapeutic community initiating the relationship is key, being able to be with the person in the emotional place they are in, to not place significant demands or expectations on them. Within this relationship forming phase there is a focus on holding the young person in mind and providing unconditional positive regard. It is the security and trust that is developed from these relationships that allows the young person to develop relationships with peers and other community members. With secure relationships being formed there is a base from which the meaning of behaviour can be explored, understood, challenged, and redirected. The fundamental principles of the therapeutic community model help to provide healthy attachments and interdependence between people, recognising the importance of mutual need, and an understanding of wider social relationships. They provide a safe, supportive, and containing environment to help the individual to develop, grow, and change by actively being involved in decision-making, sharing responsibility, and ownership. They encourage behaviour to be understood as a means of communication.

Another advantage of the therapeutic community model is the use of group process and peer challenge. The notion of the young people being experts by experience means that the feedback they provide to each other has significant power and impact. The sense that they understand and have commonality aids connection and attachments between the young people and a voice that can be heard in a different way to the professionals around them.

Therapeutic Community, Emotional Regulation, and the Development of Empathy

Primary attachment and early child development provide children with a schema for managing their emotions. Some abused adolescents may not have the skills to manage their emotions appropriately and therefore may displace these emotions into destructive or harmful sexual behaviours. Gillespie, Mitchell, Fisher, and Beech (2012) suggest that adolescents who display harmful sexual behaviours often display difficulties with appropriate regulation of their emotions. They highlight how developing the control of this maladaptive emotional arousal, originally developed as a survival strategy, needs to be part of intervention. Hunter, Figueredo, and Malamuth (2010) highlight how children growing up in environments where there is trauma and abuse can develop a sense of the world as being highly sexualised and/or hostile. These unsafe environments can lead to heighted emotions, poor emotional literacy, and self-regulation difficulties.

The therapeutic community's emphasis on the community as container provides a safe space for emotions to be expressed and understood by the group. The slowing down of responses allows for consideration of what the meaning(s) of the behaviour exhibited is and what emotions may be driving the behaviour. Rapoport's four cornerstones model gives a structure that reinforces the containment process and the need for taking a tolerant approach in responding to challenging and emotionally led behaviour. This tolerance allows the young person the opportunity to process their emotional experiences and undertake intervention around developing emotional literacy; they are able to share experiences with other young people within the community and receive feedback in relation to impact of their behaviour on others. These factors support and promote behavioural change. One Glebe House young person spoke about his experiences struggling with his emotions, describing:

> Emotions are a bit like sticky mud, it feels like you get stuck in it and you keep falling down. Glebe is helping me to control my emotions, I have emotion cards to help me say how I am feeling when I can't find the words, and I am also learning to talk to staff and to get support.
>
> *Young Person SP*

255

Empathy is a crucial element of work with young people who display harmful sexual behaviour; being aware of their own emotions enables them to understand and respond to the emotions of others. An advantage of the therapeutic community model is the focus given to understanding meaning(s) of behaviour, attending to the emotional responses of the individual and the group, and reflecting the experiences of others.

Therapeutic Community and Working with Power and Responsibility

Adult sexual offending is often identified as having compensatory motives (Prentky, Cohen, & Seghorn, 1985). It can be motivated by anger and sadism (Knight, 1999), power and control issues (Robertillo & Terry, 2007), antisocial tendencies or high levels of impulsivity (Hazelwood, 1995; Knight, 1999). These drives can have origins in developmental deficits and trauma, such as those identified by Ward and Siegert's (2002) Pathways Model. Trauma impacts on the young person's sense of safety, choice, trust of others, and feelings of empowerment, as highlighted in the principles of trauma-informed care. When these key developmental needs are not attended to, this can lead to maladaptive behaviours forming where these needs are met inappropriately through the misuse of power and control.

Glebe House explores the use of power and control, understanding it as a key therapeutic tool – starting from a point of having a flattened hierarchy between young people and the staff, with all community members having an equal voice, sharing responsibility and control over the day-to-day running of the community. Democratic communities often use a sociological framework called *Interaction Ritual Chain Theory* (IRCT: Collins, 2004), which suggests that people seek the emotional energy that others provide, creating ritual in mutually focused emotion and attention and that this creates a shared reality. This theory considers how community expectations are negotiated, challenged, and enforced and does so by observing and analysing the power dynamics within the lived experiences rather than the structured therapy spaces. This model looks at the fluidity of power and how it moves and changes with group dynamics. It also focuses on how power is experienced by group members, considering exclusion and inclusion within those dynamics.

Bloor, McKeganey, and Fonkert (1988) highlight how power is an inherent part of social interaction. Haigh (2013) describes how power within social interactions can be both creative and destructive. When an individual experiences positive power-related interactions (such as holding a position of responsibility) they can experience motivation to repeat the behaviour, however unsuccessful or negative power-related interactions (such as bullying, using power at the expense of others) can lead to feelings of alienation and despair. Using the group process inherent in the therapeutic community model, the group can reinforce positive interactions and provide feedback and challenge to unwanted power dynamics.

Understanding power and control is a key therapeutic aim in working with young people who display harmful sexual behaviour, with feelings of inadequacy and rejection from adverse childhood experiences fuelling anger and power and control issues. It is important that young people are given opportunities to receive feedback and learn to differentiate between negative and positive power interactions, recognising that micro-aggressions in everyday life are important learning opportunities. However, macro-aggressions need to be responded to robustly. Other young people can help them to understand the difference between being feared and being respected; this is crucial and is an area that IRCT can help. It is also important that the young people experience the trust and respect that comes from having positive power interactions. There are roles within Glebe House that have status such as "chairman", which provide opportunities for this to be achieved. A Glebe House young person described his experience of the chairman role, stating:

> I have been a chairman twice, I was fired and had to work to get the role back. I lost the role for trying to manipulate a member of staff into giving me their keys. I have learnt that this was not OK, I talked to the member of staff afterwards about this, I apologised and took responsibility for my actions and how it left her feeling. I wouldn't have been able to have done this before; I would have just flounced about for a bit.
>
> *Young Person DK*

The Glebe House therapeutic community model also provides opportunities to experience offence paralleling behaviour. Offence paralleling behaviour is behaviour that mirrors the offending behaviour cycle without an offence being committed. This could be behaviour that displays issues relating to power and control, spite and jealousy, or risk-taking behaviours. This type of behaviour is connected to individual experiences, often relating to the creation of certain stressors such as thoughts, situations, emotions, and reactions that mirrored those connected with their offending (Jones, 2004). The notion of offence paralleling behaviour raises significant issues in relation to relapse, or more importantly the difference between lapse and relapse. Pithers, Marques, Gibat, and Marlatt (1983) highlight that the experience of lapse is often beneficial for the offender, as they learn to manage struggles and grow in confidence and control. It is important to recognise that the offence paralleling behaviour is likely to be rooted within complex trauma paralleling behaviour, reactive enactments of past trauma (McMackin et al., 2002).

The living/learning experience of Glebe House allows for observation and comment on these paralleling behaviours. These behaviours provide opportunities to highlight both the offending and/or trauma pattern without the intense emotions and defences that are connected to the original events. For example, jealousy within relationships in the community may provide an opportunity to make links to primary relationships, past motivations to offend, maladaptive attachment behaviours, and the impact of ACEs.

Therapeutic Community and Understanding Normative Social Behaviour

In thinking about normative social behaviour, Bandura's (1977) Social Learning Theory is key, with its notion that young people learn social behaviour through observation and imitation of social interaction, experiencing reinforcement and punishment for behaviour.

In relation to sexual offending, the role of attachment and early child development are helpful in exploring how children develop working models of social relationships and intimacy, as well as cognitive skills and moral awareness (Craissati, 2009; Rich, 2003). For young people who display harmful sexual behaviour, their childhood experiences have often involved ACEs that have shaped their view of the world, with them perceiving the world as highly sexualised and/or dangerous. The difficulty with growing up in hostile and unsafe environments is that the young person is unlikely to have positive life or sexual experiences to compensate for the trauma, and this can result in a distorted understanding of social and sexual behaviours. Young people need to experience a social environment where there is security, safety, and containment. The therapeutic community model's use of community helps the young person to understand normative social behaviour through role modelling and reinforcement.

Pearce & Haigh (2017) explore relational properties of reinforcement stating:

> This is a central mechanism in the way TCs operate. In a TC that is running well there are multiple feedbacks to members from other members and staff in every meeting, and therefore multiple opportunities for vicarious learning. This is likely to be more effective when a member identifies with the person being observed, as is common in the TC when there are personal similarities in problem type or demographics.
>
> *Pearce & Haigh, 2017; p. 87*

At Glebe House community meetings are used as a space to help think about how behaviour in the community affects others. One young person spoke about this stating:

> I am learning that if there is a problem it is helpful to talk. I can call a communications meeting; this is a special community meeting because things feel unsettled. This helps everyone to have a space to talk about what is happening; these meetings help me to feel heard.
>
> *Young Person SC*

Interaction Ritual Chain Theory aids the development of morals, values, and social rules, using the power of the group to explore the impact of behaviour on others and continuously negotiating group boundaries and expectations. IRCT is typically characterised when the young people come together, sharing experiences and emotions. This repetition generates feelings of belonging and has a longer-term impact in relation to positive emotion, and it encourages the shared values of the group to become morally charged (Collins, 2004). The process of modelling is crucial in changing behaviour through observing others undertake behaviour, being encouraged to undertake the behaviour and being provided with the opportunity to reflect and gain feedback on that behaviour. Summers-Effler (2002) highlights how not conforming to community values and expectations can lead to a lack of emotional positivity and exclusion from the group. This is often a didactic process, with overt teaching; however, within the therapeutic community model this process is embedded in the culture.

Therapeutic Community, Independence, and Transition into the Wider Community

Adolescence is a time when independence and responsibility are striven for. However, young people may not have the skills or emotional capacity to manage these changes in responsibility and independence. It is widely recognised that adolescents who display harmful sexual behaviour experience deficits in the areas of intimacy and social skills which may affect the development of independence and responsibility. When left unresolved, these deficits can lead to difficulties in regulating emotions, resulting in trust issues and maladaptive relational behaviours. Maturation is a key part of developing these skills. However, individuals with harmful sexual behaviour also need to have intervention around their sexual offending and have positive aspirations about their future in order to make the necessary changes (Farmer, McAlinden, & Maruna, 2015). A Glebe House young person spoke about their journey through Glebe House:

> I have been in care for 5 years because of my sexual behaviours, I have been at Glebe House for 2 years and 1 month and am due to leave soon. When I first came to Glebe, I was very scared about going out on my own without staff supervision because of my risks. Now I feel more confident that I can manage myself and not get into tricky situations. I have also found appropriate coping strategies. My future looks a lot brighter than it used to.
>
> *Young Person TS*

Altschuler and Brash (2004) identify seven transition domains that need to be considered: family/living, employment, peer groups, substance misuse, mental health, education, and leisure. The therapeutic community model can respond to many of these identified domains. Uggen and Staff (2001) consider the importance of employment for offenders in helping them desist from offending, concluding that work programmes appear to be more useful for adults than for adolescents, and that the quality of this employment plays a significant role. Therapeutic communities provide within their structure opportunities for individuals to take roles and responsibilities. Within Glebe House there is a role of *chairman*, a mentoring role in which young people are given the opportunity to support others, be given greater responsibility and trust, and to take responsibility, and have input into the day-to-day running of Glebe House. This role is a paid role with a clear job description and accountabilities and is regularly reviewed and appraised. This gives young people the opportunity to develop a work ethic and a sense of achievement.

Beresford and Cavet (2009) highlight how young people leaving care are particularly vulnerable during transition. Boswell, Wedge, Moseley, Dominey, and Poland (2016) undertook a 10-year longitudinal evaluation of the effectiveness of the Glebe

House therapeutic community approach. The research explored the experiences of young people in transitioning from Glebe House into adulthood and independence. Boswell et al. reported that young people often experience difficulties with physical and mental health issues, echoing the earlier research in relation to the impact of adverse childhood experiences. They also highlight how there is often a lack of support services for young people to aid them with this transition. In response to this deficit in transition support, Glebe House developed a transition service that provides support for young people for 18 months after leaving Glebe House. The *Circles of Support and Accountability* model (Nellis, 2009) was adopted as a framework to provide this support. Dominey and Boswell (2018) undertook an evaluation of the Glebe House Circles Project and highlighted how the Circles of Support and Accountability model is a useful model for young people to aid them transition from services.

Is the Therapeutic Community Model Effective?

In considering the treatment of harmful sexual behaviour, Silovsky et al. (2018) highlight how targeted intervention with young people can have a significant impact in reducing harmful sexual behaviour displayed by young people. It is important that any programme has a focus on sexual concerns, such as sexual deviance, victim profile, and the use of threat and harm (Seto and Lalumiere, 2010). In addition to sexual concerns, there also needs to be a focus on non-sexual antisocial behaviours such as aggression (Righthand et al., 2005), as well as on developmental factors, such as trauma and abuse experience, domestic violence, and mental health (Hackett et al., 2013). In order for young people to benefit from the therapeutic support available and to develop the skills necessary to lead an offence-free lifestyle, there needs to be a readiness for change. Glynn (2014) highlights in the *New Moons Model* how individuals need to build on social capital, having a network of relationships that aid the development of pro-social lifestyles. The therapeutic community model can provide a framework where these factors are addressed, both within a structured therapeutic space but also in a lived experience, as highlighted throughout this chapter.

Vanderplasschen et al. (2013) describe how therapeutic communities come with a considerable history and a long research tradition, though research into their effectiveness is limited. Malivert, Fatséas, Denis, Langlois, and Auriacombe (2012) suggest that therapeutic communities are considered effective treatment methods. However, the research evidence for them is often derived from poorly controlled studies. Condelli and Hubbard (1994) highlight that therapeutic communities are effective for reducing criminal behaviour and suggest that the length of time spent in treatment is a clear predictor of outcomes.

Boswell et al. (2016) undertook a ten-year longitudinal evaluation of Glebe House. This study reported on the effectiveness of the Glebe House model; it found a notable reduction of some very serious problems identified by its residents on arrival. The research followed 43 young people from Glebe House over a period of ten years, together with a comparison group of 43 young people who were identified as having similar issues but who were not placed at Glebe House. Boswell et al. found that

84% of young people admitted to Glebe House were not subsequently re/convicted, compared to 56% of the comparison group. Of the Glebe House cohort only one person had re/offended sexually and one violently, compared with five each of the comparison group.

The therapeutic community model at Glebe House appears to be an effective approach to address harmful sexual behaviour in older teenagers, particularly where there are issues with attachment, emotional regulation, power, and control. However, the model is intensive and needs a commitment over time. For some young people the two- to three-year placement within an environment where the primary lived experience is therapeutic is necessary to rebuild relationships and address the impact of entrenched adverse childhood experiences. However, it is important to recognise that this level of intervention is not necessary or appropriate for all and that for some young people whose experiences are less entrenched, these needs can be addressed through a less intensive therapeutic approach. The assessment of suitability into a therapeutic community is crucial to ensure that young people are appropriately placed and able to make use of the therapeutic programme so to minimise the potential for further rejection and trauma if the placement was to be unsuccessful.

Further Reading

Bion, W. R. (1961). *Experiences in groups.* For readers wanting an understanding of group process and dynamics.

Kennard, D. (1998). *An introduction to therapeutic communities.* For readers wanting an introductory text on the principles of therapeutic communities.

References

Altschuler, D. M., & Brash, R. (2004). Adolescent and teenage offenders confronting the challenges and opportunities of re-entry. *Youth Violence and Juvenile Justice, 2*(1), 72–87. doi:10.1177/1541204003260048

Asmumssen, K., Fischer, F., Drayton, E., & McBride, T. (2020). *Adverse childhood experiences: What we know, what we don't know, and what should happen next.* Early Intervention Foundation. Retrieved from www.eif.org.uk/files/pdf/adverse-childhood-experiences-report.pdf

Bandura, A. (1977). *Social learning theory.* Englewood Cliffs, NJ: Prentice Hall doi:10.1177/105960117700200317

Bath, H. (2008). The three pillars of trauma-informed care. *Reclaiming Children and Youth, 17*(3), 17–21.

Beresford, B., & Cavet, J. (2009). *Transitions to adult services by disabled young people leaving out of authority residential schools.* University of York: Social Policy Research Unit. www.york. ac.uk/inst/spru/pubs/pdf/resident.pdf

Bion, W. R. (1961). *Experiences in groups.* Tavistock Publications. doi:10.4324/9780429491986-3

Bloom, S. L. (2010). Organizational stress as a barrier to trauma-informed service delivery. In M. Becker & B. Levin (Eds), *A public health perspective of women's mental health* (pp.295–311). Springer. doi:10.1007/978-1-4419-1526-9

Bloor, M., McKeganey, N., & Fonkert, D. (1988). *One foot in Eden: A sociological study of the range of therapeutic community practice.* Routledge. doi:10.2307/2073386

Boswell, G., Wedge, P., Moseley, A., Dominey, J., & Poland, F. (2016). Treating sexually harmful teenage males: A summary of longitudinal research findings on the effectiveness of a therapeutic community. *Howard Journal of Crime and Justice, 55*, 168–187. doi:10.1111/hojo.12165

Bowlby, J. (1969). *Attachment and loss volume 1: Attachment.* Basic Books. doi:10.2307/588279

Braga, T., Goncalves, L., Basto-Pereira, M., & Maia, A. (2016). Unravelling the link between maltreatment and juvenile anti-social behaviour: A meta-analysis of prospective longitudinal studies. *Aggression and Violent Behaviour, 33,* 37–50. doi:10.1016/j.avb.2017.01.006

Collins, R. (2004). *Interaction ritual chains.* Princeton University Press. doi: 10.1515/9781400851744

Condelli, W. S., & Hubbard, R. L. (1994). Relationship between time spent in treatment and client outcomes from therapeutic communities. *Journal of Substance Abuse Treatment, 11*(1), 25–33. doi:10.1016/0740-5472(94)90061-2

Craissati, J. (2009). Attachment problems and sex offending. In A. Beech, L. Craig, & K. Browne (Eds), *Assessment and treatment of sex offenders: A handbook* (pp. 11–35). John Wiley & Sons Ltd, 2009. doi:1002/9780470714362.ch2

Crittenden, P., & Ainsworth, M. (1989). *Child maltreatment and attachment theory.* Retrieved from www.patcrittenden.com/include/docs/Crittenden_Ainsworth_1989.pdf   doi:10.1017/cbo9780511665707.015

Dockar-Drysdale, B. (1990). *The provision of primary experience. Winnicottian work with children and adolescents.* Free Association Books. doi:10.1111/j.1469-7610.1966.tb02252.x

Dominey, J., & Boswell, G. (2018). *'Why wouldn't you have a Circle?'– An evaluation of the Glebe House Circles Pilot,* Centre for Community, Gender and Social Justice, Institute of Criminology, University of Cambridge.

Elliot, D., Bjelajac, P., & Fallot, R. (2005). Trauma-informed or trauma-denied: Principles and implementation of trauma-informed services for women. *Journal of Community Psychology, 33*(4), 461–477. doi:10.1002/jcop.20063

Farmer, M., McAlinden, A-M., & Maruna, S. (2015). Understanding desistance from sexual offending: A thematic review of research findings. *Probation Journal, 62*(4), 320–35. doi:10.1177/0264550515600545

Felitti, V. J., Anda, R. F., Nordenberg, D., Williamson, D. F., Spitz, A. M., Edwards, V., ... & Marks, J. S. (1998). Relationship of childhood abuse and household dysfunction too many of the leading causes of death in adults: The adverse childhood experiences (ACE) study. *American Journal of Preventive Medicine, 56*(6), 774–786. doi:10.1016/s0749-3797(98)00017-8

Gil, E., & Cavanagh-Johnson, T. (1993). *Sexualised children, assessment and treatment of sexualised children and children who molest.* Launch Press.

Gillespie, S., Mitchell, I., Fisher, D., & Beech, A. (2012). Treating disturbed emotional regulation in sexual offenders: The potential applications of mindful self-regulation and controlled breathing techniques. *Aggression and Violent Behavior, 17*(4), 333–343. doi:10.1016/j.avb.2012.03.005

Glynn, M. (2014). *Black men, invisibility and crime: Towards a critical race theory of desistance.* Routledge. doi:10.1080/17440572.2014.932538

Hackett, S., Phillips J., Masson, H., & Balfe, M. (2013). Individual, family and abuse characteristics of 700 British child and adolescent sexual abusers. *Child Abuse Review, 22* (4), 232–245. doi:10.1002/car.2246

Haigh, R. (2013). The quintessence of a therapeutic environment. *Therapeutic Communities, 34*(1), 6–15. doi:10.1108/09641861311330464

Hazelwood. (1995). Analyzing rape and profiling the offender. In R. Hazelwood & A. Burgess (Eds), *Practical aspects of rape investigation: A multi-disciplinary approach* (pp. 155–181). CRC Press. doi:10.1201/9781315316369-7

Horvath, A., Del Re, A., Fluckiger, C., & Symonds, D. (2011). Alliance in individual psychotherapy. *Psychotherapy, 48,* 9–16. doi:10.1037/a0022186

Hunter, J. A., Figueredo, A. J., & Malamuth, N. M. (2010). Developmental pathways into social and sexual deviance. *Journal of Family Violence, 25*(2), 141–148. doi:10.1007/s10896-009-9277-9

Jones, L. F. (2004). Offence paralleling behaviour (OPB) as a framework for assessment and interventions with offenders. In A. Needs & G. Towl (Eds), *Applying psychology to forensic practice.* Blackwell Publishing. doi:10.1002/9780470693971.ch3

Jones, M. (1968). *Social psychiatry in practice: The idea of the therapeutic community.* Penguin. doi:10.2307/2093903

Kennard, D. (1998). *An introduction to therapeutic communities.* Jessica Kinsley Publishers. doi:10.1192/pb.23.8.511

Knight, R. A. (1999). Validation of a typology for rapists. *Journal of Interpersonal Violence, 14,* 297–323. doi:10.1177/088626099014003006

Lanyado, M. (2001). Daring to try again: The hope and pain of forming new attachments. *Therapeutic Communities, 22,* 5–18.

Longo, R. (2008). Risk in treatment: From relapse prevention to wellness. In M. Calder (Ed.), *Contemporary risk assessment in safeguarding children.* (pp.254–265). Russell House Publishing Ltd.

Main, T. F. (1946). The hospital as a therapeutic institution. *Bulletin of the Menninger Clinic, 10,* 66–70.

Malivert, M., Fatséas, M., Denis, C., Langlois, E., & Auriacombe, M. (2012). Effectiveness of therapeutic communities: A systematic review. *European Addiction Research. 18,* 1–11. doi:10.1159/000331007

Mallinckrodt, B. (2000). Attachment, social competencies, social support and interpersonal process in psychotherapy. *Psychotherapy Research, 10,* 239–266. doi:10.1093/ptr/10.3.239

Marshall, W. L. (1993). The role attachment, intimacy and loneliness in the etiology and maintenance of sexual offending. *Sexual and Marital Therapy, 8,* 109–121 doi:10.1080/14681990903550191

McMackin, R., Leisen, M, Cusack, J, LaFratta, J., & Litwin, P. (2002). The relationship of trauma exposure to sex offending behaviour among male juvenile offenders. *Journal of Sexual Abuse, 11*(2), 25–40. doi:10.1300/J070v11n02_02.

Nellis, M. (2009). Circles of support and accountability for sex offenders in England and Wales: Their origins and implementation between 1999–2005. *British Journal of Community Justice, 7*(1), 23–44.

Pearce, S., & Haigh, R. (2017). *The theory and practice of democratic therapeutic community treatment.* Jessica Kingsley Publishers. London.

Pithers, W. D., Marques, J. K., Gibat, C. C., & Marlatt, G. A. (1983). Relapse prevention with sexual aggressives: A self-control model of treatment and maintenance of change. In J. G. Greer & I. R. Stuart (Eds), *The sexual aggressor: Current perspectives on treatment* (pp.214–239). Van Nostrand Reinhold.

Prentky, R. A., Cohen, M. L., & Seghorn, T. K. (1985). Development of a rational taxonomy for the classification of sexual offenders: Rapists. *Bulletin of the American Academy of Psychiatry and the Law, 13,* 39–70.

Rapoport, R. N. (1960). *Community as doctor: New perspectives on a therapeutic community.* Tavistock Publications. doi:10.5694/j.1326-5377.1961.tb69703.x

Rich, P. (2003). *Understanding, assessing and rehabilitating juvenile sexual offenders.* Wiley. doi:10.1002/9781118105887

Righthand, S., Prentky, R., Knight, R., Carpenter, E., Hecker, J., & Nangle, D. (2005). Factor structure and validation of the juvenile sex offender assessment protocol (J-SOAP). *Sexual Abuse, 17*(1), 13–30. doi:10.1177/107906320501700103

Robertillo, G., & Terry, K. J. (2007). Can we profile sex offenders? A review of sex offender typologies. *Aggression and Violent Behavior, 12,* 508–519. doi:10.1016/j.avb.2007.02.010

Rogers, C. R. (1957). The necessary and sufficient conditions of therapeutic personality change. *Journal of Consulting Psychology, 21,* 95–103. doi:10.1037/h0045357

Seto, M. C., Lalumiere, M. L. (2010). What is so special about adolescent sexual offending? A review and test of explanations through meta-analysis. *Psychological Bulletin, 136* (4), 526–575. doi:10.1037/a0019700

Shonkoff, J. P., Garner, A. S.; Committee on Early Childhood, Adoption, and Dependent Care. (2012). The lifelong effects of early childhood adversity and toxic stress. *Pediatrics, 129*(1), e232–e246. doi:10.1542/peds.2011-2663

Silovsky, A., Albers, B., Tolliday, D., Wilson, S., Norvell, J., & Kissinger, L. (2018). *Rapid evidence assessment: Current best evidence in the therapeutic treatment of children with problem or harmful sexual behaviours, and children who have sexually offended.* Royal Commission into Institutional Responses to Sexual Abuse.

Smallbone, S. W. (2006). Social and psychological factors in the development of delinquency and sexual deviance. In H. E. Barbaree & W. L. Marshall (Eds), *The juvenile sex offender* (2nd ed., pp.105–127). Guilford Press. doi.org/10.1002/cbm.744

Summers-Effler, E. (2002). The micro potential for social change: Emotion, consciousness, and social movement formation. *Sociological Theory, 20*(1), 41–60. doi:10.1111/1467-9558.00150

Tominson, P. (2004). *Therapeutic Approaches in work with traumatized children and young people: Theory and practice.* Jessica Kingsley Press.

Uggen, C., & Staff, J. (2001). Work as a turning point for criminal offenders. *Corrections Management Quarterly, 5*(4), 1–15.

Vanderplasschen, W., Colpaert, K., Autrique, M., Rapp, R., Pearce, S., Broekaert, E., & Vandevelde, S. (2013). Therapeutic communities for addictions: A review of their effectiveness from a recovery-oriented perspective. *The Scientific World Journal,* 427817. doi:10.1155/2013/427817

Ward, T., & Siegert, R. J. (2002). Towards a comprehensive theory of child sexual abuse: A theory knitting perspective. *Psychology, Crime and Law, 9,* 319–351. doi:10.1080/10683160208401823

Zaniewski, B., Dallos, R., Stedmon, J., & Welbourne, P. (2019). An exploration of attachment and trauma in young men who have engaged in harmful sexual behaviours. *Journal of Sexual Aggression, 26* (3), 405–421. doi:10.1080/13552600.2019.1678688

15

CONTAINING DISTRESS

Working with Compassion in a Prison-Based Democratic Therapeutic Community

Geraldine Akerman and Nathan Joshua[1]

This chapter explores the impact and challenges of adopting a trauma-informed approach in a prison-based democratic therapeutic community (DTC) at HMP Grendon, from the perspectives of those who live and work there. Those in custody may well have experienced adversity which impacted on their life pattern. The context in which each person is located can affect their ability to address their past and process any unresolved trauma. By providing structure and, most of all, safety, the residents in a DTC can consider their previous responses and what has led to their present situation. A more naturalistic setting can allow previous problematic behaviour patterns to be demonstrated and alternatives practised. A DTC provides a culture of enquiry in which decisions can be considered and their consequences tolerated. Therapy within a custodial setting allows for the exploration of the meaning of previous responses and the impact they had on others in a safe environment. One resident will illustrate this through his journey in a DTC. The chapter will also discuss the challenges of a compassion-focused approach within a custodial setting and with residents who, although they volunteer for the intervention, would rather not be incarcerated.

The DTC model works on the premise that the environment and social relationships provide the optimal conditions for change. The DTC aims to provide a pro-social, supportive, and caring environment in which all individual, residents, and staff reach their full potential. This requires ongoing monitoring and attention. To do this while feeling constantly under threat is not an easy task. Haigh and Pearce (2017) describe how compassion and kindness are basic tenets of a DTC. It is important to create a safe environment in which people do not feel the need to be hypervigilant (Akerman, Needs, & Bainbridge, 2018).

The structure of the day provides numerous opportunities for therapeutic interactions from which to learn more about the nature of relationships. The community itself is the primary therapeutic instrument (Rapoport, 1960) and so all aspects

DOI: 10.4324/9781003120766-20

of it are under consideration (see Akerman, 2019 for further details). The DTC environment provides a corrective emotional environment in which such experiences can be processed. The importance of maintaining a trauma-informed approach to supervision, as highlighted by Varghese, Quiros, and Berger (2018), is emphasised. It is vital for staff to be able to continue their work in such stressful conditions that they have regular supervision to help process their own fears. Furthermore, the increased emotional load of containing the fear and anxiety within the community needs to be explored and processed.

The Democratic Therapeutic Community at HMP Grendon

HMP Grendon opened in 1962 as an experimental psychiatric prison and remains unique in that the whole institution is a dedicated DTC. It has been documented extensively (Genders & Player, 1995; Shine & Morris, 1999; Shuker & Sullivan, 2010).

Compassion-focused therapy (CFT) is based on the evolutionary and neuroscientific models of emotional regulation (LeDoux, 1998; Gilbert, 2010a, 2010b). Panksepp (1998) described emotions that are the most primitive and shared with other species, such as proximity seeking, panic, play, fear, and rage, which, when evoked, lead to defensive emotions (including anxiety and anger). The threat response evokes the fight, flight, or freeze reaction. CFT suggests that the second system, the drive system, motivates us towards resources. The third system is the drive for safety and contentment, soothing, and affiliation. Cozolino (2008) considers that the key to regulation of the threat system is by activation of the soothing system, which generally happens at early stages of development. This is central to the work of DTCs. Residents whose habitual response has been to react and then regret it later are encouraged to slow down their responses and consider what is happening for them in the very moment emotions are evoked. Gilbert (2010b) posits that mental health difficulties happen when the threat system is poorly regulated. This can develop from a hostile and unsupportive environment when growing up. The threat system can then be overly sensitive and continually activated. Self-criticism is a common response in this situation. Therefore, one aim of the DTC is to help move from shame to guilt, which can then lead to reparation (Taylor, Akerman, & Hocken, 2020).

The CFT approach provides a non-judgemental environment which supports personal development. Residents in the DTC at HMP Grendon have all committed interpersonal violence and coming to terms with feelings of having done this can be hard to navigate. When the victim has died it is particularly painful, especially if the victim was a loved one. It is a journey of faith that the resident is going to be able to tolerate the emotions evoked. A compassionate, containing supportive, environment is vital to enable this work. There is a fine line between accepting responsibility, living with the consequences of one's own actions, and being aware of the impact this has had on the remaining family and friends. Lucre and Corten (2012) found that CFT had a beneficial impact on those with personality problems. Finding ways to ameliorate feelings of shame and self-criticism, and to calm and sooth the threat system, is vital in this intervention.

The Structure of the DTC at HMP Grendon

When residents first arrive at HMP Grendon they spend 3–6 months on the Enhanced Assessment and Preparation Unit (EAPU) to allow them to acclimatise to the environment. The EAPU is integrated by offence type, so those with sexual and other violent convictions work together. Although they do not speak about the details of their offences, they do state what they are convicted of. A number of groups within the DTC experience increased stigmatisation, for instance those who are convicted of killing children (Jacobs & Shuker, 2019), and those who perpetrate sexual offences (Kotova & Akerman, in press). Residents learn to overcome their prejudices towards others based on their offence, but this can take some time to achieve. There are two community meetings a week and one therapy group. There are other courses to help residents to understand their emotions and the DTC processes.

Residents on therapy wings at HMP Grendon have groups every morning, generally lasting one and a half hours. The whole community meets twice a week to discuss the current business, which could involve seeking jobs, explaining behaviour, or resolving conflict. As it tends to be a large group (approximately 40 residents and 4/5 members of staff) attention is paid to group dynamics. These meetings can be loud and contentious or deep and reflective all in the space of one session. Constant attention is paid to the emotions evoked for all those present, and how it may impact then and later. Those in the room will be aware as the meeting draws to a close of the need to contain the emotions, and the importance of not taking these back to the wing. There is an inherent tension between providing the opportunity for residents to learn to express their emotions and resolve their differences, and the risk of this escalating to "anarchy" (Shine & Morris, 1999). Residents can be struck by their own ability to shout at a member of staff or another resident and then continue with the relationship, which in the past has not been the case and, at worst, has ended in violence. After the community meeting the staff team meet to debrief and consider the dynamics of the community. This provides the opportunity to draw aspects of the individual together that have previously split off, and hold them in mind, just as should have happened in their early lives. The discourse between the multi–disciplinary team contributes to a powerful inclusive environment. The difference of opinion is tolerated and modelled to residents (one of the underlying principles of a DTC, see below for further details) without recourse to acting out. The input from the residents is integral and valued alongside that of staff, as meaningful and relevant experts by experience.

Small groups (comprising eight to ten residents, and two members of staff) meet three times a week to explore the unconscious material of the group members and how it impacts throughout their lives. Much of the work includes reintegration of aspects of self that have been split off. For instance, if the person had committed a violent crime against a loved one, the emotions that led to and resulted from the offence may have been repressed and these can be felt and expressed in these small groups. This is a tentative process, as the individual takes responsibility for their actions while being able to tolerate the immense feelings evoked. Further, the understanding of why the incident happened is also vital to help ensure it does not happen again. In a

DTC, everyday events are explored in depth to understand what is being re-created. For example, a comment made in a community meeting about how those who need drugs may commit all sorts of acts to fund their habit can evoke shame in a community member who has committed acts of violence against a loved one to gain money. One individual swears at the person speaking and storms out of the room. He would be encouraged to explore this in his therapy group and express his feelings about his actions in the past and how these feelings drive him to respond in the present day. In therapy groups residents have feelings, both positive and negative, towards staff (known as transference) as they would have had in the past towards various people in their lives. The groups present the opportunity to expose and explore these feelings so they hold less heat and fire and can be seen for what they are, rather than continuing to unconsciously drive their behaviour. The staff discuss their responses to individuals (countertransference) in supervision and reflective practice.

Gilbert (2010a) encourages the cultivation of compassionate states of mind, and the DTC offers support in accessing safety and soothing. The therapy naturally encounters the hurdles, fears, and resistance to these ways of relating and feeling and seeks to overcome them. CFT promotes the giving and receiving of compassion and care, and it can be as hard for staff and resident to receive it and overcome self-criticism. The DTC and CFT aim to develop the *compassionate self* and use this as a *secure base* from which to engage with, and integrate, previous experiences which have been fragmented when in a threat-based situation (Gilbert & Irons, 2005). Gilbert (2017) suggested the use of compassion to create a safe space to enable this integration.

Traditionally, DTCs have encouraged the expression of anger and other strong emotions, but more recently Veale et al. (2014) have questioned this, arguing that this is unhelpful because it triggers other threat systems and hinders feelings of safety which are crucial for opening up and encouraging exploration. For residents who have experienced an upbringing with high expressed emotions, such as critical comments, hostility, emotional over-involvement, with a lack of positivity and warmth, this can impact on their mental health or emotional management. Therefore, Veale et al. recommend that DTCs work towards an environment of relatively low expressed emotion and trying to prevent unnecessary activation of the threat system. For this reason, DTCs, along with other accredited programmes, have moved away from discussing offences in detail, due to the levels of emotions evoked.

Nathan's Story

Introduction

With infant memories of blood on the walls, mother's screams and broken glass on the floor, my early years were scarred with the violent breakdown of my parents' marriage. Following our move to the big city, with promises of prosperity, we soon got a new stepdad, who did not drink, clearly loved my mum and, it turned out, worked hard and put food on the table. They soon married and my brother was born and along with my older sister our new family unit spelt out an idyllic childhood for most.

I was a very emotional child, struggled to settle and was needy from an early age. I have one recollection of my mother smacking me with a wooden spoon so hard that the spoon broke, although she never did anything like that again. I stole sweets and food as a child, then pinched money from my mother's purse and my stepdad's pockets. These occurrences met with attention and chores for punishment. I have recollections of him giving me the silent treatment and although I remember some good role models, I ended up in the Criminal Justice System (CJS) after stealing a car on my paper round. Whilst in no doubt that my family loved me, I already felt unable to express my feelings of abandonment and separation and by the time I was 16 my problems outgrew my family unit. At this age I was already heavily using drugs and alcohol to cope with my reality, which culminated into 30 years of addiction, homelessness, several unhealthy relationships, progressively more serious acquisitive criminality, violence and years and years of prison time. My family and authorities offered me all interventions known to the western world. These included children's homes, moving house, 12 steps, rehab, NLP, counselling, joining sports clubs, school, home-school, work programmes, financial support, detachment with or without love, anti-psychotics, opiates replacements, DTTOs[2], young offenders institutes, Enhanced Thinking Skills ad infinitum.

Research has shown that spanking children is a risk factor for violence (Straus, 2000) and when residents are asked about childhood experiences they tend to use excuse the behaviour, stating "I was naughty", or "I was always playing up", sounding as if that is how they have rationalised it in later life.

Eventually prison became a welcome break for the family and a place where I had rules and conformed, would detox, attend the gym, and plan 'going straight' with all the passion I had to muster for a better life.

Thing is, prison never facilitated tangible, compassionate change. It just reinforced submission. Prison, by its very nature, suppressed my problems. The courts, with limited options, often take traumatised offenders[3] and send us to further traumatising environments to serve our punishments, never truly addressing the root cause of my behaviour. Rather, facilitating a gradual worsening of my criminality, and the way in which I struggled to form meaningful relationships with anyone significant, led to distinct loneliness and eventual lack of empathy for victims while committing acts of robbery. All that follows is by no means written to seek to justify my behaviour, somehow setting myself up as a victim, but does intend to demonstrate that through the compassionate and safe environment, insight into one's personhood can be gained and maladjusted coping strategies challenged, replaced with healthier, more nurturing alternatives.

Sign Up and Assessment

I will now describe my stay as a resident of Grendon. Whenever I use the term 'other prisons' I mean it to encompass experience of all other interventions. These include hostels, mainstream prisons, offending behaviour programmes, etc. Whilst all of these experiences had benefits and limitations, none offered the environment of compassionate safety I believe I required for me to open up unreservedly for the therapeutic process to heal in the ways I hope to do justice to here. A bold statement I could not have made with any authority until now.

Stevens (2013) describes a common theme in presentation of offenders as "hypermasculinity" where the traits of manhood (aggression, toughness, guarded emotions) are intensified to establish dominance within the closed community group (imagined or real). Compassion Focussed Therapy (CFT) would view this as an evolutionary process to stay safe. There has been no institution where I have witnessed this presentation more evidently than the Enhanced Assessment Unit at Grendon. The contrast between senior Therapy Awareness Course (TAC) mentors[4] who were years into therapy and those newly arrived from long-term prisons was glaringly obvious. Furthermore, the commonly passive, timid polite traits I witnessed in my early days in many of those arriving from prisons having been convicted of sexual crimes and those against children, compared to many long-term violent offenders was stark. Over time, the environment is the catalyst for some to allow defences to drop and others to gain in confidence to share experiences too.

The assessment unit process was at times an overwhelming experience where two worlds collided, in contrast to the mainstream, where the written and unwritten rules are set. A hierarchy for all its hypocrisy is familiar (Joshua, 2019), and, despite its flaws, bearable. This new world is where everyone is equal, people here represent both a crime and its victims, but also as a son, father, brother, musician, artist, electrician, driver or whatever. In the Grendon environment we learn to tolerate and respect one another and seek honesty and patience with a genuine human connection built through these mutual tenets amongst others. My first impressions hooked me in.

The first meeting involved a round robin[5] in which everyone introduced ourselves by our first name, our sentence and our index offence charge. The most poignant example of one beginning the road of taking full responsibility for our criminality, creating victims, though also recognising, sometimes for the first time, we all have a voice. Despite how others feel about our crimes, people can no longer hide from their past, nor do we need to. A wholly compassionate and empowering act, whether I recognised it initially or not! Other prisons, however, are traditionally places crimes are not fully disclosed (unless it is to gain notoriety, imagined or real), even on offending behaviour programmes, when open discussions are part of the model. Meeting honest unguarded responsibility in people was rare, usually due to real fear of retribution through bullying, intimidation, and of course violence.

Managing Conflict Differently

My first conflict arose following a visit. Strong family relations are seen as an indication of desistance post-release, and so Grendon makes the visits centre a huge part of the compassionate work we do here. Sitting outside on a picnic table in the sun, I went up to the counter to buy an ice cream for my niece, my sister and me. This would be unusual in another establishment, but part of the culture here. My attention, having sat down and enjoying a moment with my family, was drawn to a yelp by a young lady being inappropriately touched by the man she was visiting. The look on my niece and sister's face, of concern and fear, left me feeling very angry. Recognising him as a resident who was here for a sexual assault, who I knew from earlier days in Grendon, left me with the urge to protect the lady. This is a very natural evolutionary response. A problem, I later discovered, was a primal need to protect the females in my family from my father and his drunken rages. I had been in Grendon a month and I recognised how traumatised I was, hypersensitive and on guard, ready to snap. I had 3 weeks to wait until I was given the opportunity to challenge the resident, in what is known as a Minute Meeting[6]. When this occurred I lacked the skills to resolve the incident directly with the man. It could have resulted in violence, however, by the time the minute came to the top of the list the powerful feelings had subsided.

In placing a minute, I was going against other prison values of 'not grassing'. I gave the other resident the opportunity to hear the impact his behaviour had on my sister and niece and was able to reflect how I felt guilty for the victims of my robberies over the years, which included females, and the deep shame I felt about that. The whole community asked questions. The experience allowed me to begin to trust the therapeutic process, for all its alien nuances, thereby learning to sit with powerful, previously destructive emotions. I developed insight into my reasons for such a primitive response beyond the trigger.

Commitment

On the morning of my move from the assessment unit to C wing, where I was to continue my therapy, having already visited twice, for a meal and for association, I hand the assessment unit officer, Vernon, my key and remote control. I thanked him for all his help, whilst lying to him that the missing batteries were my own. The induction rep from C wing arrives to escort me down and help me to carry my belongings to my beautiful new room, a carpeted cell with a million-pound view and I breathed a sigh of relief because of the welcome I received…

Meeting my group on C wing was nerve wracking. Talking about my offending history for all to judge, was not easy, but for most, with differing periods of experience of therapy, (due to the rolling nature of Grendon), they expressed compassion, understanding and a sense of genuine honesty, unrecognisable in other prisons.

The following week I brought to the group that I have a problem I want to discuss. I explained that while shaking the hand of an officer I lied about stealing some batteries from a TV remote control. Trivial to most, judging by their initial response, though I knew as a life-long offender this incident lay at the core of my problems. While smiling at the nice man (who of course represented authority, fatherhood, mentors, etc.) I was hypothetic- ally picking his pocket; this was my work. My commitment was met with mixed responses, by most, "are you a screw boy[7]?"; "What are you doing?"; "What is really going on?" were some of the questions asked. I explained to the whole community that prior to my latest relapse and arrest, my grandad lent me a substantial amount of money to help me in a business venture, and I never got the chance to pay him back before he lost his life to cancer. His final memories of his grandson were of me ripping him off and being locked up again. At the roots of my offending, and despite how much I loved my grandad, I was unable to demonstrate that through empathy. A pattern I discuss further below. Following community and staff votes I was backed to remain in therapy[8]. As a part of my commitment I had to fulfil some forfeits selected by the community. A mixture of tasks that included writing a letter to my granddad, which I was required to read to the whole commu- nity. I also had to have a sit down with Vernon and write a piece on what stealing does for me. The sit down involved my personal officer, ('Daisy'), the wing chairman, Vernon and myself. It was a very emotional experience that I will never forget, compassionate, honest and real.

Understanding PTSD

My diagnosis of PTSD occurred some months after I was stabbed in the neck, face and head whilst walking away from a fight with a group. I was attacked by one of them, and then stabbed from behind by my newly ex- girlfriend. I collapsed after she cut the main artery to my arm in my neck. Awaking several days later in the High Dependency Unit with a paralyzed arm and a very sudden sense of impending doom, I soon became aware of what had happened. I began to spiral downwards whilst becoming used to the fear that they were coming back to finish me off, which would rule my life for a decade.

My trauma arose several times in quick succession over the first six months. Usual conflicts involved loud, aggressive people, and those who gave me the silent treatment.

One incident in particular involved a new guy who was feral, and threatened me several times, leading to him being placed on a commitment and me accountable to the community for my response. When he threatened me, I flashed back to the car park floor, scared, numb, holding my neck. After locking myself away I returned to the resident to try to resolve the issue, making the whole scenario worse. Regarding silent treatment, my Stepdad wasn't violent, but commonly used the silent treatment on me when angry. I found this behaviour as a child very debilitating and hard to manage in others. I find it unpredictable and for many years it left me anxious and hypersensitive. An experience which intensified since being stabbed.

Sitting through hundreds of crisis meetings and living on a wing which becomes a representation of a family unit was at times excruciating. I cried a lot, felt people's disdain at my apparent neediness, and at times felt singled out, mirroring my childhood home. Of course, I was on my therapeutic journey. I felt safe to open up completely and this was to change my life, in which compassion made it possible to be me unreservedly and honest for once in my life.

As explained above, whatever the trigger, loud aggressive people, heated conflict, sharp objects or silent treatment, I usually ended up back in the car park, laid out on the cold floor wet with blood, holding my neck. Alternatively, I flash back to the ambulance, where I have audible hallucinations of the policeman holding my neck and the amazing paramedic shouting 'I can't get a blood pressure' or 'stay with me Nathan'. Other prisons offered visits from psychiatrists, potent anti-psychotic medication, counselling, and group work for what it's worth, when the environment was rarely safe to drop your guard and process the PTSD.

Meeting Geoff[9] however changed my standpoint. In many ways Geoff and I could be no further different as people, though within an hour of talking to him about his PTSD in group and all the things that eased his trauma, felt as though I was no longer alone; the TC principle of universality and community. I completely understood what he described, how he suffered, and how alone the episodes can make us feel. However, our reactions could be distinct. For Geoff, feeling threatened provoked an intense need to lash out in extreme violence. For me however, I either freeze or run away, the classic responses. For many years since diagnosis I have kept everyone at arm's length as a result. Relationships were based on my needs only and attachments have either been overbearing, unhealthy and borderline obsessive, or not at all. The working relationship with Geoff though was built on the basis of honesty and equality. From this mutually compassionate healthy situation, endorsed by our environment, I have been allowed, over a three-year period, to be open about exploring all the complex issues I have touched on in my writing here, thereby, replacing maladjusted reactions to problems (namely obsession, violence, drug use, and criminality) with a balanced set of coping strategies when my trauma arises. For example, self-searching, sharing my feelings with others and if I do have an episode, which is rare, I implement learned strategies. These grounding exercises, (although I prefer the term "calming" because of my association, with PTSD, of laying on the floor helpless), I usually take myself to safety. I also use breathing and meditation techniques. With these interventions I tend to come out of it within half an hour, although the last time this occurred was longer ago than I can remember.

Psychodrama Therapy and Art Therapy

Augustus and Jefferies (in press) describe how core creative psychotherapies (CCP) were introduced to Grendon in the 1980s in the form of psychodrama and, later, art therapy. There are now three core creative modalities practiced at Grendon, including music therapy, which is undertaken on the wing for men with learning difficulties. The core creative psychotherapies are considered a central component of group work that takes place on each DTC. The CCP groups are once weekly for two hours, and the membership of each group is between six and eight residents. Case and Dalley (1992) state that art therapy involves the use of different media through which the participant can express and work through the issues and concerns that have brought them to therapy. The therapist and participant are in partnership in trying to understand the art process and product of the session. For those taking part it can be easier to relate to the therapist through the art object which can then provide a focus for discussion, analysis, and self-evaluation. As it is more concrete, it stays as a record of the therapeutic process and cannot be denied, eased, or forgotten, and offers a chance for reflection later. The transference that develops within the relation between the therapist and client, and is discussed in all aspects of the DTC, extends to the artwork. The participants engage with art materials, producing artwork and reflecting on the thoughts and feelings that arise in relation to both the work produced and the process itself.

The work undertaken in core creative therapy groups is fed back to the small group and community meetings. Nathan participated in art therapy and describes this below, but first a note on psychodrama psychotherapy.

Psychodrama is an action-based group psychotherapy (for more details see Augustus and Jefferies, in press). It employs action methods to encourage the expression of suppressed emotions and introduces the possibility of change by correcting the earlier responses that have taken place. It uses dramatic format, theatrical terms, and role analysis for participants to explore, in the context of the group, how his/her modes of dealing with significant others is influenced by their internal world and how their dysfunctional *internal working models* (beliefs of self and others) have been brought about by early childhood experiences. The participant is encouraged to find new ways of perceiving and reacting to past and present life experiences and to understand the process of how he/she has come to offend. The technique of role reversal increases victim empathy and provides the opportunity to explore the perspective of others by standing in their shoe and exploring their state of mind. The physical setting of scenes and the use of group members to play significant characters in their lives brings the "there and then" of the past into the "here and now" of the session. This process provokes memories and strong feelings from the past and the present and allows the protagonist[10] to examine the distorted belief systems that have influenced his/her behaviour and how unexpressed feelings of anger have been displaced onto the innocent victim. Internal working models and dysfunctional attachment strategies are understood and challenged.

I am talkative, always have been, and art therapy (AT) offered a way of communicating my life in pictures, allowing me to explore aspects of my experience in a way I could not articulate as a child. An early picture I showed the group, depicted my family on arrival in London. It illustrated my sixth birthday, a hedgehog shaped chocolate cake (which I had completely forgotten about) and how I had waited the whole day for my father to arrive to watch me blow out the candles. He never arrived, a man I was only to meet three more times before his death at the beginning of this sentence.

Through AT as a medium I processed all my relationships, the shame I felt for my victims and family, my trauma and how these problems affect my relationships today. The message absorbed from my birthday I took to every relationship I ever went into after that. There I discovered the truth; that deep down inside, people abandon you and let you down and eventually reject you. Looking back through my life, much destructive behaviour had its roots in the belief that I had no value and so I shall give everyone a reason to believe this. It's the safe and compassionate environment that eventually led me to that core truth.

Critics may disagree with a compassionate approach. My hard-earned experience, however, depicts a different standpoint. Perhaps short, sharp, shocks work for some. I've been a cog in the CJS since I was a child. The only intervention that has worked has been the compassionate, conflict-facing long-term resolution model I have now completed.

Resistance to Change

Whilst the discussion so far has focussed on upholding a safe and compassionate atmosphere to facilitate the processing of trauma, meeting and getting to know 40 men with varying maladjusted traits is difficult.

Violence is rare here, threats more common, though mostly a lot of acting out is done anonymously. Whether the incidents are directed towards the select few or the whole community, occurrences such as blocking locks, notes in the mailbox, deliberate vandalism of artwork, fittings or furniture usually trigger a crisis meeting, which all residents must attend. Sometimes it can be a witch-hunt and people's frustrations spill out in abusive language, either designed to quieten less assertive residents or to shame some. These interactions would be met with challenges of their own. We are not in the business of naming and shaming. The majority of our community have experienced the most horrendous humiliating sexual, physical or emotional abuse and seeking to shame has no place in this environment. Even those who are loud and verbally abusive usually calm down once they recognise the individual struggles with an open honest compassionate approach to our work here. Whereas other prisons would quickly expel disruptive people, Grendon tolerates a great deal of risky behaviour presented, demonstrating that where people like me would expect rejection, there are other ways to resolve conflict.

Having a wide-ranging timetable of stimulus, beyond therapy groups, empowers ownership for our environment, teaching the importance of timekeeping, upholding commitments and social interactions, whilst focussing on our trauma, rehabilitation and healthy boundaries in relationships, both personal and professional.

Over time the interactions have helped form part of my identity, relieving shame, turning guilt into positive restoration for the harm caused, and ultimately building self-esteem and self-worth, towards a prosocial future as I work towards release.

Whilst the Covid regime was restrictive compared to my time in therapy, it was the compassionate response to my problems that I feel was the catalyst of my transformation. No longer riddled with the stigmatised shame, loneliness, and fear my life in institutions helped to mould; instead, I'm proud of who I am and excited to meet the people I am yet to share my life with.

Conclusion

Whilst definite conclusions are difficult to draw from the experiences of a single staff member and a single resident, some encouraging points are raised on the effectiveness of CFT and taking a trauma-informed approach to containing distress.

Firstly, Nathan's experience is not unique. He observed that when immersed in a more supportive environment, where boundaries and living conditions are compassionate and enable the development of trust to occur over an extended period, the CFT approach can alleviate the destructive defensive barriers that many residents experience when their threat system is overactive. In the first six months there can be a period of adjustment and, over an extended period, as discussed, the ability to self-sooth increased and the threat system decreased significantly. *This made my day-to-day experience more manageable, allowing healing.*

Secondly, identifying terms such as "dropping your guard" and "feeling safe enough to share" – in addition to not having to endure the overarching threat of persecution, ridicule, and further punishment through violence, bullying, and intimidation of others – appears in stark contrast to other prisons, where experience of culture on the whole was unsafe. This appears to indicate that, among other things, CFT and having a trauma-informed approach alter the culture to a more considerate, mature and healthy one.

Thirdly, during the Covid-19 pandemic, much of the usual groups and staff supervisory meetings have inevitably reduced. Whilst there have been major challenges across the six communities, incidents of crisis have still been very rare. Since Grendon houses some of the most dangerous men serving long sentences, this appears to support the use of the CFT and DTC approaches. Although there has been distress for residents and staff (who have inevitably had their own challenges, balancing work/life commitments during the pandemic), this has not been evident in their treatment of residents. This demonstrates the multi-disciplinary approach to crisis has been humane and camaraderie has developed.

Fourth, a huge part of the work of a DTC is working through denial and developing invaluable insight through reality confrontation in a compassionate manner. As discussed, much of this work was the catalyst for change, although facing the trauma in the beginning was difficult. During the assessment period only the "here and now" is discussed, and eventually, when each individual feels ready, the move forward happens organically. Within small groups the past offending and experiences are examined. While this is done carefully, in a CFT manner, working through the past experiences helps alleviate the long-held distress. Some struggle with this, and either take time away from the group, which is very intense, or decide they have gone as far as they can on the journey and leave. They can return sometime later to continue the work. Often the defences relate to aspects of offending. One group member could not remember details of his offence, but in psychodrama, when describing the scene, recalled there was a clock in the room which had its face lit up, and he could "see" what happened for the first time. This was in a safe and secure environment, when he felt able to confront what he had done. Recalling events can also link to empathy for victims, through the resident exploring the events from the perspective of others involved. For some this is too much to tolerate and they leave.

Grendon opens its doors to many visitors. One couple who are regulars are Ray and Vi Donovan (see Donovan & Donovan, 2018), whose son Christopher was murdered by a group of young men. They speak of the impact this had on them, and the pain and distress they went through. They describe the journey through restorative justice and the impact this had on all concerned. Those listening cannot help but be moved by their response and relate to how they impacted on their own victims, without the need for individual confrontation. Through all this work it is possible to see people find the person they once were, process the extreme hurt they have carried, and tolerate the pain they have caused others.

In conclusion, whether best practice for other establishments is to take a more trauma-informed approach is outside the remit of this chapter. However, collaborative responses to debate and sharing perspectives between all who live and work in a setting is a great place to start, empowering those who otherwise have not had a voice provides autonomy. This collaborative chapter is a prime example of giving a voice to an expert by experience, thus giving value to their experience. Including and empowering those who have experienced trauma, exclusion, and disempowerment is surely a compassionate place to start, wherever therapy and trauma work is taking place.

Notes

1 Nathan Joshua is the nom de plume of a former Grendon resident.
2 Drug Treatment and Testing Orders (DTTO) are imposed by courts where someone's offending is linked to drug misuse. The focus of a DTTO is to address drug use to reduce the risk of further offending and harm.

3 Nathan uses the term "offender" whereas the preference is to use person-first language.
4 The TAC course is co-facilitated by residents from therapy wings who have experience of the process and can give a lived experience to new residents.
5 A Round Robin is when each person in the community introduces themselves in turn.
6 In a Minute Meeting residents hold others accountable for their actions, and are also held to account for what they have done and the impact it has had. This could vary in seriousness from snapping at someone to, as in this case, a fairly serious incident.
7 A "screw boy" is a resident who spends a lot of time with staff.
8 In the process described, if a person is thought to have broken the rules of the community they would explain themselves to the group and wing, and they would vote whether the rules had been broken, and also whether they would still be willing to work with the resident. If they are allowed to remain, there are generally sanctions to undertake, which can be punitive, therapeutic, and restorative.
9 Not his real name.
10 The term used for the person who is undertaking the psychodrama.

Further Reading

Akerman, G., & Shuker, R. (In press). *Interventions in forensic therapeutic communities.* Taylor & Francis Group. This volume describes various interventions in DTCs, which add to their effectiveness and enhance the progress made by residents. These include core creative therapies, working with gangs and working with mothers of young babies.
Gilbert, P. (2010). *Compassion-focused therapy. Distinctive features.* Routledge. As with all Paul Gilbert's books, this one is written in an accessible manner and explains the evolution and development of the brain and how to implement more compassion focused approaches for ourselves and those we work with.
Rothwell, K. (Ed.) (2019). *Forensic arts therapies. Anthology of practice and research.* Forensic Arts Therapies Advisory Group. This book explains the range of creative therapies and the settings in which they are practiced.

References

Akerman, G. (2019). Communal living as the agent of change. In D. Polaschek, A. Day, & C. Hollin (Eds), *The Wiley international handbook of correctional psychology.* Wiley Blackwell. doi:10.1002/9781119139980.ch37
Akerman, G., Needs, A., & Bainbridge, C. (Eds). (2018). *Transforming environments and rehabilitation. A guide for practitioners in forensic and criminal justice.* Taylor & Francis Group.
Augustus, J., & Jefferies, J. (In press). Evaluating the efficacy of core creative psychotherapies within therapeutic communities at HMP Grendon. In G. Akerman & R. Shuker (Eds), *Interventions in forensic therapeutic communities.* Taylor & Francis Group.
Case, C., & Dalley, T. (1992). *The handbook of art therapy.* Routledge.
Cozolino, L. (2008). *The healthy aging brain: Sustaining attachment, attaining wisdom.* Norton.
Donovan, R., & Donovan, V. (2018). *Restored and forgiven. The power of restorative justice.* Bridge Logos.
Genders, E., & Player, E. (1995). *Grendon: A study of a therapeutic prison.* OUP.
Gilbert, P. (2010a). *Compassion-focused therapy: Distinctive features.* London: Routledge.
Gilbert, P. (2010b). Compassion-focused therapy: Special issue. *International Journal of Cognitive Therapy, 3,* 95–201. doi:10.1111/j.2044-8341.2012.02068.x
Gilbert, P. (2017). Compassion: Definitions and controversies. In P. Gilbert (Ed.), *Compassion: Concepts, research and applications* (pp.31–68). Abingdon, Oxon: Routledge.
Gilbert, P., & Irons, C. (2005). Focused therapies and compassionate mind training for shame and self-attacking. In P. Gilbert (Ed.), *Compassion: Conceptualisations, research and use in psychotherapy* (pp.263–325). London: Routledge.

Haigh, R., & Pearce, S. (2017). *The theory and practice of democratic therapeutic community treatment.* Jessica Kingsley Publishers.

Jacobs, L., & Shuker, R. (2019). The experiences of perpetrators of filicide participating in treatment within a prison therapeutic community. *Therapeutic Communities: The International Journal of Therapeutic Communities. 40.* 66–76. doi:10.1108/TC-08-2018-0018

Joshua, N. (2019, September). Hierarchy of hypocrisy. *Inside Time.* Retrieved from www. insidetime.org Accessed on 14 August 2020.

Kotova, A., & Akerman, G. (submitted). 'There's always this strange tightrope' – The experiences of men who were sexually victimised serving prison sentences for sex offences in a therapeutic community.

LeDoux, J. (1998). *The emotional brain.* Weidenfeld and Nicolson.

Lucre, K. M., & Corten, N. (2012). An exploration of group compassion-focused therapy for personality disorder. *Psychology and Psychotherapy: Theory, Research and Practice, 86, 4,* 1–13. doi:10.1111/j.2044-8341.2012.02068.x

Panksepp, J. (1998). *Affective neuroscience.* Oxford University Press.

R. Shuker, & E. Sullivan (Eds). (2010). *Grendon and the emergence of forensic therapeutic communities: Developments in research and practice.* John Wiley and Sons.

Rapoport, R. N. (1960). *Community as doctor.* London: Tavistock.

Shine, J., & Morris, M. (1999). *Regulating anarchy. The Grendon programme.* Leyhill Press. Available from HMP Grendon, Grendon Underwood, Aylesbury, Bucks, HP18OTL.

Stevens, A. (2013). Offender rehabilitation and therapeutic communities: Enabling change the TC way. *The British Journal of Criminology, 54,* 972– 975. doi:10.1093/bjc/azu029

Strauss, M. A. (2000). Corporal punishment and primary prevention of physical abuse. *Child Abuse & Neglect, 24,* 1109–1114. doi:10.1016\soi45-2134 (00)00180-0

Taylor, J., Akerman, G., & Hocken, K. (2020) Cultivating compassion focussed practice for those who have committed sexual offences. In H. Swaby, B. Winder, R. Lievesley, K. Hocken, N. Blagden, & P. Banyard (Eds), *Sexual crime and trauma* (pp.57–84). Palgrave Macmillan. doi:10.1007/978-3-030-49068-3_3

Varghese, R., Quiros, L., & Berger, R. (2018). Reflective practices for engaging in trauma-informed culturally competent supervision. *Smith College Studies in Social Work,* 1–17. doi:10.1080/00377317.2018.1439826

Veale, D., Gilbert, P., Wheatley, J., & Naismith, I. (2014). A new therapeutic community: Development of a compassion-focussed and contextual behavioural environment. *Clinical Psychology and Psychotherapy, 22*(4), 285–303. doi:10.1002/cpp.1897

16

ADDRESSING TRAUMA WITH YOUNG ADULT MALES IN CUSTODY

Implementing a Stepped Care Trauma-Informed Approach in a Young Offenders Institution

Kate Geraghty and Chantal Scaillet

An Overview of the Complex Needs Service

The Complex Needs Service (CNS) is a day centre, located in a Young Offender Institution (YOI) for young adult men aged 18–21 presenting with complex needs borne out of early, disruptive developmental experiences. Established in 2013, the CNS sits within the overall national provision of Offender Personality Disorder Pathway (OPD)[1,2] services in the UK (Joseph & Bennefield, 2012). The evidence-base underpinning the psychosocial interventions of the CNS derives from three areas: factors involved in supporting desistance from offending, the impact of relational and developmental trauma[3] on the development of personality, and the link between complex trauma and offending or increased risk.

Desistance Factors

Desistance is a main objective for the CNS. Agencies promoting desistance from offending in young people (e.g., Youth Justice Board; Youth Offending Teams) recognise that services need to be age-appropriate and trauma-informed, that is, based on a thorough understanding of the young person's needs in context of their developmental history, psychological and social experiences. As such, treatment mapping in the CNS is sequenced, structured, and premised on the same guiding principles as other phased trauma-informed treatments, such as the Trauma Recovery Model (Skuse & Matthew, 2015) and Golding's (2015) Pyramid of Needs. More specifically,

DOI: 10.4324/9781003120766-21

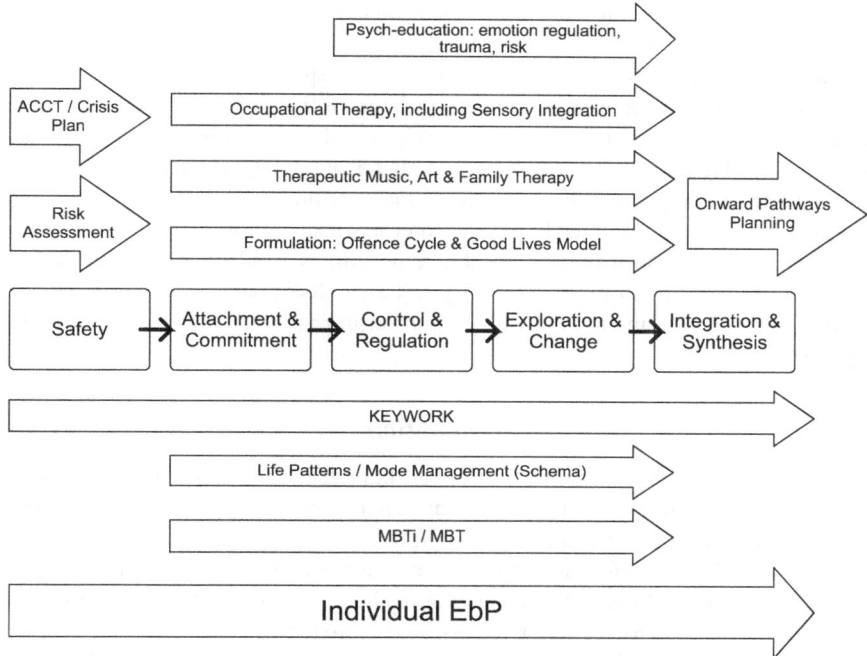

Figure 16.1 The complex needs service treatment framework

Livesley's (2015) framework for personality disorder treatment proposes integrating common elements supportive of change from a diverse range of interventions. Livesley describes five phases: safety, containment, regulation and control, exploration and change, and integration and synthesis (Figure 16.1).

Drawing from Livesley's framework, interventions in the CNS take account of individuals' readiness and *capacity to self-soothe* and *feel safe* in the present (safety, attachment, containment, control, and regulation). In particular, and highly relevant to delivering trauma interventions in environments that have the potential to re-traumatise individuals, *safety* and *stabilisation* are essential phase 1 tasks, before progressing to processing the trauma. *Exploration* and *change* (Formulation) focus on the past and making sense of difficulties. *Integration* and *Synthesis* (Onward Pathway planning, ongoing keyworks) focuses on the future and the support available in identifying positive goals, as well as areas of vulnerability and obstacles to achieving goals.

Attachment

A second objective of the CNS is developing relationships with family and the wider community, as well as developing a more hopeful, internalised self-view. This is done through regular, consistent, face-to-face meetings with the young person. Key staff (keyworkers) will *re-parent* (Treisman, 2016) and offer a relational experience that invites the young person to be curious about their difficulties within the context of a safe therapeutic relationship.

Individuals might have learned to adapt and respond to dangerous environments with trauma-related responses such as hyperarousal, hypervigilance, and mistrust (Fonagy et al., 2002; Perry et al., 1995), which may impact on their ability to mentalise (Huang et al., 2020; Fonagy & Bateman, 2008) rendering them more prone to misreading intentions of others and situations. As described in earlier chapters, betrayal trauma severely impairs interpersonal relationships and "epistemic hypervigilance, distrust or outright epistemic freezing is an adaptive consequence of the social learning environment" (Fonagy & Target, 2008; p.694). Furthermore, the need to adapt to ongoing trauma will also further impact on individuals' mentalising capabilities.

Formulation

A third objective of the CNS is to develop self-knowledge and a meaningful personal narrative. This is achieved through co-creating an understanding of the young person's life from the past to the present (psychological formulation). This personal narrative then forms the backdrop for the integration of a more realistic self-appraisal in relation to difficulties past and present, contributing to the development of a hopeful future orientation. The CNS focuses on strength-based approaches that promote growth and seeks to rebuild trust within context of a *curious culture* (e.g., Good Lives Model; Ward & Brown 2004), Mentalisation-Based Therapy (MBT: Bateman & Fonagy, 2006) and Schema Therapy (Young & Klosko, 1993). In addition, the CNS is an accredited enabling environment (EE),[4] which plays a key role in supporting the young men's learning and psychosocial development, as well as providing a safe, containing, therapeutic space to minimise re-traumatisation. In conclusion, interventions delivered within the CNS are aligned to trauma-informed ways of working and are premised on a fundamental shift from thinking "What's wrong with you?" to "What happened to you?" (Covington & Rodriquez, 2016).

An Overview of the Complex Trauma Presentations within the CNS

Having described the main aims and treatment framework of the CNS, this section will report on the diverse range of trauma experiences. In terms of reporting past distressing experiences, the young men in the CNS are no different from their peers across the wider prison estate, where trauma often goes unidentified (Boswell, 1991), with direct or witnessed trauma ranging from one single incident (PTSD, single event) to multiple exposure and type (poly-victimisation, developmental/complex, cultural and racial trauma).

The recording of the types of trauma serves the purpose of identifying complexity in the young person rather than any attempt at diagnosis. This point is important, as the CNS does not routinely administer psychometric testing in order to determine the presence of PTSD or complex trauma.[5] The identification of trauma follows a

Table 16.1 Breakdown of the types of trauma experiences taken from a sample of 38 young men from the CNS

Severely distressing bad experiences	*Event description*	*Percentage (N=38)*
	4 or more	*66% (25)*
Poly-victimisation	Witness others being assaulted	89% (33)
	Own violent assault	63% (24)
	Group assault	39% (15)
	Witness murder	26% (10)
	Shootings/riots/bombing	13% (5)
	Exposure to war	5% (2)
	Racial attack	8% (3)
Other type of trauma	Bereavement	34% (13)
Cultural/Psychosocial trauma	Gang exploitation	39% (15)
	Cultural adversity	15% (6)
	County lines	24% (9)
	Immigration/refugee	13% (5)
Perpetrator trauma	Trauma from offence	42% (16)

less rigid, more inclusive, and contextual approach than the diagnostic approaches found in the psychiatric/medical field and incorporates a range of distressing negative experiences.

As indicated in Table 16.1, 66% of the young men from the CNS have experienced four or more severely distressing negative experiences prior to age 18. As stated earlier, exposure to these initial traumatic experiences results in poorer ability in regulating emotions, significantly impacting on the young person's sense of safety and ability to manage relationships and stress. This manifests in challenging institutional behaviours such as aggression towards peers or staff.

The term "poly-victimisation" (Finkelhor, Turner, Ormrod, & Hamby, 2009) is described in detail elsewhere in this book. Certainly, within the CNS, the higher the number of different types of adversity experienced, the more pervasive and persistent are psychological problems across the domains of cognitive schemas, affecting dysregulation and relationships. Poly-victimisation is represented in Table 16.1 with very high numbers having witnessed others being assaulted (89%). Cumulative trauma impacts on the young person's affective responses, which often appear blunted in range. For example, when reporting on their histories, the young men frequently respond with blunted affect, asserting that "it is what it is", while expressing a belief in a foreshortened future. In addition, the young men appear to minimise the impact of violence on themselves (and others) and to normalise it. Some authors (e.g., Salzinger, Feldman, Stockhammer, & Hood, 2002) propose that this is as a result of the poly-victimised young person's frequent exposure to violence and trauma and defence against feelings of vulnerability and fear. Linked to this is "offence-related trauma", which refers to the experience of trauma symptoms such as intrusive, unwanted thoughts, excessive rumination, guilt, and shame as a result of committing their index offence (Mrug, Madan, & Windle, 2016).

It is well documented that childhood adversity, trauma, and violence blight the lives of young people who are more at risk of joining gangs.[6] In our sample, 39% reported gang exploitation and 24% were groomed into "county lines".[7] Young people caught up in these are likely to experience intimidation, exploitation, and violence by older gang members (Wigmor, 2018).

Systemic Issues in Delivering Trauma-Focused Treatment in a YO

Treatment in prison has predominantly focused on offender rehabilitation, and much of this has focused on the area of risk reduction and public protection (McGuire, 2013). It is widely recognised that the needs of young people in prison are different from those within the adult estate. Young people are still developing in psychosocial maturity, which affects how they engage and respond. It is also recognised that young adults can be harder to engage and have poorer outcomes in prison in comparison with older adults (NOMS, 2015). As mentioned previously, young incarcerated men have a high prevalence of complex trauma. However, prisons themselves can cause ongoing traumatisation. They can be volatile environments with concerning living conditions. There are well-known difficulties with violence, rates of assault and self-harm, particularly within the youth custody estate (Ministry of Justice, 2020). There are also issues of overcrowding in prisons, with nearly 50% of prisons being reported as being over capacity (Sturge, 2020). These living conditions do not provide humane, validating environments for people and pose numerous challenges for staff trying to implement trauma-focused interventions.

Some of these challenges are practical issues. This includes the movement of individuals to different departments in the prison. At times, individuals are kept in their cells due to their involvement in an incident, a wing or prison lockdown, or security searches. If individuals are not on the relevant list for the department or area they are due to attend, they may not get permission to go there. They may also be prevented from attending therapy sessions because of low staffing levels or security concerns. These issues may also prevent therapy being provided in a consistent and reliable way, which may undermine the basic requirement of trauma therapy in facilitating client safety. Other issues include sudden endings to therapy, which the therapist has no control over. It is common practice in prison settings that individuals deemed a security risk are moved to another prison. While this may help alleviate some of the prison disruption, it may also lead to an unplanned ending of therapy.

Prisons have been noted to exacerbate previous experiences of trauma (Bradley, 2017). Trauma can occur within prison settings (Jennings, 2004) and mental health services can inadvertently re-traumatise people through a lack of awareness of the impact of trauma (Bloom & Farragher, 2011; Davidson, 1997). Staff may adopt more punitive responses and/or experience vicarious trauma. Jennings (2004) outlines how institutional re-traumatisation can also manifest in staff practices for those with complex trauma histories. For example, those with sexual abuse histories may be re-traumatised by the experience of being strip searched or restrained by staff.

Additionally, some individuals in prison can be in physical danger from other residents, have a perception of danger or feel psychologically unsafe around key dates such as anniversaries. Furthermore, the ability to develop an appropriate attachment to staff (therapeutic relationship) is compromised due to the nature of the volatile environment, staff levels, inconsistency in staffing and the delivery of interventions. There is also a tension between confidentiality (a key requirement for therapy) and risk management. Working in a prison environment requires therapists to be attentive to both issues. It is recognised that there is a need to achieve a balance, albeit a delicate one, between managing risk and maintaining trust between the therapist and young person (Harvey & Smedley, 2017).

The implications of these systemic issues for delivering trauma therapy are significant, but not impossible to overcome. They highlight the need for offering more long-term rather than short-term therapy. Positive experiences have been reported when the conditions of confidentiality are openly discussed and shared at the start of therapy (Harvey & Smedley, 2017). Furthermore, others have reported the value that such tensions can provide as important learning experiences and used as metaphors for change. For example, in spite of these challenges progress and change can still be possible and "imperfect" situations can still be valued (Haley, 2017).

Raising Awareness of Complex Trauma Presentations Among YOI Staff

As alluded to above, not only are service level approaches needed to address trauma but also system level approaches. Staff education and training in trauma-informed care is considered fundamental to treating complex trauma services (Kezelman & Stavropoulos, 2012). This enables an organisational understanding of trauma responses, how to work with those with complex trauma presentations as well as the importance of maintaining personal and professional boundaries. Within mainstream prisons, the majority of staff will predominantly be prison officers, with clinical staff operating from other departments delivering 1:1 assessments/interventions, group work, and consultation to the wider prison. HMPPS is increasingly recognising the importance of staff-resident relationships through the introduction of initiatives such as the Five-Minute Intervention (FMI). It is also recognising the role of trauma through introducing the Trauma Risk Management (TRiM) scheme, a staff support programme designed to help staff deal with the impact of traumatic events. Additionally, HMPPS are also beginning to roll out other trauma-informed approaches, including a trauma awareness group for residents. The introduction of these initiatives is extremely positive, but there is some way to go before mainstream prisons can be considered to comply with the guidelines for developing a trauma-informed culture such as those outlined by Kezelman and Stavropoulos. As such, although the prison could not be considered to be trauma-informed, it is moving towards creating environments that are trauma informed.

As the CNS is non-residential, no CNS staff are available freely on the wing to service users. Additionally, the therapists facilitating trauma-focused treatment are not the young person's main support worker for the service. This has required the therapists to educate staff working with the young person about the trauma therapy, what is involved and, importantly, the impact this could have, both positive and negative. Adopting a multi-systemic approach to working with young people is crucial (Squire, Jefford, & Cupit Swenson, 2015). Some understanding of the systems working with the person is needed. This includes systems directly in contact with the person but also wider organisational systems. Discussions were held with other departments including HMPPS Psychology and the prison Mental Health teams about the trauma treatment, what would be involved, and how the young person would be supported through this. Additionally, staff working in the complex needs service directly with the person were given some training on what the therapy would involve. Regular discussions were held with the key workers and within service team meetings to review the person's progress, appropriateness of trauma therapy, and to raise any concerns.

Open discussions were also held with the residents about the importance of informing some wing staff and having support from staff on the wing outside of the session. This raised some initial anxiety, with concerns about confidentiality and personal information being shared. To support this the residents were asked to identify a limited number of wing staff who would be aware that they were engaging in trauma therapy, but not the content of what was discussed in therapy, so they would be aware if the resident was acting differently on the wing. Informal staff training was offered to these staff on the therapy, covering what it involved and what behaviours staff might see if the resident was struggling. It also involved advising staff on how to support the resident during these times, such as reminding them of positive coping strategies and important people in their life. Consultancy was also offered on how to maintain boundaried discussions of residents' pasts for those who may be vulnerable to adverse reactions to such discussions, crisis management, and informing staff of other agencies in the prison who could support the resident if needed.

Reflections on EMDR

Service User (AO) Reflections

I want everyone to understand my trauma; in order to do that firstly I need you to understand who I am.

Like most of kids, I also had a terrible childhood. It's not because of my family or someone, it's 'cause of where I am from. I was born during a civil war in my country where most of the kids don't even know what a good life is. At the age of seven, I lost everyone I know, even my parents and my brothers and I ended up in a refugee camp with other kids. I spent a couple of years in the camp where everyone knew there was no future for them 'cause we saw people got beaten to death. People did terrible things in order to see another day. We were assaulted every day – mostly they want to show us they are in charge. I prayed to God asking him to take me away from this war because I couldn't live anymore. In order for us to survive someone was to die. Then, one day out of the blue, the officers came to me and told me "your grandfather is here to see you". I honestly didn't know what to say. I was happy and angry because he came after all these years. Then I saw him through the fence. I felt like it's miracle day. Inside of me I had so many questions – but my grandfather told me "don't worry, I'm getting you out soon". I was emotionally over the moon. I went back to the camp and told everyone "I'm getting out!" Everyone had a smile on their face, but I know that inside of everyone, they felt sad as they didn't get the same luck. I was so happy I'm gonna leave this life and start afresh – at the same time, I know I'm gonna miss every single one of them, because, for a long time, they are the only family I had. A couple of weeks later, I left the horrible life to move to the UK to start a fresh life with my mum's family, who is my auntie. She welcomed me with open arms into her family. Then a couple of months later, my grandfather found out my mum and my brothers are in a camp and we managed to get them out. When I heard the news, I couldn't move and no words came out of my mouth – then my life in the UK was perfect.

When I got... my GCSE, I was over the moon. At the time, I know why I left my old life behind, it happened for a reason. I then started "A" levels in a college where I made friends and enjoyed my life. I went to parties, met new people, and had confidence. And I started drinking soon after that. Alcohol brought my old life memories back. I felt like the scar being ripped open. That's when I used alcohol as a medicine to help the pain go away. My alcohol use became a problem. That's when I left the college and started hanging around with the wrong people – that's when I met my uncle who is an extended family member. I trusted him and he looked after me as, when I say something, he will listen to me, so, as a human being, I trusted him. Then one day he comes to my place where I was staying, with his friends. Soon after that, he came to the house, he opened a bottle of whisky, and I started to drink as always. He got me involved in the conversation that led to a man being assaulted, then again my uncle got me involved in the assault. Then we left the house and went to a park where the assault continued. He and his friends left the victim with me and went to a shop. I spent about 30 minutes with him. The frequent thing he said was "let me go young brother". I honestly don't know why I didn't let him go. Then the assault continued. Then I left. The next thing I know he was dead. When I heard the news, I was scared of who I am, I couldn't believe I took someone's life. Even though my assault didn't kill him, I felt responsible. Then I came to jail where all these traumas keep coming in my mind. I couldn't deal with it – it's like a spider web with one thing connecting to another and I was stuck in a hole where I couldn't get up. I felt like I'm losing my mind.

That's when I started getting involved in the Prison Complex Needs Service. First, I couldn't trust anyone 'cause in my mind, people gonna take advantage of me and use me, so therefore, it's hard to trust anyone. Then I joined the MBT group with two other inmates. First few sessions, I don't know whether to trust anyone or not. Then I realised the other two inmates were sharing things that are very personal to them and they are trusting staff with it, so I questioned myself whether I should trust them. So I told myself "let myself in one by one". It took some time for me to be open about my life. So, I start trusting them. My mind became peaceful. However, the scars are still very painful. I know I need a way to get the pain out of my body and I know for certain I'm not gonna use alcohol. Why? Because it's gonna help me for some time by hiding it, not solving it. That's when I started doing EMDR. First I thought, "it's weird", 'cause someone moving their fingers from right to left. Then I know the purpose of the eye movement, which makes me focus on my issues. Then I need to know which trauma to focus on because I have so many and all of them from different situations. That's when I did the questionnaire, which helped me to understand which trauma I need to work on. That's when I know I'm living with the guilt of my victim (as I said before, I spent 30 minutes with the victim) – I had the chance to let him go, which I chose not to, and if I had, he would be alive. So I know for certain this trauma is making my day like a hell. Then every week, I did the questionnaire regarding the trauma. That's when I realised this trauma is very heavy. We then used lights instead of fingers, which was great as it did the same job as the fingers. The more I work on EMDR the better it gets. Unfortunately, because of COVID-19, we stopped the EMDR. But I can say it did help my mind a lot; it did help me with most of the questions I have asked myself for a long time.

Firstly, I would like to say EMDR is great. However, in order to get into EMDR, you need to trust the people who are trying to help you. If you can't trust them, it will be very difficult to solve your issues. As I say, that was the only thing I find very difficult. I know it's very hard to trust someone with your personal trauma. Once you trust the people who's trying to help you, then you know someone's out there who will do whatever it takes to help you.

Laura Vahabzadeh, Art Therapist for Pathways, was asked to work with AO in order to create a visual representation of his experience of earlier trauma and what his future may look like in relation to this trauma. Figure 16.2 shows the image that Laura and AO created. What is seen at the centre is a beating heart, representing the present that is vulnerable but alive. The images surrounding the heart represent past traumas that are set against the sky which, for AO, represents a view of hope and his future.

Author 2 (CS) Reflections

Prior to delivering EMDR in the YOI, both authors sought to contact prison-wide colleagues delivering or thinking of delivering EMDR. At the time we found it was delivered across the estate by a range of commissioned services (OPD) services such as Psychologically-Informed Planned Environments (PIPES) and Therapeutic Communities (TCs), and NHS (mental health in-reach teams) and prison services (HMPPS Psychology) with each service operating under their respective commissioning agendas and operational frameworks. The feedback discussions were largely influenced by how sensitive their establishments were to individuals' trauma histories and what structures (leadership, governance) were in place to implement TICP safely and ethically.

In terms of my own experience, I work with a young man (AO) following a year with the CNS, so we had already established a strong therapeutic attachment. AO has complex trauma linked to growing up during a civil war and, as a very young child, exposure to extreme violence, witnessing death and being separated from his family. As an adolescent, he was further re-traumatised by the commission of his offence while under the influence of heavy drinking, and was then a victim of an incident of severe violence while in custody. AO was ready to work on his trauma

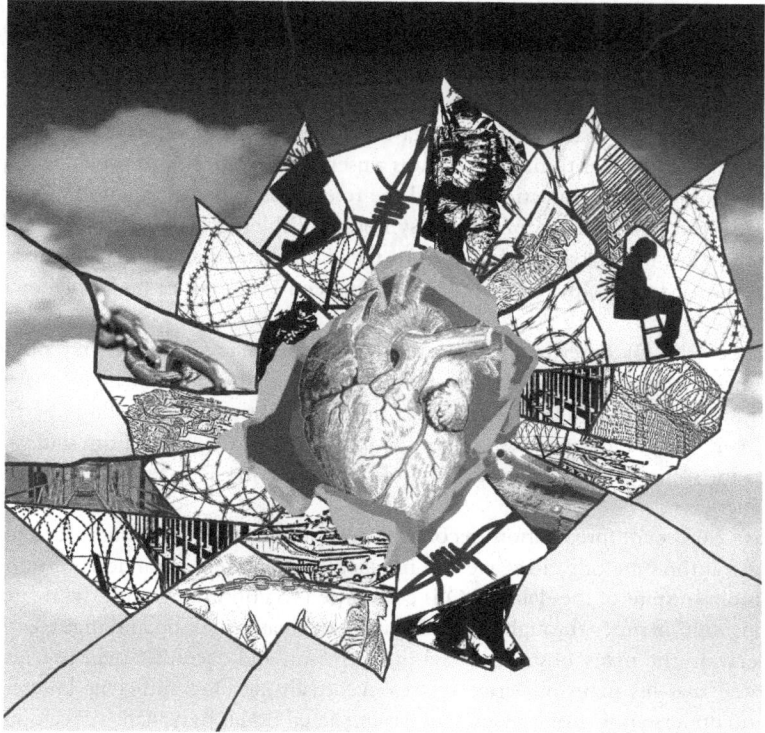

Figure 16.2   AO trauma depiction drawn by Laura Vahabzadeh, Art Therapist in CNS

as he was experiencing nightmares, intrusive thoughts about his offence, flashbacks, and somatic symptoms. Linked to his complex trauma was a daily struggle to feel safe, a deep mistrust of others, an inability to modulate stress and regulate emotions. AO's self-view was largely negative, with shame taking centre stage. Reflecting on his presentation at the time, my main concern was to "do not harm", and whether it was ethically sound to offer trauma intervention work within a custodial environment that has the potential for re-traumatising individuals. I shared this ethical dilemma with AO as I wished to be transparent about what the process would entail in terms of working through traumatic material and what may happen in-between sessions as well as during sessions. He understood the potential side effects and wanted to work on his trauma as he described his current life as "a living hell". On reflection, this is an important aspect of introducing trauma work within a custodial setting as it provides essential preparation. Another benefit of sharing my concerns was the positive impact on the therapeutic relationship and the building up of trust. Having been part of the MBT group for one year, AO had developed his mentalising capacity and made positive gains in trusting others linked to an increased sense of agency and active collaboration in sessions. As discussed in earlier sections (Figure 16.1), the introduction of any trauma work needs to scaffold on top of other interventions that promote safety and the development of strong therapeutic alliance with professionals. In other words, EMDR forms part of a toolbox of other interventions rather than a stand-alone treatment.

The initial history taking of the phase 1 took longer than anticipated as AO appeared to be easily distracted by trauma-related ruminating within sessions, leading to unproductive circular thinking. This was a useful observation, as it provided opportunity for some psychoeducation around the role of excessive rumination (about the trauma) in the maintenance of trauma symptoms (Ehlers & Clark, 2000), and how this rumination impacted on his ability to focus on the actual trauma situation. AO chose to process the shame and guilt he experienced as a result of his involvement in the offence.

Author 1 (KG) describes in her reflections the many barriers and obstacles experienced when providing therapy within a prison environment, which I share too. In addition to this, COVID-19 created a major disruption in providing any therapeutic work safely. However, the prison was able to offer in-cell calls from staff, which allowed for some continuation of the work, especially in the safety and stabilisation skills practice.

Phase 2 protocol (preparation) recommenced face-to-face following three months delay and at the time of writing we had installed a safe place and carried out resource installation. In spite of the delays, AO is committed to continuing with the treatment in a consistent manner through the phase at a pace that is realistic and that takes into consideration the many obstacles faced in the prison and current Covid restrictions. AO stated that his main objective was to eventually develop sufficient knowledge, skills, and understanding of how trauma has impacted on his personality development, mental health and behaviour, so that he can look to a future with greater hope and optimism.

BD Reflections

Unfortunately, BD was unable to contribute to this book chapter as he was transferred from the prison prior to completing this.

Author 1 (KG) Reflection

My experience of introducing EMDR in a YOI has felt slow, frustrating at times, but an incredibly rewarding experience. We were very mindful of how difficult this type of therapy can be and acutely aware of the importance of responsive approaches to addressing complex trauma. BD wished to process a time when he was stabbed in the past due to the lifestyle he led. This event left him hypervigilant to his environment and experiencing repetitive nightmares and flashbacks. BD also reported some earlier developmental trauma in terms of immigrating to the UK and parental divorce.

During the earlier sessions (Phase 1) two therapists initially worked jointly to undertake the history taking. This was part of our local protocol and not a necessary requirement of EMDR therapy. Nonetheless, it felt important given that we were introducing EMDR in the YOI for the first time. This allowed us to work together to assess BD's readiness and suitability as well as enabling a space for reflecting with another clinician. BD found it very difficult to allow himself to become vulnerable in the sessions and transference to female figures in his life was noted. BD was engaging very well in schema therapy in the service, so I was aware of his ability to reflect on past difficulties. Focusing on the emotions behind some of these was more difficult for him. Time was spent exploring this, allowing him to feel safe in expressing his vulnerability during EMDR sessions. I found it incredibly helpful for BD to use a structured intervention to explore his experience of trauma in more depth. This appeared to enable him to share his experiences in a way that felt containing, as it was a phased intervention using a semi-structured interview and psychometrics.

One source of frustration was working within the prison systems as part of a non-residential, day service. It was disheartening when I could not continue with planned sessions. This could happen for numerous reasons, for example, operational issues, which delayed the regime and being unable to bring BD to the service. This raised tensions between delivering therapy and the prison regime (which ultimately ensures the safety of staff and residents). Equally, there were challenges working with clients whose default response can be antisocial behaviour. There were times when BD was involved in fighting which meant he was located in the segregation unit and sessions could not continue. The therapy required some flexibility. I also found it hard to continue with EMDR sessions on the wing where he was located due to high levels of disruption there. There was a lot of noise on the wing. During one session another member of staff came into the room! These disturbances need to be avoided, as they are not conducive for facilitating trauma interventions. Sudden interruptions that may occur at any moment do not enable the establishment of emotional safety and may act as trauma triggers for some clients. The hour-long sessions offered did not allow flexibility for any difficulties that may arise on the day in seeing the person at the allocated time. There were times when I noticed myself being more attentive to time keeping and the prison regime rather than the therapy space. On reflection, I would allocate a minimum of 90 minutes to allow for any practical difficulties that may arise and also to enable sufficient time to achieve the aims of the session. Additionally, BD was transferred from the prison prior to processing his trauma. Time was spent managing this. However, it is vital that therapists anticipate any prison moves and respond to this prior to progressing with EMDR.

EMDR can be a very useful trauma intervention within prisons for individuals who are motivated and ready to explore their trauma. However, it should be part of an overall package of interventions offered by a trauma-informed service rather than a stand-alone intervention. It is possible to deliver trauma-specific interventions in prison settings, albeit in an adapted way. If, as a therapist, you can tolerate the inevitable challenges that arise when working in prison environments, and if you can adapt your approach to accommodate these and the needs of the person, then EMDR may be possible to offer. There is something therapeutically rich in being able to offer a trauma-informed intervention in imperfect therapeutic conditions. While it can act as a barrier, it can also act as a source of learning of how to heal trauma, as well as how to continue to change and grow within inevitable challenges.

Implications for Practice
Managing Systemic Issues

Prisons hold a dual role of custody (public protection) and rehabilitation. These roles can often conflict and create tension in trying to achieve progress. As mentioned previously, talking in a safe therapeutic environment promotes integration of fragmented memories but this can be undermined if attention to the somatic experience in which therapy is delivered is overlooked. For example, by not being attuned to the psychological and physiological experiences of undertaking therapy in prisons and the prison environment itself. For the YOI context, not only could individuals experience ongoing traumatisation and continue to experience psychological distress, where offending behaviours may be partly a consequence of past trauma, the offending behaviours could go unaddressed potentially creating future victims if trauma is unaddressed.

The importance of this systemic approach to delivering therapy is widely understood in numerous treatment modalities and other clinical and forensic settings. However, the utility of delivering interventions using a systemic approach is noted to be "the invisible problem" within prison settings (Clements et al., 2007). Creating a culture of physical and emotional safety is a key component for safe delivery of trauma interventions (Golding, 2015; Herman, 1992). Nonetheless, it is our experience that elements of safety can be achieved. This is primarily through the therapeutic relationship. It can also be achieved through attention to practical issues such as conducting therapy in rooms off-wing that minimise noise and distraction levels. Furthermore, it is vital that detailed safety plans and consideration for the individual's protective factors are formulated prior to progressing to trauma processing. This can be achieved through structured worksheets and staff training to ensure the individual has a support network they need. We found it particularly helpful to identify one member of staff who was regularly on the wing, as well as one or two senior wing staff, and to inform them, *briefly*, that the individual was engaging in EMDR therapy and what they may expect to see on the wing if the young person was struggling. We spent time with the young person exploring how their trauma may present and what aspects to share with staff before this was disclosed to the staff. One aspect we did not get to deliver due to COVID-19 was formal awareness training for staff. We would recommend this is also achieved. Additionally, we adapted the traditional EMDR protocol (Shapiro, 2018) for working with younger clients to allow more flexibility with introducing different psychoeducational tools and to allow for their suitability for the therapy to be considered. We also created an EMDR resource activation workbook for the creation of the safe place and installing resources.

Managing Self as Therapist

Professional skills need to be developed to take into account these systemic issues. A key skill for therapists is tolerance to these systemic issues. A major part of the work involved building trust and adapting the protocol to the environment. How we manage our own emotions around delivering interventions in a non-linear way can seem at odds with our own goals as the treatment provider. For instance, wanting to progress therapy sequentially in a rigid manner through the stages of the model. The therapeutic model needs to adapt its approach, and model to the client that compromise is acceptable, and more importantly needed. Tenacity and resilience will be key qualities. Professional skills need to be developed alongside this through training, supervision, and reflective spaces with others working in the field. Positively, it can challenge us to be creative in working with rather than against the processes and systems. It can also contribute to our growth as professionals. More importantly we can offer interventions to those who need it, and which may contribute to public protection in the long term.

It is also important to judge the pace of therapy, balancing the client's wish to progress to processing trauma and the therapist's anxiety about moving too quickly. Here, being attuned to the individual's needs and adopting attachment-informed approaches can support the formulation of this. Addressing trauma in a YOI requires avoiding temptation to adhere to a therapy model in prescriptive ways (where this is unhelpful) and working with the person in an integrative, attuned way while maintaining fidelity to the treatment model.

The Utility of the EMDR Protocol in a YOI

The EMDR protocol has many benefits and the potential to heal trauma in a YOI setting, for those who may need it. EMDR may support people with histories of complex trauma to heal their pasts and contribute to their readiness to then explore their offending and risks. It can support people in making sense of their past in a non-verbal way. This is particularly important for young people in prison whose executive functioning is still developing and may therefore not have developed the skills necessary to engage in talk therapies. Young people in prisons can also present with strong defences that may act as a barrier to talking trauma treatments. EMDR-informed interventions may therefore offer another non-verbal intervention to process trauma. Furthermore, it may be that aspects of the protocol may be beneficial for some. For example, it may be possible to install the safe place and offer resource installation even where a clinical decision is made not to progress to processing a memory. As such, EMDR skills may be offered as a treatment intervention.

Ward and Maruna (2007) have suggested that addressing non-criminogenic needs may be a necessary prerequisite to addressing criminogenic needs. Additionally, there are suggestions that people in prison are eager to receive more interventions that help them more generally, rather than interventions that just focus on offending only (Harvey & Smedley, 2017). There may therefore be benefits in not only engaging in risk reduction work, and internalising this change to prevent future harm, but also supporting people to address their trauma and have meaningful lives. People with trauma histories are more likely to have the cognitive, biological, and emotional capacity to engage in other interventions and learn new skills when their trauma is no longer a present-day threat for them. If we attempt to address the risk without addressing the trauma, we may be inadvertently re-enacting aspects of the trauma through dismissing, silencing, and ignoring the experience. There is also a growing body of evidence indicating the utility of EMDR in addressing adverse experiences that may contribute to offence pathways as well as targeting factors that drive offending for those who have committed sexual offences (Ricci & Clayton, 2016). As such, EMDR has utility in reducing risk as well as in healing the past.

EMDR should be delivered as part of a holistic package brought by a trauma-informed service where the individual is meaningfully engaged and has developed strong therapeutic relationships with staff. The majority of young people in prison will be experiencing complex trauma reactions related to histories of adverse experiences. These developmental considerations should be taken into account within direct trauma interventions. It is recognised that direct trauma therapies should not be viewed as the primary intervention when working with complex trauma (Rogers & Law, 2017) and as such should be delivered as part of a structured framework of therapies. This view is consistent with our experience. Effective trauma interventions in a YOI require focusing on relationship building, psychoeducation, self-regulation skills, working with rather than against systems in which the young person lives, and system level advocacy on behalf of the young person before any specific trauma processing begins. Once these are being responded to, more specialised trauma treatment, such as EMDR, may be possible.

Notes

1 The OPD pathway programme is a jointly commissioned initiative between NHS England and Her Majesty's Prison & Probation Service (HMPPS).
2 Across the wider Offender Personality Disorder pathways, the term Personality *Disorder* has been modified to Personality *Difficulties* in recognition of stigmatising terminology and growing trauma-informed research.
3 These types of childhood traumas have been named in the scientific literature with different but partially overlapping terms: early relation trauma, developmental trauma, complex trauma, or attachment trauma (Schore, 2009; Isobel et al., 2019).
4 An "enabling environment" is defined by the Royal College of Psychiatrists' (RCP) Centre for Quality Improvement (CCQI) as a place in which "participants feel safe enough to develop relationships and to share experience and ideas with others". The CCQI runs an "Enabling Environment Award" scheme, to recognise environments that meet a critical set of standards. The CNS is accredited with this award.
5 However, were we to put a diagnostic slant on the cohort, evidence corroborated by medical notes, psychiatric/psychology reports, risk assessments (OASYs and ASSET) and self-reporting, would indicate a high proportion of those young people as meeting diagnosis for PTSD, complex PTSD, and/or complex trauma.
6

> A group of three or more people who have a distinct identity (e.g., a name/badge/emblem) and commit general crime or anti-social behaviour as part of their identity. This group uses (or is reasonably suspected of using) firearms, or the threat of firearms when carrying out these offences
>
> *Home Office, 2008; p.23.*

7 Criminal exploitation is also known as "county lines" and is when gangs and organised crime networks groom and exploit children to sell drugs. Often these children are made to travel across counties, and they use dedicated mobile phone "lines" to supply drugs.

Further Reading

Harvey, J., & Smedley, K. (2017). Psychological therapy in prisons and other secure settings. For readers interested in understanding more on the range of therapeutic approaches used in prisons and other secure settings.

Joseph, N. & Bennefield, N. (2012). 'A joint offender personality disorder pathway strategy: An outline summary'. Criminal Behaviour and Mental Health, 22, 210–217. For people who want to understand more about the Offender Personality Disorder (OPD) Pathway.

Shapiro, F. (2018). Eye movement desensitisation and reprocessing (EMDR) therapy: Basic principles, protocols and procedures. A key book for people interested in reading more about the development and principles of EMDR.

References

Bateman A., & Fonagy P. (2006). *Mentalization based treatment: A practical guide*. Oxford: Oxford University Press.

Bloom, S.L. & Farragher, B. (2011). *Destroying sanctuary: The crisis in human service delivery systems*. Oxford University Press.

Boswell, G.R. (1991). *Waiting for change: An exploration of the experiences and needs of Section 53 offenders*. The Prince's Trust.

Bradley, A. (2017). *Trauma informed practice: Exploring the role of adverse life experiences on the behaviour of offenders and the effectiveness of associated criminal justice strategies* (Unpublished doctoral thesis). Northumbria University.

Clements, C.B., Althouse, R., Fagan, T.J., & Wormith, J.S. (2007). Systemic issues and correctional outcomes. *Criminal Justice and Behaviour, 34*, 919–932. doi:10.1177/0093854807301561

Covington, S.S., & Rodriquez, R. (2016). *Exploring trauma: A brief intervention for men*. Hazelden.

Davidson, J. (1997). *Every boundary broken: Sexual abuse of women patients in psychiatric institutions*. NSW Department for Women and the NSW Health Department.

Ehlers, A., & Clark, D. (2000). A cognitive model of posttraumatic stress disorder. *Behaviour Research and Therapy, 15*(3), 249–275. doi:10.1016/S0005-7967%2899%2900123-0

Finkelhor, D., Turner, H.A., Ormrod, R., & Hamby, S.L. (2009). Violence, abuse, and crime exposure in a national sample of children and youth. *Pediatrics, 124*(5), 1–13. doi:10.1542/peds.2009-0467

Fonagy, P., Gergely, G., Jurist, E.L., & Target, M. (2002). *Affect regulation, mentalization, and the development of the self*. Routledge. doi:10.4324/9780429471643

Fonagy, P., & Bateman, A. (2008). The development of borderline personality disorder – a mentalizing model. *Journal Personality Disorder, 22*(1), 4–21. doi: 10.1521/pedi.2008.22.1.4.

Fonagy, P., & Target, M. (2008). Attachment, trauma, and psychoanalysis. In E.L. Jurist, A. Slade, & S. Bergner (Eds), *Mind to mind* (pp.15–42). Other Press.

Golding, K.S. (2015). *Meeting the therapeutic needs of traumatised children*. Retrieved from https://kimsgolding.co.uk/resources/models/meeting-the-therapeutic-needs-of-traumatized-children/

Haley, M., (2017). "Attachment-based psychodynamic psychotherapy". In Harvey, J., & Smedley, K. (Eds). *Psychological therapy in prisons and other secure settings*. Routledge.

Harvey, J., & Smedley, K. (2017). *Psychological therapy in prisons and other secure settings*. Routledge.

Herman, J. (1992). *Trauma and recovery: The aftermath of violence*. Basic.

Home Office (2008). *Tackling Gangs: Practical Guide for local authorities, CDRPS and other local partners*. Home Office.

Huang, Y.L., Fonagy, P., Feigenbaum, J., Montague, R., & Nolte, T. 2020. Multidirectional pathways between attachment, mentalizing, and posttraumatic stress symptomatology in the context of childhood trauma. *Psychopathology, 53*(1), 48–58. 5. doi:10.1159/000506406

Isobel, S., Foster, M.K., Goodyear, J. M. (2019). Psychological trauma in the context of familial relationships: a concept analysis. *Trauma Violence & Abuse, 20* (40), 549–559. doi:10.1177/1524838017726424

Jennings, A. (2004). *Models for developing trauma-informed behavioral health systems and trauma-specific services.* National Association of State Mental Health Program Directors and the National Technical Assistance Center for State Mental Health Planning.

Joseph, N., & Bennefield, N. (2012). A joint offender personality disorder pathway strategy: An outline summary. *Criminal Behaviour and Mental Health, 22,* 210–217. doi:10.1002/cbm.1835

Kezelman, C., & Stavropoulos, P. (2012). '*The last frontier'. Practice guidelines for treatment of complex trauma and trauma informed care and service delivery.* Adults Surviving Child Abuse (ACSA).

Livesley, J. (2015). *Practical management of personality disorder.* Guilford.

McGuire, J. (2013). 'What works' to reduce re-offending: 18 years on. In L.A. Craig, L. Dixon, & T.A. Gannon (Eds), *What works in offender rehabilitation: An evidence-based approach to assessment and treatment* (pp.20–49). Wiley Blackwell. doi:10.1002/9781118320655.ch2

Ministry of Justice. (2020). *Safety in custody statistics, England and Wales: Deaths in custody in prison custody to December 2019 assaults and self-harm to September 2019.* Ministry of Justice.

Mrug, S., Madan, A., Windle, M. (2016) Emotional desensitization to violence contributes to adolescents' violent behavior.. *Journal of abnormal child psychology, 44*(1), 75–86. doi:10.1007/s10802-015-9986

National Offender Manager Service. (2015). *Better outcomes for young adult men: Evidence based commissioning principles.* NOMS.

Perry B.D., Pollard R., Blakely T., Baker W., & Vigilante, D. (1995). Childhood trauma, the neurobiology of adaptation and 'use-dependent' development of the brain: how "states" become "traits". *Infant Mental Health Journal, 16*(4), 271–291. doi:10.1002/1097-0355(199524)16:4<271

Ricci, R.J., & Clayton, C.A. (2016). EMDR with sex offenders: Using offence drivers to guide conceptualisation and treatment. *Journal of EMDR Practice and Research, 10*(2), 104–118. doi:10.1891/1933-3196.10.2.104

Rogers, A., & Law, H. (2017). Working with trauma in a prison setting. In Harvey, J., & Smedley, K. (Eds). *Psychological therapy in prisons and other secure settings.* Routledge.

Salzinger, S., Feldman, R.S., Stockhammer, T., & Hood, J. (2002). An ecological framework for understanding risk for exposure to community violence and the effects of exposure on children and adolescents. *Aggression and Violent Behavior, 7*(5), 423–451. doi:10.1016/S1359-1789(01)00078-7

Schore, A. N. (2009). Attachment trauma and the developing of right brain: origin of pathological dissociation. In P. Dell and J. A. O'Neil (Eds). *Dissociation and dissociative disorders: DSM-V and beyond.* Routledge.

Shapiro, F. (2018). *Eye movement densensitization and reprocessing (EMDR) therapy* (3rd Ed). Guildford Press.

Skuse, T., & Matthew, J. (2015). The trauma recovery model: Sequencing youth justice interventions for young people with complex needs. *Prison Service Journal, 220,* 16–25.

Squire, B., Jefford, T., & Cupit Swenson, C. (2015). Whole systems approaches. In A. Rogers, J. Harvey, & H. Law (Eds), *Young people in forensic mental health settings: Psychological thinking and practice* (pp.123–142). Palgrave Macmillan.

Sturge, G. (2020). *UK prison population statistics, July 2020.* House of Commons briefing paper. Retrieved from https://researchbriefings.files.parliament.uk/documents/SN04334/SN04334.pdf

Treisman, K. (2016). *Working with relational and developmental trauma in children and adolescents.* Routledge.

Ward, T., & Brown, M. (2004). The good lives model and conceptual issues in offender rehabili-tation. *Psychology, Crime & Law, 10*, 243–257. doi:10.1080/10683160410001662744

Ward, T., & Maruna, S. (2007). *Rehabilitation: Beyond the risk paradigm.* Routledge.

Wigmor, J. (2018). Recognising & acting on signs of 'county lines' child exploitation. A case study. NHS England.

Young, J., Klosko, J., (1993). *Reinventing your life: The breakthrough program to end negative behaviour and feel great again.* Plume.

17
TRAUMA AND THE EXPERIENCE OF IMPRISONMENT

Kerensa Hocken, Jon Taylor, and Jamie Walton

The presence and prevalence of trauma and adversity in the histories of people in prison present an important factor in understanding the trajectory to offending. Trauma and adversity demand survival responses which become learnt ways of living. We propose that these survival responses give rise to the psychological characteristics conceptualised in the forensic literature as criminogenic needs (or dynamic risk factors for offending). Changes to these criminogenic needs are a key target of rehabilitative efforts and we argue that for long-lasting change to occur, the survival responses that underpin them need to be addressed. However, an individual is only likely to succeed at changing their survival responses in a stable non-threatening context in which they are no longer needed. This chapter explores the traumatic origins of criminogenic needs and the subsequent experience of imprisonment, arguing that the prison environment can act as a threat-based context for some, which demands previously learnt survival responses not only from those living, but also those working in prison. As such, the prison environment can be viewed as is a co-produced (staff and prison resident) threat-sensitive context where survival (physical and psychological) is the priority, creating conditions for (re)traumatisation and restricting the ability of residents to engage with and benefit from rehabilitative efforts. We examine the possible pragmatic responses to facilitate context change in the prison environment, focusing on the concept of Procedural Justice as an opportunity to intervene with and modify a threat-based environment to create optimum conditions for rehabilitation efforts to flourish.

Developing a Trauma-Sensitive Framework for Prison Rehabilitation

Since the seminal publication by Felitti et al. (1998) detailing an association between various types of adversity and health challenges across the lifespan (Adverse Childhood Experiences: ACEs), various studies have extended this work and sought to investigate

298

DOI: 10.4324/9781003120766-22

the long-term consequences of various types of trauma and adversity in early life. In this section we present a brief overview of the more recent studies that investigate the relationship between trauma and adversity and one particular outcome – offending and imprisonment – before considering the pathways that may link early adversity and adult harmfulness and use this to begin to consider key features of rehabilitative environments.

Adverse Childhood Experiences and the Stimulation of Criminogenic Capacities

Prison services have been slow to respond to the growing evidence that some people who serve prison sentences bring with them stories of harsh, punitive, and neglectful early lives. In helping people to change, our focus in forensic practice has been on harm caused not harm experienced. While this is perhaps understandable given the focus on harm reduction, it is ironic, given the indications that harm experienced can contribute to the acquisition of criminogenic capacities and offending (see Chapter 1). The last decade has, however, seen an increasing willingness in general forensic practice to explore and understand the links between childhood trauma and adversity and the development of harmful behaviour. A number of studies have pointed towards an association between early adversity and offending in later life (Reavis, Looman, Franco, & Rojas, 2013; Topitzes, Mersky, & Reynolds, 2011), while some studies suggest that certain types of offending, such as sexual offending, may also be associated with particularly high rates of adverse experience (Levenson, Willis, & Prescott, 2015). Taken together, there seems to be some suggestion that people who develop their capacity and willingness to harm others are far more likely to have been subjected to various harmful experiences during their development (see Table 17.1). Furthermore, there is some evidence that increasing experience of adversity and abuse increases the likelihood of more serious offending, with men who commit the most serious offences having the most chronic exposure to abuse and neglect (DeLisi & Beauregard, 2018; Drury et al., 2017).

Although the ACE-to-offending link seems to be robust, it is nuanced with a number of factors influencing the link and a number of repercussions arising from the association. For instance, the impact of these experiences is found to emerge

Table 17.1 Prevalence of ACEs in general populations and offending groups

Study	Population	*n*	Prevalence (%)	
			1 ACE	*4+ ACE*
Felitti (2009)	US citizens	13500	52	6.2
Bellis et al. (2014)	UK citizens	3885	47	8
Reavis et al. (2013)	Convicted groups			
Levenson (2014)	Men with sexual convictions	679	84	50
Levenson et al. (2015)	Women with sexual convictions	47	80	41
Morris et al. (2020)	Adolescents in secure healthcare	36	91	58
Taylor (2021)	Men with repeat sexual convictions	21	100	83

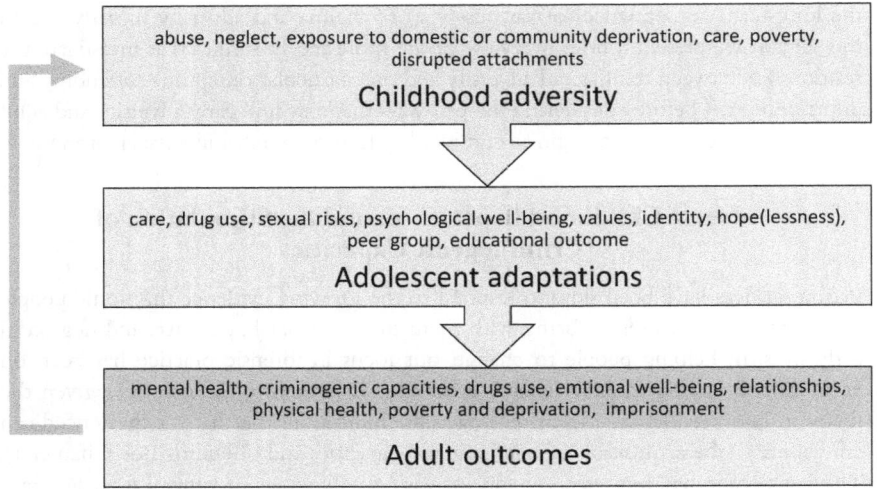

Figure 17.1 Pathways from adversity to criminogenic vulnerability and back again

during the developmental period with harmful and offending behaviour emerging by adolescence (Abram et al., 2004; Becker & Kerig, 2011; Ford, Chapman, Connor, & Cruise, 2012; Tyler, Johnson, & Brownridge, 2008). The implication here is that the effects of early adversity begin to materialise early in life and therefore such responses can be rehearsed, refined, and strengthened across adolescence and into adulthood such that they become highly resilient. It is these resilient strategies that are perhaps perceived as "treatment resistance".

Adversity also follows people into prison. It seems likely that common features of prison living, such as violence and drug use, simply repeat early life conditions. To add insult to injury, literally for some, the experience of adversity and trauma may increase vulnerability to further trauma responses once imprisoned. For example, Mandelli, Carli, Roy, Serretti, & Sarchiapone (2011) found that people in prison who had attempted suicide had significantly greater trauma histories than people who had never attempted, while repeated attempts were predicted by sexual abuse.

What this seems to suggest is a pathway from adversity to criminogenic vulnerability and back again (see Figure 17.1). If prisons contain and care for people who have followed this path then the least that these services will need to do is to witness the process, understand the impact on people, criminogenic and otherwise, and build interventions around this. With this in mind we now briefly consider this impact before moving on to discuss the nature of rehabilitative environments.

Adversity and Pathways to Offending: Epigenetic Modifications

The early ACEs studies identified a pathway between the ACE and later difficulties that was based largely on a disease model. ACEs prompt a disruption to neurodevelopment and subsequent cognitive and emotional impairment. In turn, these lead to high-risk

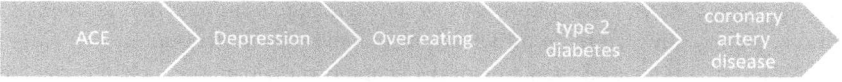

Figure 17.2 Disease model of the impact of ACEs

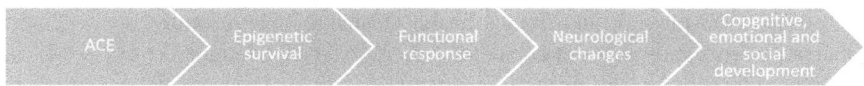

Figure 17.3 Functional adaptation in the context of adverse living conditions

behaviours that generate physical health problems, disease, and disability. Felitti (2009) proposed two broad mechanisms that may mediate the link between ACEs and bio-medical disease. First, the outcome, the disease, is a delayed consequence of various coping strategies. These include drug use, overeating, smoking, etc. Felitti provides an example of this as illustrated in Figure 17.2. Second, the disease is caused by chronic stress mediated by cortisol.

However, the regularity of the adversity to offending link begins to raise the possibility that these recurring difficulties are not diseased reactions but rather adaptive responses to adversity (Figure 17.3). There are two possible mechanisms that may explain these responses. First, human beings have evolved to respond to adversity in particular ways that are related to our threat-defence processes. This is because our ancestors evolved in an unforgiving primitive environment, where food scarcity and predation were formidable barriers to life. Only those who were vigilant survived. Human nervous systems are the result of these evolutionary pressures, and as such our brains come hardwired to prioritise our survival, automatically mobilising safety strategies such as aggression, avoidance, hiding, submissiveness, and forming useful alliances. Second, our epigenetic capacity can hardwire these responses and the learning that we take from our early experiences, into lasting phenotypes – and does so because of their intrinsic survival value. We propose that these processes represent ordered and not disordered adaptations to adverse living environments and suggest that the neurological changes that are linked to ACEs provide some evidence of a routine human response.

Offending and Pathways to Desistance: Neurogenesis and Rehabilitative Environments

So far, we can see that the experience of adversity is not just present in the lives of people who develop criminogenic capacities but is a recurring and persistent feature of many people's lives. Many people who reside in prison have grown up in a culture that allows youngsters to be harmed; neglect may be the dominant parenting style; violence is frequent; drug use is encouraged; and sexual abuse is not uncommon (DeLis & Beauregard, 2018). Accommodating the research into ACEs we are beginning to establish a model of forensic needs where early adversity is recognised as a strong predictor of survival responses that may become harmful as development continues, such as using violence to defend oneself and hostile attribution.

Although it is beyond the scope of the chapter to evaluate these changes (epigenetic, neurological, and neurogenetic) in detail, the regularity of findings suggests that there is a normal biological/neurological and psychological adaptation to adversity (sensitive to individual differences) and that criminogenic needs are as much a typical response as are physical and mental health challenges. Furthermore, the suggestion that repeated exposure to trauma (four or more ACEs; Hughes et al., 2017) and chronic adversity are the primary facilitators of this pathway would suggest that it is context, a repeated living experience, which drives such change. We suggest that a trauma-sensitive context of rehabilitation is therefore a primary agent of (re)change.

Rehabilitative Environments? Imprisonment and the Cycle of Trauma

Independent of where in the world a prison is, there are a few features that remain the same: punishment, segregation, regulation, and confinement. Critically, and because nearly all people who enter prisons at some point leave, they must be humane environments of decency, safety, healing, mentorship, hope, purposeful activity, and change. In other words, prisons must be *rehabilitative*. According to Her Majesty's Inspectorate of Prisons (HMIP, 2019), progress to create rehabilitative environments has been made, especially in some high secure prisons and women's prisons where safe, calm, and professional atmospheres have been observed. However, many English and Welsh prisons experience high through-put, much of their fabric is aging, and there have been staffing challenges to implementing purposeful activity, and managing violence (HMIP, 2019). The social disadvantages inherent in the communities of people most likely to enter prison, particularly poor living conditions, poor sleep hygiene, poor diet, overcrowding, and violence, often continue within them (House of Commons, 2018; Prison Reform Trust, 2019; HMIP, 2019).

All prisons deny people of their liberty as free citizens, but in doing so, and without a robust resolve to provide a humane environment, they can quite easily bring about physical, mental, and social harm to residents (and staff), subjecting them to basic resource deprivation. In the UK for example, HMIP and parliamentary inquires report that because of limited budgets, prisons struggle to provide appetising meal choices of adequate quantity and quality (HMIP, 2018; House of Commons, 2018). Poor sleep hygiene is another example (House of Commons, 2018), with thin mattresses, cramped rooms, and noise meaning that poor sleep can be a common experience. There are also psychological difficulties associated with prison life. For example, experiences of fear, anxiety, loneliness, depression, injustice, powerlessness, and uncertainty as well as the experience of being punished itself (Liebling & Maruna, 2005). At the very least, prison is emotionally and socially painful. People, to varying degrees, are exposed to stigmatisation, violence, intimacy deprivation, restrictive systems, and a depersonalised pattern of daily living that they must adapt to. By nature, prisons deprive liberty and freewill, but they also hold power over those living within them, and the way that power operates in prison can be a source of damage, as Auty and

Liebling (2020) observe: "Prisons are full of power, and power has inherent tendencies towards abuse, misapplication and corruption, achieving [legitimacy] is an uphill struggle" (p.20).

As practitioners working in prisons, we ought to be attuned to these realities to validate (or avoid invalidating) the lived experiences of the people who are locked up. When prison conditions are excessively unsafe, dysfunctional, or deprived, or if people are confined in prisons for extensive lengths of time, it would be unreasonable to expect them to come away unscathed. It is unsurprising then that a number of authors have commented on the traumatising effects that imprisonment has on some people (e.g., Haney, 2012; Jones, 2015), and even the identification of a *Post-Incarceration Syndrome* (Liem & Kunst, 2013). The question about labelling as a syndrome a set of behaviours that may be contextually adaptive notwithstanding, it points to the long-lasting damaging effects that prison can have on people.

We have discussed the connection between the cycles of adversity, inequality, and social disadvantage that serve as a backdrop for the development of criminogenic need. This is not *just* a social backdrop, it is a biological one too. Biological adjustments, including those at the epigenetic level, ensure that neurodevelopmental, psychological adjustment, and behaviour are all choreographed and contextualised by adverse experience such that they are calibrated to fit the harsh social pressures faced. Humans are well-equipped to respond to adversity of course, and as we have noted, we are good at adapting to adversity. When conditions are unsafe, when stimulation is low, and when resources are scarce, as can be the case in socially deprived crime-ridden neighbourhoods and in underperforming prisons, these adaptations will be common. This is often found in prison research (e.g., De Viggiani, 2006; Sykes, 1958). Residents strive to "survive" emotionally, psychologically and socially, as well as physically. However, prisons do not merely risk maintaining the experience of adversity. It has been recognised for decades now that they also "import" it (Cohen & Taylor, 1981; Ditchfield, 1990). This is because prison communities share the cultural norms of their host communities. That is to say, those who enter them bring their values, attitudes, and learnt behavioural strategies from their local social niches. When people who arrive in prison have experienced abuse, cruelty, poverty, addiction, or other trauma, which many have, these experiences and their developmental effects arrive as well. When faced with the adversity and deprivations of daily prison life, they may further manifest biologically, psychologically, and behaviourally, most likely as a heightened response to threat, with associated guardedness, suspicion, aggression, risk taking, egocentricity, and impulsivity. These strategies in turn contribute to and collectively shape the prison subculture.

This is not out of the choice of residents. As alluded to above, what we are talking about here is an evolved adaptive response to threat and adversity, from the epigenetic level upwards. Fundamentally, minds, brains, and behaviour are environmentally contextualised; they are patterned by, and attuned to, the cost-benefit pay-offs that are present in the environment that people are situated in. In turn, the "best-fit" strategies for surviving the particular pressures of the environment will emerge, etched in neurobiology, personality, and behaviour. For example, in a safe, predictable and cohesive community with good education, leisure, and healthcare infrastructure, it will prove adaptive for an individual to learn to invest in others with trust, sharing, cooperation, and care. Similarly, in safe prisons with adequate facilities and constructive activity, and staff who work diligently to be compassionate, transparent, fair, and cooperative, these pro-social strategies are at least in step with the environment. Residents can "dare to be vulnerable" and enter into a change process, because turning towards their own harm and the harm they have caused others is consistent with the safeness embedded in their immediate social surroundings. Now contrast a safe community setting with a dangerous and deprived neighbourhood, stricken with crime, violence, and drugs. The strategies of trust, sharing, cooperation, and care will be less useful in these conditions, or even disadvantageous. As such they may be down-regulated, both behaviourally and biologically. This down-regulation will occur at various levels through different mechanisms and processes, from the biomolecular regulation of gene expression (*epigenetic modifications*, see Leshem & Weisburd, 2019; Walton, in press) to the shaping and reshaping of brain circuitry (*neuroplasticity*); and at the behavioural level, through basic observational learning process such as modelling and imitating, and direct contingency learning including classical and operant conditioning. At a cultural level too pre-existing in the norms, social rules, and niche language of deprived crime-ridden communities, caring and cooperative pro-social strategies are unlikely to be reinforced, and in fact, may even be punished. As a result, in many cases, brains and behaviour will not be attuned to pro-social strategies because the experiences of safeness, care, forgiveness, and nurturement required for them to flourish biologically and psychologically have been severely lacking. Instead, the high risk, self-focused, and exploitative strategies associated with criminogenic need are more likely to emerge as the best fit. These may include aggression, insensitivity, exploitation, excessive risk taking, disinhibition, and impulsiveness.

Now consider the poor levels of safety and substandard living conditions in an underperforming prison. Such high-risk, self-focus, and exploitative strategies can be of best fit in these conditions as well, predominantly because they are similar in dangerousness, adversity, and deprivation. Use of these strategies is not without consequence. Adaption to adverse conditions simply enables individuals to survive in chronically stressful circumstances, even though the emerging best-fit strategies are destructive (or criminogenic). Under these conditions, pro-social change that society seeks from all residents is, at best, extremely hard to achieve. Instead, brains and bodies will continue to be calibrated by adversity, threat, and danger, and they will continue to optimise and select the (criminogenic) strategies needed to survive in the face of it.

The way in which prison choreographs brains, minds, and bodies is of course not limited to residents. Prison staff, particularly prison officers, are also embedded in the institutional culture. They are exposed to prison life in lower doses than residents, but they still spend substantial amounts of time immersed in the physical environment. Unsurprisingly, stress and adverse effects on well-being are well-noted among prison staff (Bierie, 2012; Stöver, 2017). The same harsh conditions, that recruit and heighten threat responses in residents, can also call for them in prison staff. The human response to threat is ubiquitous, meaning the side of the "prison bars" a person finds themself on is not necessarily the key determinant in how the prison takes its toll on them. In an unsafe prison, staff must learn to stay safe. Their brains and bodies must deal with the threat of danger just as much as the residents they supervise. When the minds and bodies of residents and prison staff are both severely threatened, there is little biological space for connection, let alone the social space for decency and change. We mean "biological space" in real terms. When under strongly perceived or actual serious threat, the parts of the nervous system which enable openness and social engagement as the basis for giving and receiving care, connecting and co-regulating are at best dampened or at worst turned off by a heightened threat system which (rather adaptively to aid survival) keeps minds on high alert, suspicious and cautious, and bodies guarded, tied to the safety *within* the identified in-group (residents vs. officers), and if needed ready to attack. In short, people's threat systems reinforce each other, creating staff-resident division and strengthening a "them-and-us" culture. In this context, it is easy to see why staff might adopt punitive and authoritarian strategies, which in turn create feelings of injustice and powerlessness within residents and reinforce previous trauma experiences.

Trauma-Sensitive Practice in Prison

So far, we have discussed the biopsychosocial origins of criminogenic needs, understanding their beginnings as an early survival response to adversity, the capacities for which are inbuilt within all humans at a biological level and shaped by environmental context. We have further discussed how a threat-based context of prison can maintain rather than reduce the need for behavioural strategies linked to criminogenic needs and its capacities for (re)traumatisation. The important question is how we begin to change the prison context such that it is trauma informed, to acknowledge the trauma and adversity experiences of prison residents (and staff) and respond to these in ways that create the best physical and relational environment to support long-term change of criminogenic needs, and towards a non-offending life for those living there.

Experiences of unjust, illegitimate power are a key feature of adverse and traumatic experience (Johnstone & Boyle et al., 2018), and if prisons are to be spaces of rehabilitation and positive change, they ought to start by breaking cycles of powerlessness, inequality, and disadvantage. There are several examples where prisons have created trauma-informed contexts such as Therapeutic Communities (TC; see Chapters 14 and 15 for a detailed review of TC practice), Psychologically-Informed Environments (PIPE), Procedural Justice (PJ), and Rehabilitative Culture (RC) (Akerman & Andrews, 2020; Bennett & Tilt, 2019; Kordowicz, 2019; Rawlings & Haigh, 2017; Turley, Payne, & Webster, 2013). Such initiatives provide psychologically healthier environments that are sensitive to people's adverse life experience, reflected in regimes that strive to be constructive, prison infrastructure that is sympathetic, and training to ensure staff are equipped to be agents of change. The golden thread within these models is the operation of power between staff and residents, exemplified in the democratic TC model where the hierarchy is flattened, power democratised (Rapoport, Rapoport, & Rosow, 1960), and prison residents and staff function together as a community and make decisions jointly. This democracy provides a basis for power that is recognised by residents as legitimate, safe, and allows them to feel humanised, valued, and autonomous (see Armstrong and Ludlow, 2019; Davis, 2019; Shah, Allen, Peters, & Bennett, 2019 for review of resident TC experiences). The democratic TC model demonstrates that legitimate and safe use of power in prison is possible, but the challenge is to apply this learning from a small number of specialist prisons, to prison environments more broadly. We will now review one approach to creating legitimate authority, Procedural Justice, and consider how it might be understood as a trauma-informed practice in prison.

Procedural Justice

Procedural Justice (PJ) originates from court settings and is a relatively simple concept referring to the perceived fairness by which the process of justice is conducted, not the fairness of outcome (Lind & Tyler, 1988). Much has been written about the relationship between perceived fairness increasing feelings of confidence in the legitimacy of the authority and this being essential for effective justice (see Laxminarayan, 2012; Tyler, 2010). An important influence on perceptions of fairness is that the authority or decision-maker is acting legitimately in the best interest of the individual without other agenda (Levi, Sacks, & Tyler, 2009). Lind and Tyler (1988) cite three features of PJ that facilitate acceptance by and identification with the decision-maker: standing within one's social group (that is, respect), trust in the decision-maker, and neutrality of the decision-maker. These features with the addition of voice (having a chance to contribute opinions and to be heard) make up the four principles of PJ. PJ, as conceptualised by Tyler (1989), emphasises a relational premise in which group belonging is considered to be at the heart of feeling fairly treated. The authority figure, as an agent of society, recognising the harm caused to someone and acting to do something about it, validates an individual's value and status as a member of society, which signals group belonging. This facilitates feelings of identification with the decision-maker. The relational premise that PJ rests upon reflects mammalian evolved motives for group belonging, an important signal for safety; when in the presence of an "in group", we are more likely to feel safe and able to recuperate (Baumeister & Leary, 1995). Involvement in decisions is a cue for cooperation and therefore safety.

Wells (2007) reported that where people feel decisions have been made in fair and just ways, they experience the decision-makers as legitimate and are therefore more able to cooperate with that decision-making. Court processes which provide positive experiences of PJ for victims of crime are less likely to leave them feeling coerced by the justice system (Winick, 2006) and can provide therapeutic value. Elliott, Thomas, and Ogloff (2014) found that validation and acknowledgement that wrong had been done was a key therapeutic factor for victims. Their research participants judged that the way police responded to them was a reflection of how the community saw them, and where it was positive it was received as a proxy means of community validation. Elliott et al. (2014) propose this can strengthen the link between individual

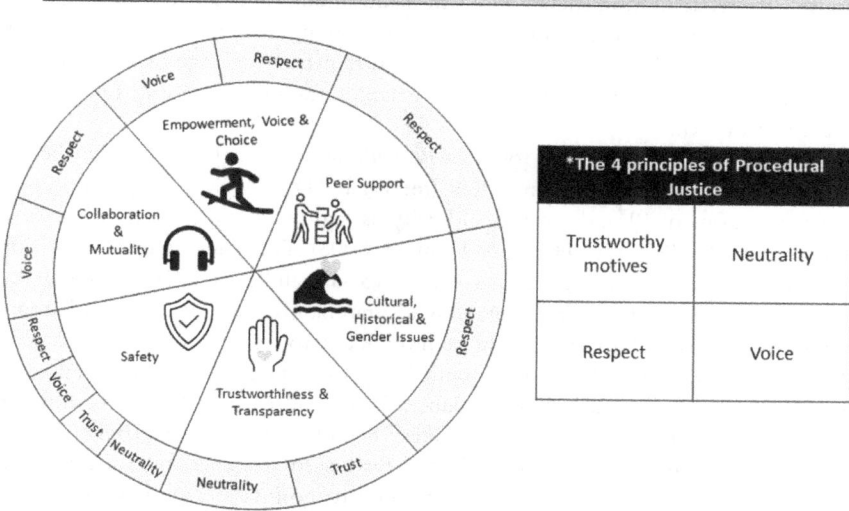

How Trauma Informed and Procedural Justice* Principles Fit Together

*The 4 principles of Procedural Justice	
Trustworthy motives	Neutrality
Respect	Voice

Figure 17.4 How trauma-informed and procedural justice* principles fit together

and community. When conducted in this way, the justice process is hypothesised has having a therapeutic value, known as *Therapeutic Jurisprudence* (Winick, 2006).

PJ in the court system is well recognised as a trauma-informed concept, implemented largely as a response to the recognition that criminal justice processes, with the imbalance of power, can re-traumatise victims of crime (Laxminarayan, 2012). McKenna and Holtfreter (2020) draw attention to the overlap between PJ principles and trauma-informed principles as defined by Substance Abuse and Mental Health Services Administration (SAMHSA, 2014) (see Figure 17.4). The PJ model of giving voice and respect to individuals creates a feeling of group belonging and safety, and is a move towards a trauma-informed way of working, especially with people who have experienced repeated patterns of powerlessness, illegitimate authority, and decisions made about them, not with them. Such people are primed to feel unjustly treated by authority including the Criminal Justice System. For example, Penner, Shaffer, and Viljoen (2017) found that a history of trauma in young defendants is associated with negative perceptions of legitimacy of law, underscoring the need for criminal justice processes to be trauma informed.

Procedural Justice in Prison

In the UK, HM Prison and Probation Service (HMPPS) use the term Rehabilitative Culture (RC) to describe the optimal prison environment to support rehabilitation activity (Mann, Fitzalan Howard, & Tew, 2018). RC is a relational concept, acknowledging the relationship between staff and residents as an agent of change, creating

a safe, decent, and respectful environment which is hopeful and provides opportunities for rehabilitation such as education and offending behaviour interventions.
However, feelings of safety and control are prerequisites for positive change to
occur (Allcock, 2015) and a rehabilitative culture can only thrive in the context of
a safe and decent environment in which harmful, trauma learnt survival strategies
become redundant.

HMPPS have identified the role that Procedural Justice (PJ) can have in the creation of a safe and decent environment (see Figure 17.5). Where people have positive perceptions of PJ and see the authority as legitimate, they are more likely to
follow the rules (Murphy, Hinds, & Fleming, 2008). This has obvious applications
for prisons where following rules is central to safe and decent environments but
where there are elevated rates of people with trauma histories (e.g., Ford, Chapman,
Connor, & Cruise, 2012) who might be more likely to have negative perceptions of
PJ (Penner et al., 2017). PJ has been applied to prison environments in several countries and shown improved rule compliance (Reisiga & Mesko, 2009) and although
a small effect, reduction in recidivism rates 18 months post-release (Beijersbergen,
Dirkzwager, & Nieuwbeerta, 2016). Several further studies have found decreases in
official and self-reported offending in response to positive perceptions of PJ with
police encounters (Paternoster, Bachman, Brame, & Sherman, 1997; Penner, Viljoen,
Douglas, & Roesch, 2013; Tyler, Sherman, Strang, Barnes, & Woods, 2007; Sunshine &
Tyler, 2003) suggesting the potential for PJ to have rehabilitative capacities.

In UK prisons, PJ is being implemented into daily practice, most notably in relation
to the way adjudications (prison-based hearings for rule breaking) are run. Fitzalan
Howard (2017) argues that the typically punitive process of adjudications can have
greater rehabilitative gain and increase intention to comply with rules when those

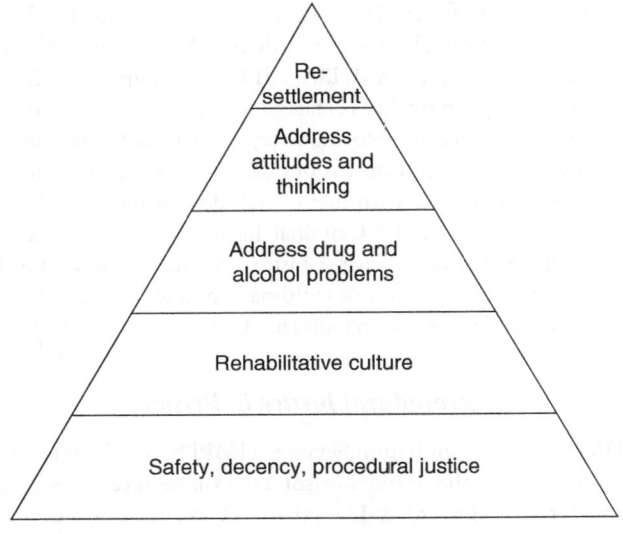

Figure 17.5 Hierarchical components of a rehabilitative prison

Table 17.2 Examples of procedural justice practice adjudications

Procedural Justice Principles	Procedural Justice Practice
Respect	Being courteous, maintaining eye contact, using preferred names, communicating that the person and their rights are important
Neutrality	Explaining how rules are being applied and why, explaining how decisions have been made, referring to rules and evidence rather than personal views
Trustworthy motives	Explaining reasons for all decisions, consciously being approachable and not intimidating, being sincere and caring, and offering support where appropriate
Giving voice	Accounting for their views in the decision, active listening, asking for an individual's view of the problem and possible solutions

performing them use PJ principles. So-called Rehabilitative Adjudications (RA) involve adjudicators (typically prison governors) explicitly and deliberately adopting PJ principles in the adjudication process. In RA, adjudicators are specially trained in the principles of PJ and how to adopt them in practice, shown in Table 17.2.

Compared to the experience of a typical adjudication, Fitzalan Howard and Wakeling (2020) found both prison residents and adjudicators experienced RA as procedurally just. Residents experienced them as fair, with greater increased positive perceptions of staff and the wider system and showed an increased intention and commitment to comply with rules. Adjudicators viewed RA as more constructive, productive, and meaningful.

Expanding from judicial prison processes, PJ can be the basis for other processes and policies such as cell searching (Mann, 2019) and decision-making. The way these decisions are communicated also needs to reflect PJ principles. Figure 17.6 shows an example of a notice to prison residents at HMP Leicester which demonstrates PJ ways of communicating.

This illustrates that fairly simple changes to the way prison processes are conducted could have positive outcomes for perceptions of PJ and therefore feeling fairly treated. This has important implications for improving prison safety. Fitzalan Howard and Wakeling (2019) found that people in prison who perceive their treatment as unfair and disrespectful reported higher rates of self-harm and attempted suicide, and in some prisons it was associated with higher assaults and disorder. Similarly, staff who perceived themselves as treated unfairly and unjustly were more likely to have higher sickness rates and a more punitive orientation towards prison residents. Conversely staff who had positive perceptions of PJ were less stressed, had greater overall rehabilitative orientation, less punitive views, and were more trusting of and compassionate towards residents. PJ perceptions between staff and residents were linked; where staff had less punitive attitudes and were more orientated towards helping and trusting residents, residents perceived their treatment to be fairer and more just. This speaks to the co-produced nature of the prison environment in which behaviours are

---

Reducing Reoffending: Updated Prisoner

Pay and Activity Allocation Policy

At HMP Leicester, we are committed to supporting you to address the issues that led to you coming into custody.

It is our aim to provide paid activities, to enable you to gain experience of work, training, and life skills in preparation for your release. The attached Prisoner Pay and Allocation to Activities Policy intends to support you to make positive choices about which activity to apply for by making our best paid jobs those that are linked to gaining formal qualifications and skills linked to employment on release. You will notice that college is now one of the best paid activities per session. This is because attaining qualifications along with work experience increases your chances of getting a job on release.

Some of our sessional payments are lower than last year. This is so that we can offer more activity spaces across the prison, so that more of you can be in activity. When preparing the policy, the prison council were consulted and some changes were made to the policy in line with feedback.

Figure 17.6 Notice to prison residents

interdependent; where there is trust and a care-focused, cooperative mentality from staff, residents are less likely to need trauma learnt survival strategies and are able to reciprocate a cooperative rather than defensive behavioural response, resulting in a safer place to live and work.

Characteristics of prison staff are highly relevant to resident perceptions of PJ. In a large-scale Dutch study, Beijersbergen, Dirkzwager, Molleman, van der Laan, and Nieuwbeerta (2013) found that staff who had more positive views towards rehabilitation, female staff, and higher staff to resident ratios were all associated with positive perceptions of PJ by prison residents. Beijersbergen et al. speculate that traits typically associated with the female social identity such as caregiving, empathy, and bonding account for these findings. The availability of staff is also likely to counterbalance early neglectful experiences from caregivers. This points to the importance of the social mentality of staff; staff perceived as operating from a caring social mentality are associated with positive experiences of PJ. It is likely that staff groups who operate from competitive social mentality, featuring dominance and punishment, are less able to notice distress and suffering in others.

In order for PJ to be successfully adopted, its implementation must be consistent with the PJ principles. In an evaluation of PJ in policing, MacQueen and Bradford (2017) found that a lack of transparency about the aims of PJ from managers created a subsequent lack of trust in the motives for its implementation by policing staff resulting in their negative perception of PJ and translating into poor application. The study clearly highlights the importance of organisational leadership in the success of any PJ implementation; for PJ to be effective it must take place in a context in which staff also feel treated in procedurally just ways (Fitzalan Howard & Wakeling, 2019). If staff feel they are treated unjustly and in punitive ways, they will more naturally respond by treating residents in this way. Drawing on broader leadership literature, Mann (2019) proposes that PJ and rehabilitative culture must be situated with a rehabilitative leadership.

Procedural Justice as a Trauma-Informed Practice in Prison

It is clear that, when implemented correctly, PJ has the potential to improve safety and perceptions of safety of prison environments as well as rehabilitative practice and relationships between staff and residents. This has significant implications not only for creating a rehabilitative environment but for trauma-informed practice. Literature on the benefits of PJ in prison have focused on safety, compliance, and staff/resident relationships and there has been little attention given to the trauma-informed benefits, despite this being recognised as a benefit for victims in court processes (Elliott et al., 2014). We speculate that this reticence is in part explained by scepticism that prison staff will be welcoming of an approach that rests on the acknowledgement of previous trauma and the possibility of prison-induced trauma. However, the explicit implementation of PJ as a trauma-informed practice may bolster its benefits. For example, if PJ can be implemented with a caring social mentality on the part of the prison, it is more likely to foster a spirit of alliance rather than compliance between residents and staff.

For PJ to be effective it must become embedded in the day-to-day culture of the prison and not be seen as an additional task (Jackson, Tyler, Bradford, Taylor, & Shiner, 2010). This can be hard to achieve in very large organisations where the messaging about change in practice can get lost. Consequently, the implementation of PJ as a trauma-informed approach in prisons might best be supported by psychologists and other mental health practitioners bringing a trauma-informed understanding to the PJ model. This could include training staff about the role of trauma and adversity in the perpetration of harmful behaviour and criminogenic need and the ways in which prison can hinder and help, as well as coaching or supervision of staff. Staff at all levels should be supported to recognise the nature of humanity as outlined in the first section of this chapter, and to understand their own reactions and human tendency for punitiveness towards each other and towards residents. The Power Threat Meaning Framework (Johnstone & Boyle et al., 2018) may have some utility as a model on which to train staff and orientate them to the significance of how power operates in people's lives and the role prisons should have by providing safe, legitimate power and create optimal conditions for engagement and response to rehabilitative efforts.

Conclusion

Many people in prison have histories characterised by adverse experiences and in this chapter we have illustrated the relationship between experiences of adversity, the biopsychosocial responses to these, and the development of criminogenic need. It follows that the way we treat people in prison should acknowledge and account for these experiences of adversity and trauma to support long-standing change. This chapter has outlined procedural justice as one promising approach in bringing about culture change within prisons. A rehabilitative culture is often considered to effect change at cultural, social, and behavioural levels, but as we have discussed, epigenetic change is a dynamic process and as such there is the potential to think of rehabilitative environments as effecting change at a biological level. So far, the benefits of procedural justice as a trauma-informed practice in prison have not been widely recognised and this is something we propose could bolster its effectiveness to create an environment which supports change and rehabilitation at a biopsychosocial level.

Further Reading

Liebling, A., & Maruna, S. (Eds). (2005). *The effects of imprisonment.* Willan. A comprehensive exploration of the internal workings of prisons and the effects on those who live and work there.

Sapolsky, R.M. (2017). *Behave: The biology of humans at our best and worst.* Penguin Press. An accessible examination of the multitude of influences on human behaviour, including evolution, neurobiology, and culture. A good start for those who are new to the biology of behaviour.

References

Abram, K.M., Teplin, L.A., Charles, D.R., Longworth, S.L., McClelland, G.M., & Dulcan, M.K. (2004). Posttraumatic stress disorder and trauma in youth in juvenile detention. *Archives of General Psychiatry, 61(4),* 403–410. doi:10.1001/archpsyc.61.4.403

Akerman, G., & Andrews, T. (2020). Abuse, offending and addressing this in therapy: A staff and service user's perspective on the journey to self-acceptance and a crime-free life. In Swaby H., Winder B., Lievesley R., Hocken K., Blagden N., & Banyard P. (Eds). *Sexual crime and trauma* (pp.175–196). Palgrave Macmillan. doi:10.1007/978-3-030-49068-3_7

Allcock, A. (2015). *Developing a trauma informed approach to rehabilitative group work in prisons.* Winston Churchill Travelling Fellowship. Retrieved from www.wcmt.org.uk/sites/default/files/reportdocuments/Allcock%20A%20Report%202015%20FINAL.pdf

Armstrong, R., & Ludlow, A. (2019). Rehabilitative culture part 2: An update on evidence and practice. *Prison Service Journal, 244,* 3–10.

Auty, K.M., & Liebling, A. (2020). Exploring the relationship between prison social climate and reoffending. *Justice Quarterly, (37)2,* 358–381. doi:10.1080/07418825.2018.1538421

Baumeister, R.F., & Leary, M.R. (1995). The need to belong: Desire for interpersonal attachments as a fundamental human motivation. *Psychological Bulletin, 117*(3), 497–529. doi:10.1037/0033-2909.117.3.497

Becker, S.P., & Kerig, P.K. (2011). Posttraumatic stress symptoms are associated with the frequency and severity of delinquency among detained boys. *Journal of Child & Adolescent Psychology, 40,* 765–771. doi:10.1080/15374416.2011.597091

Beijersbergen, K.A., Dirkzwager, A.J.E., Molleman, T., van der Laan, P.H. & Nieuwbeerta, P. (2013). Procedural justice in prison: The importance of staff characteristics. *International Journal of Offender Therapy and Comparative Criminology, 59*(40), 337–358. doi:10.1177/0306624X13512767

Beijersbergen, K.A., Dirkzwager, A.J.E., & Nieuwbeerta, P. (2016). Reoffending after release: Does procedural justice in prison matter? *Criminal Justice & Behaviour, 43*(1), 63–82. doi/10.1177/0093854815609643

Bellis, M.A., Lowey, H., Leckenby, N., Hughes, K., & Harrison, D. (2014). Adverse childhood experiences: retrospective study to determine their impact on adult health behaviours and health outcomes in a UK population. *Journal of Public Health, 36*(1), 81–91.

Bennett, J., & Tilt, M. (2019). Creating an enabling environment. *Prison Service Journal, 244,* 11–16.

Bierie, D.M. (2012). The impact of prison conditions on staff well-being. *International Journal of Offender Therapy and Comparative Criminology, 56(1),* 81–95. doi:10.1177/0306624X10388383

Cohen, S., & Taylor, L. (1981). Psychological survival: *The experience of long-term imprisonment.* Penguin Books Ltd. doi:10.1177%2F089124167300200111

Davis, B. (2019). Rehabilitative culture part 2: An update on evidence and practice. *Prison Service Journal, 244,* 3–10.

DeLisi, M., & Beauregard, E. (2018). Adverse childhood experiences and criminal extremity: New evidence for sexual homicide. *Journal of Forensic Sciences, 63(2),* 484–489. doi:10.1111/1556-4029.13584

De Viggiani, N. (2006). Surviving prison: Exploring prison social life as a determinant of health. *International Journal of Resident Health, 2(2),* 71–89. doi:10.1080/17449200600935653

Ditchfield, J. (1990). *Control in prisons: A review of the literature.* HMSO. doi:10.1080/23761407.2016.1166844

Drury, A., Heinrichs, T., Elbert, M., Tahja, K., DeLisi, M., & Caropreso, D. (2017). Adverse childhood experiences, paraphilias, and serious criminal violence among federal sex offenders. *Journal of Criminal Psychology, 7,* 105–119. doi:10.1108/JCP-11-2016-0039

Elliott, I., Thomas, S., & Ogloff, J. (2014). Procedural justice in victim police interactions and victims' recovery from victimisation experiences. *Policing and Society, 24(5),* 588–601. doi:10.1080/10439463.2013.784309

Felitti, V.J. (2009). Adverse childhood experiences and adult health. *Academic Pediatrics, 9(3),* 131–132. doi:10.1016/j.acap.2009.03.001

Felitti, V.J., Anda, R.F., Nordenberg, D., Williamson, D.F., Spitz, A.M., Edwards, V., Koss, M.P., Marks, J.S. (1998). The relationship of adult health status to childhood abuse and household dysfunction. *American Journal of Preventative Medicine, 14(4),* 245–258. doi:10.1016/S0749-3797(98)00017-8Fitzalan Howard, F. (2017). *Investigating disciplinary adjudications as potential rehabilitative opportunities.* HMPPS.

Fitzalan Howard, F., & Wakeling, H. (2019). *Resident and staff perceptions of procedural justice in English and Welsh prisons. HMPPS Analytical Summary.* Retrieved from https://assets.publishing.service.gov.uk/government/uploads/system/uploads/attachment_data/file/771324/resident-staff-perceptions-procedural-justice-research.pdf

Fitzalan Howard, F., & Wakeling, H. (2020). Evaluating 'Rehabilitative Adjudications' in four English prisons. *Ministry of Justice Analytical Series.* Retrieved from www.justice.gov.uk/publications/research-and-analysis/moj

Ford, J.D., Chapman, J., Connor, D.F., & Cruise, K.R. (2012). Complex trauma and aggression in secure juvenile justice settings. *Criminal Justice and Behavior, 39(6),* 694–724. doi:10.1177%2F0093854812436957

Haney C. (2012). Prison effects in the era of mass incarceration. *The Prison Journal.* http://dx.doi.org/10.1177/0032885512448604

Her Majesty's Inspectorate of Prisons. (2018). *Annual report 2017–18.* HM Chief Inspector of Prisons for England and Wales. London. HMIP. Retrieved from www.gov.uk/government/publications/hm-chief-inspector-of-prisons-annual-report-2017-to-2018

Her Majesty's Inspectorate of Prisons. (2019). *Annual report 2018–19.* HM Chief Inspector of Prisons for England and Wales. London. HMIP. Retrieved from www.gov.uk/government/publications/hm-chief-inspector-of-prisons-annual-report-2019-to-2020

House of Commons Health and Social Care Committee. (2018). Prison health. *Twelfth Report* (HC2017–19). The Stationery Office.

Hughes, K., Bellis, M.A., Hardcastle, K.A., Sethi, D., Butchart, A., Mikton, C., & Dunne, M.P. (2017). The effect of multiple adverse childhood experiences on health: A systematic review and meta-analysis. *The Lancet Public Health, 2(8),* e356–e366. doi:10.1016/S2468-2667(17)30118-4

Jackson, J., Tyler, T.R., Bradford, B., Taylor, D., & Shiner, M. (2010). Legitimacy and procedural justice in prisons. *Prison Service Journal, 191,* 4–10.

Johnstone, L. & Boyle, M. with Cromby, J., Dillon, J., Harper, D., Kinderman, P., Longden, E., Pilgrim, D., & Read, J. (2018). *The power threat meaning framework: Towards the identification of patterns in emotional distress, unusual experiences and troubled or troubling behaviour, as an alternative to functional psychiatric diagnosis.* British Psychological Society.

Jones, L. (2015). The peaks unit: From a pilot for 'untreatable' psychopaths to. Trauma informed milieu therapy. *Prison Service Journal, 218,* 17–23.

Kordowicz, M. (2019). *The perceived impact of the Enabling Environments Programme within Her Majesty's Prison and Probation Service settings.* Royal College of Psychiatrists and Her Majesty's Prison and Probation Service.

Laxminarayan, M.S. (2012). *The heterogeneity of crime victims: Variations in procedural and outcome preferences.* Wolf Legal Publishers (WLP).

Leshem, R., & Weisburd, D. (2019). Epigenetics and hot spots of crime: Rethinking the relationship between genetics and criminal behavior. *Journal of Contemporary Criminal Justice, 35,* 186–204. doi:10.1177%2F1043986219828924

Levenson, J. (2014). Incorporating trauma-informed care into evidence-based sex offender treatment. *Journal of Sexual Aggression, 20*(1), 9–22.

Levenson, J.S., Willis, G.M., & Prescott, D.S. (2015). Adverse childhood experiences in the lives of female sex offenders. *Sexual Abuse, 27(3),* 258–283. doi:10.1177/1079063214535819Levi, M., Sacks, A., & Tyler, T.R. (2009). Conceptualizing legitimacy, measuring legitimating beliefs. *American Behavioral Scientist 53,* 354–375. doi:10.1177/0002764209338797

Liebling, A., & Maruna, S. (Eds). (2005). *The effects of imprisonment.* Willan.

Liem, M., & Kunst, M. (2013). Is there a recognizable post-incarceration syndrome among released "lifers"? *International Journal of Law and Psychiatry, 36,* 333–337. doi:10.1016/j.ijlp.2013.04.012

Lind, E.A., & Tyler, T.R. (1988). *The social psychology of procedural justice.* Plenum Press. doi:10.1007/978-1-4899-2115-4

MacQueen, S., & Bradford, B. (2017). Where did it all go wrong? Implementation failure—and more—in a field experiment of procedural justice policing. *Journal of Experimental Criminology, 13,* 321–345. doi:10.1007/s11292-016-9278-7

Mandelli, L., Carli, V., Roy, A., Serretti, A., & Sarchiapone, M. (2011). The influence of childhood trauma on the onset and repetition of suicidal behavior: An investigation in a high risk sample of male residents. *Journal of Psychiatric Research, 45*(6), 742–747. doi:10.1016/j.jpsychires.2010.11.005

Mann, R.E. (2019). Polite, assertive and sensitive: Procedurally just searching at HMP Holme House. *The Prison Service Journal, 242,* 26–30.

Mann, R.E., Fitzalan Howard, F., & Tew, J. (2018). What is a rehabilitative prison culture? *The Prison Service Journal, 235,* 3–9.

McKenna, N.C., & Holtfreter, K. (2020). Trauma-informed courts: A review and integration of justice perspectives and gender responsiveness. *Journal of Aggression, Maltreatment & Trauma, 30*(4), 450–470. doi:10.1080/10926771.2020.1747128

Morris, D.J., Webb, E.L., Parmar, E., Trundle, G., & McLean, A. (2020). Troubled beginnings: the adverse childhood experiences and placement histories of a detained adolescent population with developmental disorders. *Advances in Mental Health and Intellectual Disabilities, 14*(6), 181–197. doi:10.1108/AMHID-01-2020-0003

Murphy, K., Hinds, L., & Fleming, J. (2008). Encouraging public cooperation and support for police. *Policing & Society, 18,* 136–155. doi:10.1080/10439460802008660

Paternoster, R., Bachman, R., Brame, R., & Sherman, L.W. (1997). Do fair procedures matter? The effect of procedural justice on spouse assault. *Law & Society Review, 31,* 163–204. doi:10.2307/3054098

Penner, E.K., Shaffer, C.S., & Viljoen, J.L. (2017). Questioning fairness: The relationship of mental health and psychopathic characteristics with young offenders' perceptions of procedural justice and legitimacy. *Criminal Behaviour and Mental Health, 27*(4), 354–370. doi:10.1037/lhb0000280

Penner, E.K., Viljoen, J.L., Douglas, K.S., & Roesch, R. (2013). Procedural justice versus risk factors for offending: Predicting recidivism in youth. *Law and Human Behavior, 38*(3), 225–237. doi:10.1037/lhb0000055

Prison Reform Trust. (2019). *Prison: The facts. Bromley Briefings. Factfile, Summer 2019.* Prison Reform Trust.

Rapoport, R.N., Rapoport, R., & Rosow, I. (1960). *Community as doctor.* Tavistock Publishing.

Rawlings, B., & Haigh, R. (2017). Therapeutic communities and planned environments for serious offenders in English prisons. *British Journal of Psychiatric Advances, 23*(5), 338–346. doi:10.1192/apt.bp.115.015636

Reavis, J.A., Looman, J., Franco, K.A., & Rojas, B. (2013). Adverse childhood experiences and adult criminality: How long must we live before we possess our own lives? *The Permanente Journal, 17*(2): 44–48. doi:10.7812/TPP%2F12-072

Reisiga, M.D., & Mesko, G. (2009). Procedural justice, legitimacy, and resident misconduct. *Psychology, Crime & Law, 15*(1), 41–59. doi:10.1080/10683160802089768

Shah, A., Allen, J., Peters, P., & Bennett, J. (2019). Rehabilitative culture part 2: An update on evidence and practice. *Prison Service Journal, 244,* 3–10.

Stöver H. (2017). Prison staff under stress: Causes, consequences and health promotion strategies. In Elger B., Ritter C., & Stöver H. (Eds), *Emerging issues in prison health* (pp.253–259). Springer. doi:10.1007/978-94-017-7558-8_16

Substance Abuse and Mental Health Services Administration (SAMHSA). (2014). "SAMHSA: Essential Components of Trauma Informed Judicial Practice", Crawford County System of Care Shared Resource Library.

Sunshine, J., & Tyler, T.R. (2003). The role of procedural justice and legitimacy in shaping public support for policing. *Law & Society Review, 37,* 513–548. doi:10.1111/1540-5893.3703002

Sykes, G.M. (1958). *The society of captives: A study of a maximum security prison.* Princeton University Press. doi:10.2307/j.ctv14164hw

Taylor, J. (2021). Compassion in custody: developing a trauma sensitive intervention for men with developmental disabilities who have convictions for sexual offending. *Advances in Mental Health and Intellectual Disabilities.*

Topitzes, J., Mersky, J.P., & Reynolds, A.J. (2011). Child maltreatment and offending behavior: Gender-specific effects and pathways. *Criminal Justice and Behavior, 38*(5), 492–510. doi:10.1177/0093854811398578

Turley, C., Payne, C., & Webster, S. (2013). *Enabling features of psychologically informed planned environments.* National Offender Managed Service, Ministry of Justice Analytical Series.

Tyler, K.A., Johnson, K.A., & Brownridge, D.A. (2008). A longitudinal study of the effects of child maltreatment on later outcomes among high-risk adolescents. *Journal of Youth and Adolescence, 37*(5), 506–521. doi:10.1007/s10964-007-9250-y

Tyler, T.R. (1989). The psychology of procedural justice: A test of the group-value model. *Journal of Personality & Social Psychology, 57,* 830–838. doi:10.1037/0022-3514.57.5.830

Tyler, T.R. (2010). Legitimacy in corrections: Policy implications. *Criminology and Public Policy, 9,* 127–134. doi:10.1111/j.1745-9133.2010.00615.xTyler, T.R., Sherman, L.W., Strang, H., Barnes, G.C., & Woods, D. (2007). Reintegrative shaming, procedural justice, and recidivism: The engagement of offenders' psychological mechanisms in the Canberra RISE drinking-and-driving experiment. *Law & Society Review, 41,*553–586. doi:10.1111/j.1540-5893.2007.00314.x

Walton, J.S. (In press). Fit in your genes: An introduction to genes and epigenetics for forensic practitioners. *Journal of Forensic Practice.*

Wells, W. (2007). Type of contact and evaluations of police officers: The effects of procedural justice across three types of police-citizen contacts. *Journal of Criminal Justice, 35,* 612–621. doi:10.1016/j.jcrimjus.2007.09.006

Winick, B. (2006). Therapeutic jurisprudence: Enhancing the relationship between law and psychology. *Law and psychology: Current legal issues* volume 9. Oxford University Press. doi:10.1093/acprof:oso/9780199211395.001.0001

18

TRAUMA-INFORMED COMMUNITY SERVICES

Karen Orpwood and Sue Ryan

Service Delineation and Exclusion

This chapter is about community services that people with a forensic history may access, but not limited to community forensic services. In thinking about forensic practice in the community, the services most obviously of relevance would be community forensic services (under the NHS – National Health Service), and the Probation Service (PS – under the criminal justice system). Users of forensic services, as part of our society, should have equality of access to all services of relevance to their needs and difficulties – something that is not commonplace. It has been noted elsewhere in this book that those with forensic histories have experienced high rates of childhood adversity of all kinds, a variety of different traumatic experiences that can leave them susceptible to struggles with their psychological well-being, relationships, and social functioning. The authors will use their collective experiences of working with individuals across a range of different criminal justice services and NHS Trusts to illustrate pertinent issues and reflections. However, each "case" is a composite of a number of people who have entered community services and any resemblance to an actual person is coincidental.

We started this chapter with some uncertainty about the population and services we were going to be thinking about. Between us, we have worked in prisons, probation, adult mental health and forensic mental health settings in both community, inpatient and secure settings. Reflections about who fell within the scope of this chapter were not so straightforward, because most of the people we have worked with in these various settings had a great deal of similarity in terms of the psychological problems, trauma, and adversity they struggled with. What seemed to make the difference was where they could become a user of services. People were deemed either too risky for mental health services, not risky enough for forensic services, or not have the right "disorder" or sufficient level of "readiness" or stability to meet the different service criteria. Many people are still not reached by forensic services and fall right through the gaps, often replicating early life experiences of rejection and dismissal. Those people may often be struggling to manage substance misuse, financial

DOI: 10.4324/9781003120766-23

difficulties, and broken relationships with a lack of structure, routine, or sense of purpose. They are ultimately socially excluded.

There is a clear division between services: health and criminal justice are separate, and so people are categorised as "in" or "out" of either group, or in both (which gets complicated), or neither. The evolution of this dichotomy may be interesting to consider but falls out of the scope of this chapter. In the UK and many, though not all, other similar countries, behaviour or presenting problems are largely viewed as being *either* primarily about mental health-based problems, *or* law-breaking, criminal behaviour. This split may be considered to reflect differences in the evolution of how social groups set and perpetuate certain rules and norms and has obvious practical utility. However, there may be unintended consequences/unwelcome side effects of this split, and where the fault lines lay may be one of the most significant challenges to being "trauma informed". Why does the category that someone falls into matter? Aside from the authors' practical decisions about what services fall into and outside of the scope of this chapter, it reflects the very real decisions made every day about the people within the community at risk of offending or with a history of offending, and whether they fall into or outside of the remit of a service. It is a central problem in being truly trauma-informed with forensic clients, or indeed with people in general whenever, and however, they present with distress or distress-driven difficulties.

The degree of struggle is undoubtedly layered by the experiences of trauma in early and later life. Almost every client that we have worked with in forensic community services has experienced trauma within their early lives and often repeated incidences thereafter. These experiences are often unacknowledged by systems and families, and at times its impact is dismissed by the clients themselves. The alternative is to consider how society may have contributed to shaping individuals, compounded by culture, socioeconomic status, race, education, gender, and sexuality in addition to their family experiences. Such reflections can be emotionally difficult and draining and bring to the surface the uncomfortable fact that we are all more similar than different and, faced with similar experiences, we may too have taken similar steps.

Working with trauma in the community with forensic clients raises many dilemmas. There is often a profound sense that individuals are wholly "bad". This is often the perception of society and infiltrates into the systems that provide services, commissioning, budgets, cultures, and staff perceptions about who is "deserving" and worthy of investment. Once an individual has offended, they are often no longer described as a person, but as the sum of their offending behaviour (offender/criminal/perpetrator), which is likely to have a major impact upon their sense of self, perception of hope and may be a possibly conscious or unconscious way to humiliate or punish the individual from an organisational or societal perspective. Individuals are often raised in systems that have shaped their world view and their view of self as being wholly responsible for their childhood selves, negative self-concepts embedded at their core. This is true not only of criminal justice systems who label clients as "offenders" but also of clients who enter health systems who then become "patients". What both labels can often lead to is a distancing, where the person and their identity can become clouded and hidden behind the very label(s) that the systems place upon them. However, there is a shift in how trauma is being better understood, from "what is *wrong* with you" to "what *has happened* to you"; however, it is far from being embedded within systems and minds and feels at its infancy of development, despite its first being referenced in 1991 (Perry & Winfrey, 2021).

The splits between categories of "person" and "problem" and the "othering" of people described as "offenders" and "patients" invites or perpetuates the false beliefs that, in truth, these issues and people are "separate". Society seeks to separate themselves from individuals who commit abusive acts, who are often subject to myths, categorised and labelled (Craissati, 2019). Having both criminal justice and mental health services as well as those that appear to cross the divide or overlap should, in theory, reduce the impact of "othering" and categorising for users of these services. However, the authors' experiences in working with forensic clients are that this is seldom the case. Central to being trauma-informed is having policy, practice, and culture that places the person first and seeks to avoid re-traumatisation, as well as offering a holistic response to the complexity of an individual's experiences and difficulties (McCartan, 2020). A trauma-informed approach and service would have a compassionate curiosity about what a person has experienced which has resulted in their distress becoming unmanageable, spilling over into their functioning and relationships with others. By labelling and distancing ourselves from those who have been traumatised and become traumatising, we are failing to understand the person within their context and are at risk of relating in ways that cause re-traumatisation.

Adult Mental Health Services in the Community

Darren, who said he had an "anger management" problem as well as self-harming behaviours, was rejected from primary care mental health services as he did not fit the commissioned service criteria in terms of the nature and complexity of the issues, or what interventions they offered. As he reported increasing hopelessness and suicidal ideation, he was referred to secondary care mental health services. In assessment he spoke about his difficulties with "anger" and how these had manifested in a range of problems, including a number of criminal convictions, and that he felt "stressed" and ashamed and wanted help. As there had not been serious violence, he had no input from the probation service, and he was not sufficiently violent or "mentally ill" to be eligible for the community forensic mental health service (something many areas do not even have). He was told by community mental health team (CMHT) staff that his anger and aggression were about his choices, that he was not "mentally ill", but presented with antisocial personality traits, so he was not eligible for secondary care mental health, and he "needed to manage himself better", the subtext seeming to be that he did not "deserve" help such as medication or talking therapy. Another unhelpful implication was that, if he were considered to be "mentally ill enough", then his aggression might be judged differently and that he might be deemed more worthy of support. The CMHT did not consider the meaning of his behaviour. Darren was fundamentally invalidated by this view of him. His shame was reinforced. There was little sensitivity about how he might have heard this perspective. Services were withheld, his behaviour was judged as "wrong", and an over-simplistic perspective was provided. His self-control was assumed to be the fundamental issue and he was expected to better control his anger, and if he did not, then criminal justice was the way forward. This mirrors the cold, harsh invalidating environment of his early years. In his pain and anger, he lashed out at those he felt had hurt him, his punishment being criticism, rejection, and shame. Just as he had been frightened of his parents' rage and violence, the team were frightened of his. He felt uncontainable and the system and society further rejected and isolated him so he was left to navigate a rejecting system alone. Such re-enactment is typical in the life experiences post-trauma for people who have struggled to heal (De Zulueta, 2006).

Darren had a history of complex trauma relating to adversity and abuse during childhood, and trauma during his early adult life. What he labelled "angry", perhaps due to gendered ways of describing the difficulties of one's inner life, could also be understood as overwhelming negative affective and cognitive states, including PTSD symptoms that he was unable to regulate, and which frightened him, causing him to become harmful to himself, the environment, and others. Darren's difficulties could easily have been described instead as emotional instability, intense reactions in the context of interpersonal issues, distress, and fear, as well as rage, feelings of anxiety, depression, and hopelessness. His presentation was very similar to many of the female service users the authors have met over the years, whose difficulties have been conceptualised as complex trauma or, more contentiously, "borderline" or "emotionally unstable personality disorder" and mental health problems secondary to it.

However, in relation to other people the authors have known, a diagnosis of personality disorder too can often mean that this is a diagnosis to exclude rather than include, despite the paper *Personality Disorder: No longer a Diagnosis of Exclusion* (National Institute for Mental Health in England, 2003) and services are still failing to include and meet the needs of this population who are still viewed by some as being less deserving of support and compassion and as more responsible for their difficulties than those perceived to be "mentally ill". NHS England & NHS Improvement & the National Collaborating Centre for Mental Health have in the last few years published a series of reviews and strategies relating to adult mental health, recognising that "the model of care is not in need of fundamental transformation and modernization" (NHS England & NHS Improvement & the National Collaborating Centre for Mental Health, 2019; p.2).

Darren was offered psychological therapy with the CMHT. Psychological formulation allowed both him and the team to see what had happened to him, connecting the trauma to his distress and the difficulties this led to. This enabled the team to empathise with him, following which he received further assistance (Wilkinson et al., 2017). Darren experienced validation. He came to understand that he has been the victim of trauma, that his "anger" actually reflects complex reactions to situations that evoke past traumas and, in that context, is quite understandable. His aggressive actions have functioned to protect himself from anticipated harmful treatment by others and helped him feel a sense of power and agency in this respect. He learned to trust a little and to cope better; he developed hope, and his functioning and experience of life significantly improved. He did end up receiving what could be described as a trauma-informed service; his needs were listened to and understood, and the service responded from a position of flexibility. Furthermore, his psychological support was formulation-led, collaboratively designed, and responsively delivered. This approach would be in keeping with the Power Threat Meaning Framework (Johnstone & Boyle et al., 2018).

What might have been? Had Darren been rejected by all services, where might his deteriorating presentation taken him? Perhaps to the point that he was too risky for mental health services at all, and created another victim, and then managed under criminal justice, with his needs as a victim, subsumed under those relating to his being a perpetrator.

Other service users came to mind, from mainstream, and specialist mental health services, who have been users of multiple services, some of which can be contracted out to other providers. With each service trying to protect itself in relation to commissioning, criteria, and caseload, falling between the cracks is easy. Fragmented services use different systems and often fail to communicate effectively. Holding an individual client in mind is all but impossible sometimes, as is monitoring someone's deteriorating situation. We can both think of many people who have died or seriously harmed others as a consequence. If someone is in a mild road traffic accident, the emergency services will initially attend to deal with acute and immediate risk; then for treatment and any rehabilitation or functional or social needs, the person sees other health professionals, in order of priority and specialism. Perhaps this model works relatively well for physical health problems (ignoring the social context of the person with a physical health problem and any psychological or emotional impact of it), but for problems with psychological and emotional health, it does not. One cannot "carve up" the person and their problems to fit the organisation of services. This is fundamentally how mental health services function, using a psychiatric approach that "diagnoses" psychological and social issues and clusters them together as discrete and separate entities. This approach has been challenged by many (Bentall, 1990; Boyle, 1990; Johnstone & Boyle et al., 2018) as invalid, unreliable, and not taking account of the cause or social context of an individuals' circumstances. Kinderman (2019) has proposed a social and psychological approach to well-being and health in which the person, their difficulties, context, and history are understood and involved in consideration of what may be able to assist their needs. In this case, "person" is not "put before protocol" (McCartan, 2020).

The individuals who came to mind when considering Darren did not come under a forensic service, but they were no different from cases the authors have known in prison or secure forensic hospitals, or supervised by probation or community forensic teams following serious violent crime. If there is a difference, in addition to them crossing the barrier into offending, it is that those in prison and sometimes secure hospitals did not even make it as far as an assessment.

Forensic Services in the Community

A significant part of working in forensic services in the community involves collaborating with The Probation Service (PS), a criminal justice agency. The PS's remit is public protection through addressing the factors relevant to criminal behaviour, providing support and rehabilitation to enable offenders to desist from crime. For the last few years, people who are supervised by probation have been referred to as "offenders", with probation officers being called "offender managers". This has now been changed and users of services are now referred to as "people on probation"; crucially, their humanity is recognised. Offender managers contribute to rehabilitation and risk management, monitor and enforce or sanction breaches of requirements. McCartan (2020) suggests "a trauma informed approach … seeks not to re-traumatise with blame and sanction" (p.8), which is somewhat antithetical to what is required of PS. To what extent is it realistically possible to reconcile these positions? Consideration of being trauma informed in the context of probation is very recent, with training and guidance only just beginning to emerge.

Despite the organisational context, individuals within probation services try to relate and respond to service users in a way that is less punitive or driven by enforcement. It is not unheard of for a probation officer's phone number to be the only number, or one of very few, that a person using the service has to call, and for the probation officer to be the only visitor or correspondent they have in prison. The relationship with a probation officer may be the longest and most stable relationship that some service users have had, and the probation officer may know the most about them. The service user may experience their probation officer as a proxy-parent, with all the desires and fears of their actual primary caregivers, a vessel into which they can put their projections. The probation officer has a huge challenge to enforce, monitor, and focus on risk, as well as holding the other pole of the person, their trauma experiences, and be mindful of how their person might experience them in relation to this.

How can services divided into *Health*, *Social Care*, and *Criminal Justice* be open to hearing the shifting needs of complex individuals and to change when things are no longer working, instead of prescribing them, and requiring people to fit into boxes defined by others? (Wilton & Williams, 2019). Organisations can and do traumatise and trigger or perpetuate trauma (Goldsmith, Martin, & Smith, 2014); even when they aim to do what they feel is best by someone, there can be a paradoxical effect.

Reintegration into the Community?

Some clients within forensic community services may always have resided in the community, serving lesser sentences for less serious offending. However, many are arriving back to the community from often lengthy custodial sentences that have led to them losing many of their life skills in custody due to limited opportunities. Their ability to emotionally and relationally develop has been compromised by the loss of connections to families and society, and by exposure to prison environments where survival requires masking of real selves, vulnerabilities, and fear. They may have experienced traumatic events within the prison system and their experience of the system may have led to them becoming mistrusting and hostile, with a wariness and defence against further hurt.

Upon release, this newfound freedom can often reveal overwhelming emotions of hope and expectation of self and others. What has been yearned for is interlaced with fear of failing, disappointment, and worries about how to navigate life and where they "fit" into society that has often changed beyond recognition. The hurdles are many; basic needs are the priority, but complex issues arising from traumatic histories and traumatising patterns in relating to others can make the future feel bleak. Although some are able to find a way to be accepted back into families, into society, and find a level of self-acceptance that enables them to lead less destructive and damaging lives, many continue to live lives where they are not afforded opportunities or acceptance but are faced with a multitude of hurdles which can be hard to keep overcoming.

Forensic services in the community are one part of a multi-layered system working with individuals who have multiple needs and difficulties. A client can have physical health issues, be financially compromised, have housing difficulties (lack of adequate housing, barriers to securing private tenancies due to limited finances and lack of guarantors), substance misuse dependence, social needs, and child protection involvement. Many clients face these challenges with a traumatic history that manifests in deeply engrained emotional dysregulation and disconnection, limited ability to mentalise, and lack of sense of self and identity. Service users are referred primarily for issues relating to their offending behaviour, and therapists need to formulate how such issues link into their current struggles and how their past has contributed to their offending behaviour. This is a complex process for complex issues that must be addressed within time-limited therapies from which they may be suddenly discharged for missing appointments or misusing substances. The task can be to understand the many layers of complexity, work in the here and now, and prioritise and help scaffold agencies around a client to assist with the multi-layered needs. Many clients in community forensic services may not enter into the service to address any traumatic experiences, but to find ways to assist them to understand why their issues have developed and learn alternative ways to regulate and contain their strong feelings.

Working within such services requires a level of flexibility, awareness of the above, and willingness to try to meet a client where s/he is at and understand what may or may not be possible for them at the point they attend for therapy. This may be a different focus to what the referrer has wished for and it can mean that part of the work involves exploring how to meet the differing expectations of referrer and service user so that work can be truly collaborative, building upon their strengths and knowledge. Society, services, and therapist may have a desire to help people never offend again, which is of course a priority, but in order to do so, we also need to focus on enabling people to feel a greater level of self-understanding and self-compassion, and through this, enable them to be more attuned to the emotional and relational states of others (Bateman & Fonagy, 2016). This takes time, and for some may mean multiple contacts with services to enable them to settle into society and within themselves. It requires maintaining hope (Farrall & Calverley, 2006), despite an individual's best or less than best efforts, that they may be able to reach a more fulfilled and less destructive life at some point in their future, if not now.

Exploring trauma with a client in the community without the physical constraints of the secure setting can be challenging. The dilemmas for a therapist to consider involve considering the ethics of doing no harm and whether the client can tolerate such work without the stability of a residential environment. Can the client manage not to revert to old patterns of substance dependence, self-harm, or suicidality or acting out their fear and hate onto others? We have found that some cannot, which may mean that they disengage or are discharged from services or are returned to custody. However, many can make meaningful change, reach a degree of awareness, increase their coping and functioning, and appreciate that they can achieve a level of stability and become connected to parts of themselves that enable their value to be seen by themselves and others.

Working with Tom

Tom was 45 at the point of being referred. He had recently been released from prison after committing a violent offence against a female. He had made advances towards her and when thwarted, he had punched her in the face, breaking her nose. He was inebriated and high on cocaine at the time. She was not previously known to him and he had not committed an offence towards a female before, although had many convictions for acquisitive crime, fraud, violence towards males, and breaching previous licence conditions.

Tom had served five years in custody for this offence and, although had engaged in a specific course to address his thinking and substance misuse, he had not had any opportunity to explore his past and the impact upon his present. He had spent most of his life oscillating between custody and the community. When in the community he had always depended upon alcohol, cocaine, and cannabis to help him feel energised, confident, and what he felt was "normal". Substances also enabled him to numb the pain, to forget and detach.

Tom came to the psychology service as he wanted to stay out of custody and recognised that his behaviour at times was out of control. His risk factors included his aggression to women and substance misuse and were issues that the system and referrer felt were outstanding. He hated the system and those who worked within it and was extremely mistrustful of individuals within it. He would often inform practitioners of all the reasons why psychologists could not be trusted, how he would be unlikely to engage and was not hopeful that anything could be done. Yet he had attended and, in some respects, laid his cards on the table. Despite his wariness, mistrust, and challenge, he was open, a little unsettled and on edge, but had shared his anxieties of how he expected the therapist to be unreliable, ineffective, and damaging and was offered a space to be heard, validated, and begun to be understood. From that first session the therapist aimed to create a safe, collaborative, and "good enough" experience of therapy and felt a pull to provide a more corrective experience for him.

This was the beginning of providing a space and experience that was trauma-informed, understanding the client where he was at and appreciating why he had become so aggrieved. The assessment was to begin to understand him and his context and how this could be repeated, or not, by adapting the approach, compassionately connecting and beginning to collaborate about his hopes for the sessions, how they aligned and differed from the referrer's, and how he could be placed at the forefront of the intervention plan whilst also holding in mind the public protection and the need to share pertinent themes from discussions with the referrer. Contracting was key, openness and honesty, recognition of fallibility, and a willingness to work through those tentative moments and times when a thick skin was needed. However, the therapy was one part of a bigger picture. Had this been the whole intervention then Tom would not have continued to engage with the therapist for over 12 months. Tom shared some of his early experiences which involved deceit, abuse, and uncertainty and whilst doing so, pertinent parts of his narrative were noted on a piece of paper in the room and in doing so, a collaborative way of working was created that was visible and contained. Through reaching a collaborative understanding of what had occurred, how it had impacted upon him, and what he carried with him as an adult in his relationships and intrapersonally, he began to develop trust and hope that things could be different. There were no moments of enlightenment, quick fixes, or significant changes. Therapy involved a long period of Tom "working through" enduring pain and a toil of emotion when his trauma was triggered repeatedly by encounters that he had with people in the system, including in the therapeutic relationship which left him feeling exposed and threatened. The primary task was relational – not a series of discrete interventions but a process of relating to and "being with" him to share, understand, and notice what he did in relation to others. Additionally, therapy enabled him to develop a greater sense of who he was in relation to another and in doing so, gently enabling him to better understand what he carried with him that was helpful and what repeatedly caused himself and others distress, often by making use of moments that were live in the room. Therapy helped increase his awareness, choices, and ability to connect to himself and others and work with "the system" rather than to feel or be set up or further traumatised by it. Working in this way enabled him to experience someone in the system as being able to help rather than harm him and was an experience that he could build upon and carry forward in his future experiences of relationships.

The Offender Personality Disorder Pathway

The Offender Personality Disorder Pathway (OPD Pathway: Department of Health/ National Offender Management Service, 2011) is designed for/at the population of people within criminal justice and forensic mental health services who are likely to have a severe form of personality disorder (a controversial construct) that is clinically linked to significant risk of harmful behaviour towards others. It was developed for the many individuals within secure settings, mostly in prison, whose needs were unmet by the system. Despite the name of the pathway, there is a move away from diagnosis to formulation (Skett, Goode, & Barton, 2017) to help understand the person's needs and presenting difficulties within their context. This should include their individual experiences, social and environmental factors, protected characteristics, attachment and relationship history, and physical variations. These factors alongside temperament impact upon an individual's ability to cope with and respond to stress and can lead to overwhelming distress and unbearable feelings (British Psychological Society, 2018).

The OPD strategy pays attention to specific interventions but crucially focuses upon the environmental aspects of the system. It recognises that improving the culture, relationships, and activities in an environment can positively impact upon how individuals feel and behave, and the relationships that they form. While this may seem obvious, it appears to be missed within many prisons and secure setting that house people who have been traumatised and traumatising. Through developing psychologically informed planned environments (PIPEs) (National Offender Management Service/Department of Health, 2012), specialist intervention services in prisons and supporting and training staff, individuals may be able to make changes and begin to understand that they have potential, strengths, and contemplate hope.

The OPD strategy recognised that many individuals who would meet criteria for the OPD pathway (via a screening tool that identifies features associated with the construct of antisocial personality disorder, Mawby, Newman, & Wilkinson-Tough, 2020) would be stuck in the system, often feeling persecuted by it with little opportunity to make meaningful change. Due to capacity and demand, if an individual is not motivated to engage with interventions in the criminal justice system, they can often be left to "reconsider their position". In this position they are often unsupported and labelled "hard to reach" or "not motivated", rather than the system recognising that it has not found a way to reach or motivate them. A major asset of the pathway is that individuals are given a possible "pathway" and hope. They are understood as needing a whole system to help them to change and their engagement difficulties are understood within the systems within which they reside rather than solely within their person. The pathway is not perfect, but it provides a more realistic opportunity for some who have previously little hope of progression. Although the pathway has a whole systems approach spanning custody to community, it recognises that there is much investment needed in the community, where the vast majority of individuals with forensic histories will return.

In the community, specialist workers support offender managers to reflect upon the people they are working with in core offender management services. Through psychological formulation, offender managers are assisted to better understand what has happened in an individual's life and how such experiences may be driving unhelpful patterns of relating. Formulation also enables the worker to consider their responses to working with an individual, how they may enable the relationship to develop, and what interventions may be useful for the individual going forward. The pathway has also invested in creating Intensive Intervention and Risk Management Services (IIRMs) in the community, an acronym which coincidentally or unconsciously may suggest a more hesitant and less certain approach to this work, which may reflect the evolving and involving nature of the development of the delivery model and the recognition to the lack of evidenced-based models for working with this population.

The first IIRMs was developed and piloted in Merseyside in 2008 (Nathan, Centifanti, Baker, & Hill, 2019) although it was not referred to as such until 2014 when this name was developed. The service continues to provide a pathway out of custody towards a more hopeful future for some. Its success and support from commissioners and key stakeholders have enabled the service to mature, develop, and contribute to the growth of IIRMs nationally. There are now two IIRMs within the North West of England, *Resettle* in Liverpool and *Evolve* in Manchester. Although both are very different in their funding, resources, and intervention model, they share principles of being a shared approach between health and justice, a recognition of complexity of need and risk, and in providing intervention to offer stabilisation. There is a practical focus, opportunity for skill and relational development, and for some an opportunity to engage in trauma-focused work. IIRMs are in their infancy but working within them feels that there is a movement to do something different, away from punishing, rejecting systems, but that this is a small part of greater systemic change that is needed.

Working in forensic community services is without doubt difficult. The service and individuals within it can act as a "container" for the risk and associated anxiety. There are many factors that impact upon a person's desire to enter into working in this field and there are many which contribute to their willingness to remain working within it. We have chosen to work in services that fit our own values. Our disconnect with the medicalisation of distress has led us to ways of working that are "psychologically informed", as the OPD pathway promotes. The support, value, enrichment and safety of a team, and shared organisational approach are also factors in these innovative services. This undoubtedly brings challenges, frustration, and much need for compromise, but are invaluable to this work, provided all are signed up to the shared values and approach.

The Challenge of Change

Trauma is endemic in our society, yet people who are marginalised and disempowered in our society experience more of it (Wilton & Williams, 2019). The authors have written this chapter during the Black Lives Matters protests, and the COVID pandemic, which has disproportionately affected people of colour, and people of lower socioeconomic and health status – a population in which people of colour are also disproportionately represented. How can we effectively notice and hear the trauma-related needs of this group? We know that in the UK people of colour are more likely to suffer from poverty, poor educational and occupational opportunities, to receive criminal convictions and custodial sentences, to suffer mental and physical health problems, and to die early. How can these socially and politically derived sources of trauma be recognised by systems, both health and criminal justice, that tend to locate the main source of an individual's problems within them (De Zulueta, 2006), as if it is divorced from their context (Johnstone & Boyle et al., 2018). Furthermore, under the current systems, infused as they are by predominately white, Eurocentric philosophical assumptions, how can the traumatic experiences of the population who carry ancestral cultural and religious beliefs make use of these services, whose rigid and limited definitions and criteria exclude different expressions of trauma? Lifelong adverse experiences, commencing in childhood, are a monumental social problem, especially for the population of people minoritised in our society, that our systems seem inadequate to address in their current form (Williams, 2020).

There is a disparity between what is needed in a trauma-informed context for the cases like those discussed in either health or criminal justice services, and what is offered. There are problems with the options given to or taken away from survivors of trauma depending on how the sequelae of trauma manifests. When our services look at people with a history of violence, they rightly see the risk of further victims and "what's wrong with" them. But, in holding only that pole, they miss the other, their vulnerability, and how they have been hurt. This vulnerability, "what's happened to them", where it remains unhealed, drives or fails to regulate the part of them that can harm others, and is intrinsically linked to risk. It is a fallacy to separate the two into two different service pathways, as so often ends up being the case in the community. One wonders how many incidents of harm might have been avoided had people who were not as lucky as Darren been helped by mainstream services. Similarly, how many incidents of harm might have been avoided if people like Tom had not been worked with only in terms of his criminal behaviour as opposed to holistically, earlier in their lives. We need a cultural shift and a system level change to have trauma-informed services in our society (Kings Fund, 2019) and a trauma-informed society.

Can the culture be further changed and embedded with the development of the Power Threat Meaning Framework (Johnstone & Boyle et al., 2018) and the Manifesto for Mental Health (Kinderman, 2019) as an alternative to the medicalisation of trauma reactions? These proposed approaches mean that people's adverse experiences are acknowledged, heard, understood, and responded to from within a limited framework to be trauma-informed, as opposed to the current situation in which the reverse is true (Wilton and Williams, 2019).

This population is invariably complex; trauma may only ever be partially addressed and interventions may be insufficient to fully mitigate risk. To work with this population, staff and services need the capacity to hold the *whole* person in mind, the victim, the vulnerability, the perpetrator, and the risk. Practitioners need to be containing and contained by their team, the wider service and, on an organisational and political level, by concentric circles of containment. There have been many occasions when we or our colleagues have spoken about the impact of other people's harsh and negative comments about the population we work with, and the media often reports on individuals who have been released from prison or secure hospital and harmed someone, as well as criticism of the workers like us who try to support them. As we finish our chapter, the inquest into the deaths of two people killed in a terrorist incident in London in November 2019 by man deemed suitable for release from prison has just ended. The media have criticised criminal justice staff who held on to hope for the people they work with, perpetuating the view that the capacity for violence is something that is solely within a being, and that people like us should be infallible in our capacity to accurately discern it. It can be a very hard job.

Many practitioners leave this work, perhaps overwhelmed by how disturbing it can be, or tired of the stress of the responsibility; how much it hurts when things go wrong; the stress of the organisational response to incidents; or the pathology that can end up being re-enacted within and between teams and services. When we reflect on what enables and motivates us to stick with it, it is our enduring belief that what we do is what it is fundamentally right, even if we as individuals are not always right. We believe in each person's capacity to create a life worth living, to find a way to live with the harm done to them and to make a positive contribution to the lives of others despite the harm they have caused in the past. We have been fortunate to have received a lot of creative, evocative, and memorable learning experiences, worked with inspirational figures and skilled and supportive colleagues, and contained by quality supervision and supervisory relationships that have stretched, challenged, and been kind to us. We have reflected upon the many people that we have worked with, been impacted by them, some carried in our minds from very early in our careers. We have memories of those who did not make it, their bodies and at times their minds unable to cope with this life. We have also been shaped by others who have at times abruptly reminded us of when we have got things wrong, when the system has harmed them and those around them or been immoveable and infuriating. We have also connected with individuals who have progressed through a system that has needed many people to help them work through and towards their future.

Further Reading

De Zulueta, F. (2006). *From pain to violence: The traumatic roots of destructiveness.* John Wiley & Sons Ltd. For readers wanting to understand how trauma and violence are linked.

Dowsett, J., & Craissati, J. (2008). *Managing personality disordered offenders in the community. A psychological approach.* Routledge. For readers wanting a working understanding of the core principles of working with this complex, traumatised client group in the community, as well as references for further relevant reading, research, and theory.

HM Prison and Probation Service & NHS England. (2020). *Practitioner guide to working with people in the criminal justice system showing personality difficulties.* (3rd ed.). HM Prison and Probation Service & NHS England. For an accessible overview of the theoretical framework and associated guidance relating to the OPD strategy.

Johnstone, L., & Boyle, M. with Cromby, J., Dillon, J., Harper, D., Kinderman, P., Longden, E., Pilgrim, D., & Read, J. (2018). The power threat meaning framework: Towards the identification of patterns in emotional distress, unusual experiences and troubled or troubling behaviour, as an alternative to functional psychiatric diagnosis. British Psychological Society. For a critical and alternative perspective on conceptualising and addressing psychological problems.

Kinderman, P. (2019). *A manifesto for mental health: Why we need a revolution in mental health care.* Palgrave Macmillan. For a critical perspective and alternative to the medicalisation of psychological difficulties.

National Offender Management Service & NHS England. (2015). *The offender personality disorder pathway strategy.* National Offender Management Service & NHS England. For a description of the OPD pathway and strategy.

Williams, P. (2020). *Community empowerment approaches. The key to overcoming institutionalised racism in work with black, Asian and minority ethnic (BAME) people in contact with the criminal justice system.* Clinks. For readers who want to know more about the problems faced by racially minoritised groups in the context of criminal justice.

References

Bateman, A., & Fonagy, P. (2016). *Mentalization based treatment for personality disorders: A practice guide.* Oxford University Press. doi:10.1093/med:psych/9780199680375.001.0001

Bentall, R. P. (Ed.). (1990). *Reconstructing schizophrenia.* Routledge. doi:10.1017/S0033291700014914

Boyle, M. (1990). *Schizophrenia: A scientific delusion?* Routledge.

British Psychological Society. (2018). *'Shining lights in dark corners of people's lives', The consensus statement for people with complex mental health difficulties who are diagnosed with a personality disorder.* Retrieved from https://mind.org.uk/media/21163353/consensus-statement-final.pdf

Craissati, J. (2019). *The rehabilitation of sexual offenders complexity, risk & desistance*. Routledge. doi:10.4324/9780203703342

Department of Health/National Offender Management Service. (2011). *Consultation on the offender personality disorder pathway implementation plan*. Department of Health/ Ministry of Justice.

De Zulueta, F. (2006). *From pain to violence: The traumatic roots of destructiveness*. John Wiley & Sons Ltd.

Farrall, S., & Calverley, A. (2006). *Understanding desistance from crime*. Open University Press.

Goldsmith, R. E., Martin, C. G., & Smith, C. P. (2014). Systemic trauma. *Journal of Trauma & Dissociation, 15*(2), 117–132. doi:10.1080/15299732.2014.871666

Johnstone, L., & Boyle, M. with Cromby, J., Dillon, J., Harper, D., Kinderman, P., Longden, E., Pilgrim, D., & Read, J. (2018). *The power threat meaning framework: Towards the identification of patterns in emotional distress, unusual experiences and troubled or troubling behaviour, as an alternative to functional psychiatric diagnosis*. British Psychological Society.

Kinderman, P. (2019). *A manifesto for mental health: Why we need a revolution in mental health care*. Palgrave Macmillan.

Kings Fund. (2019). *Tackling poor health outcomes: The role of trauma-informed care*. Retrieved from www.kingsfund.org.uk/blog/2019/11/trauma-informed-care

Mawby, Z., Newman, A., & Wilkinson-Tough, M. (2020). Offender personality disorder pathway screening tools evaluation. *Journal of Forensic Practice, 22*(3), 199–211. doi:10.1108/JFP-09-2019-0043

McCartan, K. (2020). *Trauma informed practice*. HM Inspectorate of Probation.

Nathan, R., Centifanti, L., Baker, V., & Hill, J. (2019). A pilot randomized controlled trial of a programme of psychosocial interventions (Resettle) for high risk personality disordered offenders. *International Journal of Law and Psychiatry, 66*, 101463. https://doi.org/10.1016/j.ijlp.2019.101463

National Institute for Mental Health in England. (2003). *Personality disorder: No longer a diagnosis of exclusion. Policy implementation guidance for the development of services for people with personality disorder*. Department of Health.

National Offender Management Service & Department of Health. (2012). *A guide to psychologically informed planned environments*. National Offender Management Service and Department of Health, London.

NHS England & NHS Improvement & the National Collaborating Centre for Mental Health. (2019). *The community mental health framework for adults and older adults*. NHS.

Perry, B. P., & Winfrey, O. (2021). *What happened to you? Conversations on trauma, resilience & healing*. Melcher Media.

Skett, S., Goode, I., & Barton, S. (2017). A join NHS and NOMS offender personality disorder pathway strategy: A perspective from 5 years of operation. *Criminal Behaviour and Mental Health, 27*, 214–221. doi:10.1102.cbm.2026

Williams, P. (2020). *Community empowerment approaches. They key to overcoming institutionalised racism in work with black, Asian and minority ethnic (BAME) people in contact with the criminal justice system*. Clinks.

Wilkinson, H., Whittington, R., Perry, L., & Eames, C. (2017). Does formulation of service users' difficulties improve empathy in forensic mental health services? *Journal of Forensic Psychology Research and Practice, 17*(3), 157–178. doi:10.1080/24732850.2017.1297758

Wilton, J., & Williams, A. (2019). *Engaging with complexity*. The Centre for Mental Health and the Mental Health Foundation.

PART V

Organisational Issues

19

DEVELOPING TRAUMA-INFORMED YOUTH JUSTICE SERVICES

Nicola Silvester

Introduction

Safeguarding children from harm is everyone's responsibility!
Department for Education, 2018

Everybody who has ever worked in a person-facing role will have been regularly reminded that safeguarding children from harm is everyone's responsibility. Legislation sets out our responsibilities regardless of the nature of the organisation to safeguard and promote the welfare of children (Department for Education, 2018). Understandably so, as childhood is a fragile time of intense development and learning that we know helps lay down the foundations for the type of adult that child will become. Therefore, both the importance and innate vulnerability of childhood are recognised and thus must actively be preserved by protecting children from harm. However, the world is an unsafe place where many children do unfortunately experience trauma and, as a result, have their learning or development impacted upon. Adverse Childhood Experiences (ACEs) research (Felitti et al., 1998) indicates that the effect of multiple traumas within childhood can lead to poorer outcomes in adulthood, including higher levels of mental health issues, substance abuse, and aggressive behaviour, influencing educational and employment opportunities. The Department of Health (2013a) reported that children with mental health issues, and those who engage in substance misuse or aggressive behaviour are over-represented within the Criminal Justice System, as are children in care and those living in poverty or experiencing any of the factors highlighted by the ACE's research. This report suggests that, despite declining numbers, there appears to be "evidence of growing levels of multiple, complex and damaging health and social needs among those who come into contact with the youth justice system" (p.202). Therefore, it is undeniable that children who come into contact with the Criminal Justice System have often experienced (or are still experiencing) high levels of

DOI: 10.4324/9781003120766-25

childhood trauma. So a trauma-informed approach to this cohort of young people would appear essential. However, current systems and processes make this a challenge to achieve – from the sheer nature of how we define offending within an adolescent cohort, to the practicalities of arrest, police interview, bail, remand, the court process, community interventions, and detention. All of these can re-traumatise an already traumatised child or compound their traumatic experiences, going against the principle of safeguarding all children from harm (Paterson-Young, Hazenberg, Bajwa-Patel, 2019). Therefore, systems-wide change is needed in order to take a trauma-informed approach to Youth Justice. This chapter will aim to summarise the journey of one Youth Justice Service towards adopting a trauma-informed approach and give guidance as to how this was achieved, through considering how to mobilise this type of thinking initially and then how this may impact upon certain aspects of the service such as assessment and understanding of the child, the child's journey through the criminal justice process including arrest, sentencing, and intervention, as well as consider the impact on the staff team itself. This will be done through sharing the challenges and the benefits of this way of working, interweaving examples of this in action to help guide anyone wanting to adopt this within their organisation.

Mobilising Trauma-Informed Thinking in Statutory Organisations

> Trying to implement trauma-specific clinical practices without first implementing trauma-informed organizational culture change is like throwing seeds on dry land.
>
> *Sandra Bloom (2014), MD, Creator of the*
> *Sanctuary Model (Gerber, 2019)*

What is "Trauma-Informed Thinking?" What does it look like in practice and how will you know when you have it? This is an on-going debate amongst likeminded professionals across the globe and, as this approach takes traction, various terminologies are emerging to help articulate what is meant by *trauma-informed thinking*. There is an acknowledgement that a difference lies between organisations that are aware that trauma exists within their populations, those that are sensitive to, or informed about, the impact of trauma on those individuals, and those that are able to consider this impact in their response to their clients (and their staff) and offer interventions and support specifically tailored to take into account the traumatic experiences of those being served. This is the difference between knowing about trauma, thinking about the impact and doing something about it. These three processes are very different and it can be hard to know where to start, but in my experience they are the three sequential steps to becoming trauma-informed.

In Simon Sinek's seminal TED Talk (2016), he advocates to "Start with the why!" He postulates that "people don't buy what you do, they buy why you do it!" and as such "it's those that start with 'why' that inspire us or find others that inspire them". Therefore, the first step is to raise awareness within the organisation of the sheer prevalence of trauma among the people we work with, before helping the organisation to understand the impact of this. This needs to include not only what brought these children into the organisation, but also what might be keeping them there; this is key to laying the foundations for all other aspects of the process. However, often organisations such as Youth Justice are made up of overlapping, integrating organisations, each with their own overriding agendas, a range of professionals, with a range of levels and modalities of training and skill, often being governed by a range of authorities working within different legal frameworks. This often includes the Police, Crown Prosecution Service, Criminal Justice Liaison and Diversion Service, Victim Liaison Service, Courts, Youth Offending Service, remand and custodial settings, as well as peripheral partner agencies such as Health, Education, and Social Care. Creating change across these organisations concurrently would be a miracle, so aim to work by influencing the immediate system first before ideas gather traction and begin to garner more support and collaboration from those outside of the inner circle in order to begin to start a movement.

Raising awareness and understanding within an organisation takes on two distinct actions. It begins with understanding the needs of the population, requiring access to information and training in what that means for the child. Access to information is important in developing a holistic picture of what life has been like for the child growing up, thereby shifting focus to what has happened to them rather than solely what they are presenting with, allowing for better connections to be made between the experience of trauma, understanding the presenting behaviour and where it might stem from. Often this information is limited to what is held within the organisation and is directly related to the child. However, trauma can be trans-generational, societal, institutional as well as individual, so a whole-systems approach needs to be adopted. The setting or environment into which this child was born and raised is also important; understanding the childhood experiences of both the child's biological parents and other caregivers, the development of their relationship and the circumstances in which the child came into these relationships should not be underestimated, as well as the society and political climate in which they were raised. This gives a sense of not only the capacity of the parents and the community into which they were born to provide "good enough" care to the child within those formative early years of life, but also their current capacity to support any intervention the organisation attempts to offer, which can often be the first barrier to overcome.

In order to achieve this, organisations need robust information sharing agreements with key partnership agencies, both within the adult and child arena, as well as a thorough understanding of their legal responsibilities in relation to consent to gather and share information. Often the biggest challenge with this is understanding the complexity of information governance (including consent, confidentially, and disclosure) across and within statutory organisations. As such when embarking on this process it is important to become familiar with the legal frameworks governing information sharing in respect of safeguarding, alongside those relating to public protection from criminal activity, such as The Crime and Disorder Act (1998). Information including history of contact with the police, social care, and health agencies, alongside educational history, diagnoses of any additional needs or involvement with any special educational needs processes, as well as parents' involvement with police, social care, and health services, including support from domestic violence services and consideration of what might be going on in the family in relation to other siblings and the community in which they were raised will develop a richer foundation of information to work from. Best practice guidelines relating to handling and sharing sensitive and confidential information, such as the Caldecott Principles (Department of Health, 2013b), should always be applied, and motivations made clear from the outset. However, when operating from a basis of trauma-informed practice then truly understanding the "why" for a particular child or family is important in determining the "what to do about it". Similarly, operating a restorative practice approach (Costello, Watchel, & Watchel, 2009) encourages collaboration rather than subjugation or dictation. Within our organisation we set up a multi-agency partnership service involving Police, Youth Offending, Victim Liaison, Social Care, Youth & Community Development, Education and Health to intervene with some of the most complex young people entering our services to inform and coordinate a trauma-informed approach to all our services understanding of them and target the necessary support.

When it comes to raising awareness about trauma through training in Youth Justice organisations, this needs to begin with basic education on child development, including developmental milestones such as walking and talking, but also include an overview of social and sexual development. Having a basic understanding of the development of emotional regulation, empathy, self-concept, and social and sexual identity is crucial in becoming trauma-informed, as it gives a foundation of "normal" patterns of development in a population that will typically display "atypical" patterns. It also gives an understanding of the basic environment and interactions needed to promote healthy childhood development. Secondly, training in the biopsychosocial model of attachment trauma is needed to understand the impact of trauma on the child's development, whether neurological or psychological, impacting on a child's core beliefs and concept of self, alongside how it can impact on interaction within their communities. This training will lay the foundations for understanding how childhood trauma can disrupt typical childhood development and lead to atypical development often seen within Youth Justice populations.

Transforming Case Formulation

Most Youth Justice (and non-youth justice) organisations will have embedded protocols and practices around assessing risk of harm to others alongside the safety and well-being of the child, whether this be a formal process of identifying risk factors, employing a risk matrix and quantified level of risk or simple structured, clinical judgement. Most Youth Offending Services use ASSET Plus (Youth Justice Board, 2014) as standard (a comprehensive assessment based on clinical research combining both actuarial and clinical judgements regarding the likelihood of re-offending and the risk of serious harm), in addition to the AIM-3 (Assessment, Intervention, and Moving-on) Framework for cases involving Harmful Sexual Behaviour (Leonard & Hackett, 2019). However, whilst both are moving towards a strength-based approach, incorporating more protective factors, neither truly captured the essence of a trauma-informed assessment. ASSET Plus in particular is seen as a cumbersome document, taking disproportionate time to complete, incongruent to the level of risk posed, ineffective in guiding an appropriate intervention plan and not easily accessible for the child or their family (Picken, Baker, d'Angelo, Fays, & Sutherland, 2019). However, more could be done to identify the cumulative vulnerability of the child when considering wider contextual factors such as developmental trauma, understanding the impact this has on the child and their presentation and the harm that could be caused to that child through any actions taken by services failing to consider this when planning their intervention or support. Therefore, there are currently three Youth Offending Services across the country trialling alternative assessments to the ASSET Plus, including our organisation.

Given that most Youth Offending Services are now incorporated into Children's Services the Signs of Safety Model, which has been adopted throughout, Social Care appears to have been most influential here. Signs of Safety was developed by Andrew Turnell and Steve Edwards through years of practice, eventually being rolled out as a model from 1993. It "expands the investigation of risk to encompass family and individual strengths, periods of safety and good care that can be built upon to stabilise and strengthen a child's and family's situation" (Turnell & Murphy, 2017). Whilst it is more succinct and tailored to the individual child and family context, collaborative and accessible for the individuals involved and links well onto an intervention plan, leading to an evaluative process, it still does not fully utilise a trauma-informed approach to understand where the concerns arise from and therefore why some intervention strategies might be more successful than others. Therefore, a model of trauma-based psychological formulation is needed.

Formulation is the act of making sense of the information that has been gathered within the assessment phase of the process, thus creating meaning out of facets of information by hypothesising about the links between cause and effect. There are numerous models of formulation available to use, each with their own merits and limitations; however, each organisation will need to find the one best-suited for them. This might come down to the specific nature of the cohort being supported, the nature of the staff group within the organisation and their familiarity and expertise within the field of formulation, the availability of specialist knowledge or resources within the organisation or the transferability of the formulations between other organisations they work closely alongside or have partnership arrangements with. Consequently, it is advisable to collaborate closely with colleagues from psychological disciplines as formulation is a key component of their skillset, which can be useful to harness throughout this transformation.

Earliest incarnations that were used within our organisation were the Circle of Security Model of attachment trauma (Hoffman, Marvin, Cooper, & Powell, 2006), which looks at how early experiences of relational safety and security can interweave with childhood traumatic experiences to develop adaptive safety behaviours that are often seen in the presentations of the young people being supported. This enables problematic behaviours or risky presentations to be framed within the context of relational trauma and guides the intervention strategy within the context of relational repair. This has helped developed knowledge of trauma into an understanding of the impact trauma can have on the child and their family, not only in respect of what may have led to where they are now, but how to intervene effectively going forward. It also takes into account trans-generational trauma, by using the formulation model and approach to consider any caregiver within the family system and their experience of relational trauma, and thus their safety behaviours and relational approach to both their child and the professionals offering support. Within this the concept of intersectionality needs to be considered – this is not merely the understanding of how individual factors can prejudice or promote an individual or their circumstances, but how a combination of these factors can lead to situations of cumulative advantage or disadvantage in respect of a specific individual and the situations in which they find themselves (see Intersectional Theory: Burgess-Proctor, 2006).

Journey Through the Criminal Justice Process

Arrest and Interview

Understandably, children who come into contact with the police are processed differently from adults; however, there is still progress being made around how trauma-informed or trauma-responsive this is. The Police and Criminal Evidence Act (1984) sets out the police's responsibilities when it comes to processing children. These include being responsible for identifying and informing the person responsible for the child's welfare of their arrest or detention, providing an "Appropriate Adult" to be present for the child during searching and questioning, and ensuring that a child is detained no longer than necessary and, if necessary, conveyed to the Local Authority for accommodation to avoid them being held in custody overnight. Therefore, sharing information with local policing teams as well as raising their knowledge of trauma and its impact on children and childhood can be beneficial. Flags can be added to the Police National Computer (PNC) highlighting pertinent information that might aid the police in understanding the needs of a child they have detained, including known diagnoses of mental health concerns or additional needs, linked professionals or services, and risk or vulnerability markers. However, this requires partnership working. This could help to support that child being safely and appropriately arrested, interviewed and, where possible, released back into the community with support in place to manage any arising issues, thus reducing the additional trauma that this may cause to a child, especially those with traumatic histories already and/or underlying mental health and learning needs. Identifying and relaying these factors to the police has become easier since the introduction of Criminal Justice Liaison and Diversion Services, which came from a Health and Justice specialised commissioning workstream called the Collaborative Commissioning Network, following The Five Year Forward View for Mental Health (Mental Health Taskforce, 2016). This has allowed the creation of partnership arrangements to screen all consenting children in contact with the police for factors increasing their vulnerability within society and guide them to access the support they need throughout this process at the earliest opportunity. However, more progress is possible in proactively considering the needs of these children before they come into the system alongside the progressive work being done at the point of contact.

Over the years significant changes have occurred to our perceptions of children involved in antisocial or criminal activity causing changes in policies and procedures. In the UK, a number of high profile cases and reviews of critical incidents where children have come to harm (namely Rotherham, but see the NSPCC archives for other serious case reviews) have forced us into acknowledging the role of criminal and sexual exploitation within this, including radicalisation, child trafficking, county-lines, and modern day slavery. Therefore, children persistently missing from home or care providers, those engaging in criminal activity with other children or with adults known to criminal justice services, or those that meet criteria set out on screening tools for exploitation should now be flagged and investigated for links to organised crime. Within this, collating an understanding of the vulnerabilities experienced by this population is vital, as well as how these can make certain children more suscep-tible to exploitation, and how services can respond effectively. Many of the above serious case reviews around exploitation reference the need for inter-agency com-munication and collaboration on identifying those at risk, the networks maintaining the exploitation, as well as actions that disrupt and ultimately safeguard vulnerable children from exploitation. Therefore, having a child criminal and sexual exploit-ation specialist employed by organisations to collaborate with the police service and monitor cases that come through where exploitation is suspected and utilising or developing a criminal exploitation screening tool (our local example having been created by Lincolnshire Safeguarding Children's Partnership, date unknown) which is used widely across all partner services can assist with early identification of young people at risk of or being exploited.

Having a centralised coordinator for exploitation also facilitates strategically mapping the connected networks operating across the local area and will feed into the organisation's Multi-Agency Safeguarding Hubs (or equivalent). Locally, there should be processes for submitting intelligence to the police to help them build the bigger picture around exploitation; however, this needs to be promoted as colleagues need to be made aware of what to share, why, when and where – so this comes back to training in order to build awareness or processes that can support trauma-informed practice. Organisations should now have access to the National Referral Mechanism (NRM) whereby they can report and register children believed to be being crimin-ally exploited and seek support from specialists within this field, such as Independent Child Trafficking Advocates (ICTA) about measures or interventions they can put in place which may safeguard children. All these things help to foster a mindset of understanding, compassion and proactive prevention of exploitation, criminalisation and re-traumatisation of this population, whilst maintaining statutory responsibility for public protection alongside safeguarding the needs of the child. This foundation then follows the child through the entirety of their criminal justice journey and may in time prevent criminalisation of exploited individuals.

Diversion Away from Criminalisation and Sentencing

When adopting a trauma-informed approach to Youth Justice, it becomes apparent that often what these complex, traumatised children need least is criminal justice interventions. For many years now, research guiding us on reducing the risk of reoffending in adolescents has sought to include social and relational interventions (such as Desistence Theory & The Good Lives Model) alongside individual ones, which makes better sense when adopting trauma-informed practice. Desistence Theory (Mofitt, 1993) highlights levels of change including intra-psychic, interpersonal, community and societal, often encouraging education, training, and employment, eliciting a sense of achievement and responsibility as pivotal in desistence. Similarly, emotional well-being though leisure activities and social connectedness through association with pro-social peers and stable relationships with family and significant others are also considered relevant factors, none of which addresses the offence explicitly, but nevertheless are seen as successful in eliciting desistence. The Good Lives Model of offender rehabilitation (Ward & Stewart, 2003) also advocates for this, encouraging the identification of needs met by the criminal behaviour to be replaced by healthier behaviours thus preventing reoffending. Therefore, following the Legal Aid, Sentencing and Punishment of Offenders Act (2012) there was both a desire and a need across Youth Justice Services to reduce the amount of young people entering the court arena and being managed on criminal justice interventions. So, building on the strong relationships already forged across our services, we developed a Joint Diversionary Panel (JDP).

The JDP was a multi-agency collaboration that considers cases of first-time or low-level criminal activity, using a set of strict collaborative guidelines, underpinned by formulation of behaviour, for offering alternative, holistic interventions in lieu of formal criminal justice interventions. Referral to the JDP requires the admission of responsibility for the criminal activity by the young person, as any form of denial or doubt, needed to be subjected to the rigours of criminal investigation. If the young person admits responsibility, then the police officer in charge of the investigation could offer them an out of court disposal by referring them into the JDP. Subsequently, key partner agencies would gather information on the individual's behalf and consider all the information in context on aspects of both risk and vulnerability to decide on the best intervention to divert the young person away from further offending. This allowed our service to extend the scope of preventative work being offered across the cohort, holistically considering the context behind adolescent risk-taking behaviour and its links with adverse childhood experiences, as well as offering some of the more systemic preventative work out to our partner agencies. As often when operating from a trauma-informed approach, the most suitable action to take may be a social care- or health-focused approach. This resulted in a significant reduction in court orders and disposals, as well as robust multi-agency mechanism for diverting children away from the Criminal Justice System which 'just by the nature of association' can further traumatise, limit, and marginalise them.

Inevitably, there will be cases where the nature, frequency, or persistence of the offending behaviour will require statutory intervention. However, by diverting away the population that requires little or different forms of interventions to encourage desistence, specialised resources and intensive interventions can be focused on those requiring it most. However, even here, a trauma-informed approach can be adopted.

In fact, most young people coming in at this level of the organisation are already known to partner agencies. Therefore, after working collaboratively with our partner agencies on the JDP the service also underwent a restructure, in which the Youth Offending Service was incorporated into Children's Services and amalgamated with an offshoot of Early Help forming a specialist service aimed at supporting adolescents at risk, thereby discarding the unhelpful arbitrary labels of victim or perpetrator and working holistically with them and their families before, during, and after contact with the Criminal Justice System. Therefore, any young person identified as being vulnerable or at risk, by the nature of their behaviour at home or within the community, can be referred into the service and begin receiving support on a voluntary basis in an attempt to provide safety and stability or to divert them away from potential criminal activity. However, should their behaviour escalate into low-level offending behaviour, the JDP can offer an out of court disposal which, in most instances, can be assigned back to the professional that has an already established relationship with the individual and their family. Similarly, if their behaviour continues to escalate into the court arena, whilst court orders require the specialist skills of a trained Youth Offending Officer, within this model they can collaborate with the child's individual worker to understand the context behind the offending behaviour and advocate for the best possible outcome through the courts. Again, having already established relationships with that child, their network of support and a range of specialist provision from the network of professionals already in place around the child and their family can assist in being able to recommend robust community-based sentences to the court, especially as often established engagement or impact can be evidenced. Also, newer sentencing guidelines (Sentencing Council, 2020) gave greater responsibility to those sentencing children to recognise their developmental and contextual needs, thereby advocating for a more restorative and rehabilitative approach, which helps to endorse a trauma-informed approach when addressing sentencing needs.

Intervention for Both the Child and Their Family

There are many models of trauma-informed intervention, each with their own merits and challenges. Within our organisation we have found several models helpful to dip into when completing direct work with young people both within the context of addressing their offending behaviour to holistic support for their whole families or within the wider context of their lives. This has included support to our Local Authority homes, as well as rolled out an internally developed training package (Caring2Learn) across our education providers, foster carers, and care providers, enabling trauma-informed practice to be adopted across a whole spectrum of organisations coming into contact with our local population of young people:

Desistence Theory (Clarke & Cornish, 1985; Giordano, Cernkovich, & Rudolph, 2002; Laub & Sampson, 2001; Maruna, 2001) – the approach of introducing and promoting factors which are identified by research to contribute towards the desistence of offending;

Good Lives Model (Ward & Stewart, 2003) – where needs associated with problematic or criminal behaviour are encouraged to be met with healthy, pro-social behaviour;

Contextual Safeguarding (Firmin & Knowles, 2020) – creating relational safety for a child outside of their family home within the context of school, community, & peer groups;

Trauma Recovery Model (TRM) and Enhanced Case Management (ECM) (Skuse & Matthew, 2015) – incorporating psychological formulation and an understanding of the impact of developmental trauma into a tiered approach to strategic intervention to aid recovery;

Signs of Safety (Turnell & Murphy, 2017) – a strengths base approach exploring existing support and protective factors both within and around the child that can be drawn upon to create increased safety and stability for that child;

Restorative Practice (Costello, Watchel, & Watchel, 2009) – an approach that encourages sustained change to be created by collaborative action that provides both high support and high challenge, rather than taking action by doing for or to an individual;

Social Pedagogy (see Hatton, 2013 for an overview of its development) – an approach that postulates that every individual has the infinite potential to contribute meaningfully to society if supported to access that potential and channel it appropriately;

PACE Principles (Hughes, 2017) – a practice incorporate within Dialectical Behaviour Therapy encouraging Playfulness, Acceptance, Curiosity, and Empathy within all interactions with children.

Trauma-informed interventions are often based on the principle that the concerning presentation is just a manifestation of hidden unmet needs and thus a symptom of the problem, rather than the target of the solution. Historically, criminal justice interventions have often targeted the problematic behaviour directly either through educative interventions; knife crime programmes, classes around the impact of substances, or even victim empathy work or restrictive and punitive means; curfews, tags, exclusion zones, and non-association orders. However, they have rarely addressed the underlying need met by the offending behaviour, particularly now that the core population becomes more complex as efforts are made to divert first-time entrants and lower level offences away from the Criminal Justice System. Therefore, the impact of criminal justice interventions can be limited and in some cases can be seen as creating a bigger issue – such as putting restrictive measures around a young person who has engaged in harmful sexual behaviour (HSB) not to associate with peers of their own age, thus preventing them from actively being able to establish healthy peer relationships as part of their rehabilitation! Therefore, the most important part of determining the right type of intervention from a trauma-informed approach is to seek to understand the "why" behind the behaviour, not just the "what". Understanding why the child has taken this path into offending behaviour then helps to determine what needs to happen to discourage this behaviour. For example, using the example above of the child engaging in HSB, this could be for example because the child has suffered abuse themselves and is re-enacting abusive behaviour; or they may have additional needs and their behaviour is a consequence of misunderstanding social relationships; or they may be acting out in their peer group due to other underlying factors within their environment. In all these cases, restricting healthy peer relationships while attempting to prevent further victimisation does not address the underlying cause and in some instances could cause an escalation in concerning behaviour if that child is prevented through this restrictive action from developing healthy social and sexual relationships. It is therefore imperative to treat the need over the behaviour, in order to have any success in extinguishing the problematic behaviour.

When considering trauma-informed interventions for young people across the Criminal Justice System it is important to hold in mind normal child development, the building blocks of attachment and the impact of childhood trauma on the developing child, as often this can get forgotten, especially when applying adult-focused interventions adopted for and often only marginally adapted to a juvenile population. Adolescent risk-taking behaviour needs to be understood as a developmentally appropriate stage of childhood development and whilst most young people engage in this type of behaviour without being caught, some will unfortunately come into contact with the Criminal Justice System (especially those that are more highly scrutinised, such as those from black and ethnic minority communities, children with additional needs, and children in care), which is why it is important not to prematurely label these individuals as engaging in problematic criminal behaviour. Research shows that progression from adolescent contact with the Criminal Justice System to adult offending is rare (Farrington, 1986; Piquero, Farrington, & Blumstein, 2007). Therefore, operating a preventative support service and/or a diversionary process like our Joint Diversionary Panel aims to filter out those dabbling in possibly developmentally appropriate risk-taking behaviour, but unlikely to go on to become adult or lifetime offenders. This approach to giving the young person the benefit of the doubt based on a developmental understanding of the child also prevents pigeon-holing or labelling the child before they have had a proper opportunity to develop their societal or moral identities. Given that we know that group association, especially within adolescence, both physically and psychologically can have an impact on assimilation to that group's sense of identity. This may increase the likelihood of reoffending; therefore, labelling a child in this way can be counterproductive to what we hope to achieve.

Similarly, if knowledge of childhood development underpins intervention planning then aspects such as the child's developmental age and stage should be considered. Often aspects such as the developmental processes involved in the acquisition and refinement of a sexual identity, moral reasoning, perspective taking, and empathy are overlooked or over-ascribed to adolescent behaviour, despite much of the development within these specific areas being attributed to adolescent developmental processes. We cannot then expect a child to effectively employ a skill that they are still actively developing. More importantly, we cannot expect a child to actively continue developing a skill that they have shown to need developing or refining when there is a potential that the applied criminal justice intervention actively undermines or prevents opportunities for that individual to be exposed to contexts in which they can develop those skills (for example restricting a child's opportunities to associate with peers when they have engaged in harmful sexual behaviour, thus reducing their opportunities to be support to develop health sexual relationships with peers). Therefore, understanding the age and stage of the individual and how their level of adolescent development may have contributed towards their offending behaviour is useful for tailoring an effective trauma-informed intervention. This often requires a restorative approach of repeated, structured, and somewhat strategically supervised exposure to those sorts of developmental opportunities that foster learning and build skills in order to prevent further offending behaviour, such as mainstream education, extra-curricular activities, role-modelling, and pro-social relationship building. However, sometimes, this does fall into the realms of altered development rather than just delayed when acknowledging the impact of trauma and abuse. Therefore, these interventions require more of a recovery focus, whereby interventions are offered that counteract the child's previous experiences (such as abuse). Due to the nature of working with children and young people we know this often takes a whole family, if not a whole community approach.

Interventions around these areas of need often take on two forms, a retrospective and a prospective approach. Retrospectively, we need to look at what the child missed out on or is still missing out on and how that can be restored, thus creating a sense of safety for a child. This comes through a secure connection with a persistent, nurturing adult who may or may not be the child's parent, but certainly should be someone within the child's family if at all possible, as these relationships last longer than professional ones (albeit these are better than nothing if the former is not available – see Family Finding Approach – Campbell, no date). Tackling the aspects of the child's life that makes them feel unsafe, such as unstable home-life, disrupted or inconsistent education, criminality within their peer groups or communities and exploitation can help, and here is where a contextual safeguarding (Firmin & Knowles, 2020) approach can be adopted. Prospectively building positive activities into the child's life encourages positive self-esteem, healthy relationships, and a sense of achievement/fulfilment through structure and routine to give them some sense of consistency that can help to stabilise what is often a chaotic home environment. Once this is achieved, we can begin to build in restorative approaches so that the altered patterns of relating and behaving can be encouraged into more pro-social patterns of behaviour. These changes do not just need to happen for the children, who are often traumatised by their environments. Restoration and recovery also need to happen within their environment. Therefore, it is important to start from a "whole family" or "whole system" approach. Sometimes this involves taking a retrospective approach to what has happened in the past to lead the family or the community to explore what can be done to recover this or meet the needs that have been left unmet. However, sometimes this needs to take a proactive approach to addressing some of the issues that may arise from the incident, such as supporting families or the community to process the impact of the offence on them or help the systems around the child feel safe about maintaining a child within their environment who may pose a risk to others, such as within education.

Managing Vicarious Trauma within the System

Self-care is not always about being able to cope but recognising when you are struggling, we all have our limits. Giving yourself permission to be vulnerable and allowing others to see your vulnerability shows your strength. There should be a collective sense of accountability for self-care and looking after each other creates a more cohesive and connected team

Future4Me Practice Supervisor

One of the biggest challenges in developing trauma-informed services or introducing trauma-informed practice into an organisation is responding to the impact this will have on the staff team. No one who has ever worked within these services or with these populations is under any illusion that this work is not hard or stressful at times. However, developing awareness of the impact of trauma on the lives of service users undoubtedly invites reflection and insight into the impact of working with trauma on the staff team themselves. In my experience the concept of stress and burnout are familiar terms used within these settings. Understandably "the expectation that we can be immersed in suffering and loss daily and not be touched by it is as unrealistic as expecting to be able to walk through water without getting wet" (Remen, 1996). However, we need to understand what causes this impact, what consequences it has for the staff and how to mitigate or alleviate it when it happens. Therefore, an acknowledgement and understanding of secondary trauma is needed across the service, recognising that through the process of supporting people who have experienced trauma the clinician themselves may also be affected. Promoting good self-care amongst all the staff within the service, as well as modelling this throughout the organisation, is key to developing a resilient workforce. Staff that are able to acknowledge that their emotional well-being is paramount to being able to support and promote the emotional well-being of the individuals they work with within an environment that is trauma-informed is key. Therefore, they must first and foremost acknowledge the impact of this traumatic work on themselves, and model this throughout the organisation. Therefore, robust clinical supervision arrangements and safe and supportive reflective practice opportunities, as well as opportunities to debrief after high impact incidents, is paramount. However, this can only be done within an organisational culture that promotes trauma-informed practice for its employees and not just for the populations they serve (see Hawkins & Shohet, 2006).

Further Reading

A number of seminal works on understanding childhood trauma:

Burgess-Proctor, A. (2006). Intersections of race, class, gender, and crime: Future directions for feminist criminology. *Feminist Criminology, 1*(1), 27–47.

Gerhardt, S. (2004). *Why love matters: How affection shapes a baby's brain.* Brunner-Routledge.

Hughes, D. (2017). *Building the bonds of attachment: Awakening love in deeply traumatized children.* Rowman & Littlefield.

Kotter, J. (2017). *Our iceberg is melting: Changing and succeeding under any conditions.* Holger Rathgeber. A useful book on organisational change.

Porges, S.W. (2011). *The polyvagal theory: Neurophysiological foundations of emotions, attachment, communication, and self-regulation.* W.W. Norton & Company.

Sivers, D. (2010). *How to start a movement.* Retrieved from www.ted.com/talks/derek_sivers_how_to_start_a_movement?language=en. A helpful TED talk on effecting organisational change.

Smith, R. (2011). *Doing justice to young people.* Taylor and Francis.

Treisman, K. (2016). *Working with relational and developmental trauma in children and adolescents.* Routledge.

van der Kolk, B. (2014). *The body keeps the score: Brain, mind, and body in the healing of trauma.* Viking Penguin.

References

Bloom, S. (2014). *The heart of trauma theory: Sickness v's injury model: Changing the fundamental question from "what's wrong with you" to "what happened to you".* Retrieved from www.youtube.com/watch?v=X9zEb1YCprg.

Burgess-Proctor, A. (2006). Intersections of race, class, gender, and crime: Future directions for feminist criminology. *Feminist Criminology, 1*(1), 27–47. doi:10.1177/1557085105282899

Campbell, K. (No date). *The California evidence-based clearinghouse for child welfare: Family finding.* Retrieved from www.cebc4cw.org/program/family-finding/detailed

Clarke, R.V., & Cornish, D.B. (1985). Modelling offenders' decisions: A framework for research and policy. In M. Tonry & N. Morris (Eds), *Crime and justice: An annual review of research* (Vol. 6; pp.147–185). University of Chicago Press.

Costello, B., Watchel, T., & Watchel, J. (2009). *The restorative practices handbook: For teachers, disciplinarians and administrators.* International Institute for Restorative Practices.

Department for Education. (2018). *Working together to safeguard children: A guide to inter-agency working to safeguard and promote the welfare of children.* Department for Education.

Department of Health. (2013a). *Annual report of the Chief Medical Officer 2012, our children deserve better: Prevention pays.* Department of Health.

Department of Health. (2013b). *Information: To share or not to share government? The information governance review.* Department of Health.

Farrington, D.P. (1986). Age and crime. In M. Tonry & N. Morris (Eds), *Crime and justice: An annual review of research* (pp.189–250). University of Chicago Press. doi:10.1086/449114

Felitti, V.J., Anda, R.F., Nordenberg, D., Williamson, D.F., Spitz, A.M., Edwards, V., Koss, M.P., & Marks, J.S. (1998). The relationship of adult health status to childhood abuse and household dysfunction. *American Journal of Preventative Medicine, 14*(4): 245–258. doi:10.1016/S0749-3797(98)00017-8

Firmin, C., & Knowles, R. (2020). *The legal and policy frameworks for contextual safeguarding approaches: A 2020 update on the 2018 legal briefing.* The International Centre.

Gerber, M.R. (2019). *Trauma-informed healthcare approaches: A guide for primary care.* Springer.

Giordano, P.C., Cernkovich, S.A., & Rudolph, J.L. (2002). Gender, crime and desistance: Toward a theory of cognitive transformation. *American Journal of Sociology, 107*(4): 990–1064. doi:10.1086/343191

Hatton, K. (2013). *Social pedagogy in the UK: Theory and practice.* Russell House Publishing.

Hawkins, P., & Shohet, R. (2006). *Supervision in the helping professions.* Open University Press.

Hoffman, K., Marvin, R., Cooper, G., & Powell, B. (2006). Changing toddlers' and preschoolers' attachment classifications: The circle of security intervention. *Journal of Consulting and Clinical Psychology, 74*, 1017–1026. doi:10.1037/0022-006X.74.6.1017.

Hughes, D. (2017). *Building the bonds of attachment: Awakening love in deeply traumatized children.* Rowman & Littlefield.

Laub, J.H., & Sampson, R.J. (2001). Understanding desistance from crime. *Crime and Justice, 28*, 1–69. doi:10.1086/652208

Leonard, M., & Hackett, S. (2019). *AIM3 assessment model: Assessment of adolescents and harmful sexual behaviour*. The AIM Project.

Lincolnshire Safeguarding Children's Partnership (LSCP). (Date Unknown). *Multi-agency child exploitation screening tool*. Retrieved from www.lincolnshire.gov.uk/safeguarding/lscp/8

Maruna, S. (2001). *Making good: How ex-convicts reform and reclaim their lives*. American Psychological Association.

Mental Health Taskforce. (2016). *The five year forward view for mental health*. Retrieved from www.england.nhs.uk/wp-content/uploads/2016/02/Mental-Health-Taskforce-FYFV-final.pdf

Mofitt, T. (1993). 'Life-course Persistent' and 'adolescent-limited' antisocial behaviour: A developmental taxonomy. *Psychological Review, 100*, 674–701.

Paterson-Young, C., Hazenberg, R., & Bajwa-Patel, M. (2019*). The social impact of custody on young people in the criminal justice system*. Palgrave Macmillan.

Picken, N., Baker, K., d'Angelo, C., Fays, C., & Sutherland, A. (2019). *Process evaluation of ASSET Plus*. RAND Corporation.

Piquero, A.R., Farrington, D.P., & Blumstein, A. (2007). *Key issues in criminal career research: New analyses of the Cambridge study in delinquent development*. Cambridge University Press.

Remen, R.N. (1996). *Kitchen table wisdom: Stories that heal*. Penguin.

Sentencing Council. (2020). *Sentencing Act 2020*. Retrieved from www.legislation.gov.uk/ukpga/2020/17/contents/enacted

Sinek, S. (2016). *Start with WHY to inspire action*. Retrieved from www.youtube.com/watch?v= HjriwYrGL28

Skuse, T., & Matthew, J. (2015). The trauma recovery model: Sequencing youth justice interventions for young people with complex needs. *Prison Service Journal, 220*, 16–24.

Smith, R. (2011). *Doing justice to young people*. Taylor and Francis.

Turnell, A., & Murphy, T. (2017). *Signs of safety comprehensive briefing paper (4th Edition)*. Resolutions.

Ward, T., & Stewart, C.A. (2003). Criminogenic needs and human needs: A theoretical model. *Psychology, Crime, and Law, 9*(2), 125–143. doi:10.1080/1068316031000116247

Youth Justice Board. (2014). *Asset Plus: Assessment and planning in the youth justice system*. Retrieved from www.gov.uk/government/publications/assetplus-assessment-and-planning-in-the-youth-justice-system/assetplus-assessment-and-planning-in-the-youth-justice-system

20

TRAUMA-INFORMED CARE IN SECURE PSYCHIATRIC HOSPITALS

Frank McGuire, Julie Carlisle, and Fiona Clark

The enduring and often devastating pattern of psychological response to what we refer to as trauma has been recognised for centuries or even millennia. References in literature, art, history, in the everyday conversations of people from all walks of life reveal an appreciation of the enduring influence of events long past on the lives not only of people who have experienced unbearable pain and loss, but also often in subsequent generations. This concept of the transgenerational transmission of trauma finds a welcome home in systemic therapy, but often is confined to the parameters of the nuclear or extended family. Yet trauma and the trauma-genic organisation of systems is neither solely linear nor transactional, it is developed out of multiple historical contexts (Bloom, 2010; 2012). The systematic oppression and persecution of communities, of countries, of people from different racial and religious groups reverberates long beyond the lifespan of those who are oppressed, their oppressors and the systems which embolden and enable their actions. The fragmentation of a sense of belonging, of pride and values, and the usurping of culture and language eventually culminate in groups who are disenfranchised, excluded, and seen as lesser. This reality has been brought to the forefront of collective consciousness over the last 18 months, a period which has exposed damning health inequalities in a global pandemic, brought the *Black Lives Matter* campaign to global attention, and seen an increase in rates of domestic violence, and mental health and social care crises (UK Parliament, 2021; NHS Strategy Unit, 2020).

Secure hospitals are reflective of the communities they serve. In consideration of traditional models of illness, people who have experienced oppression and exclusion experience treatment in ways that reinforce exclusion and isolation, coercive control, invalidation, and a violation of boundaries. Faced with the question of whether the care they offer or the way they practice emphasises abusive and unhealthy systems, staff are likely to be dismayed and horrified. Staff offer care in a controlled environment where it is necessary to enforce treatment or perhaps physically restrain for everyone's safety. This is the critical issue: the practices, policies, and procedures of a

DOI: 10.4324/9781003120766-26

system, which are both the accelerator and the brake of the organisation function independently of the needs of all the individuals who comprise it, often at times in a manner wholly contrary to their requirements. This is the crux of re-traumatising systems, not only for patients but for staff. The axiom of trauma-informed care is that trauma–genic experiences are pervasive across, as well as within, groups. This is a fundamental aspect of secure mental health services bringing, therefore, a need to guard against the fallacy that the entirety of trauma in the system belongs to patients.

Thus, the consequences of injustice, powerlessness, oppression, and poverty are inherent in everyday life, and for millions of families their struggles within these societal systems show up in the interactions and meaning-making of their lives. The fragmentation of supportive systems, communities, and cultures makes each member of a family unit vulnerable to a range of harms that occur in their relationships; victim becomes perpetrator. Children are disadvantaged by adversity and learn to navigate their normality in ways that serve to maintain a status quo.

The significant prevalence of trauma and childhood adversity amongst people in forensic settings is increasingly well evidenced and the long-term consequences of these experiences are acknowledged (Karatzias, Shevlin, Pitcairn, & Thomson, 2019; Facer-Irwin, Karatzias, Bird, & Blackwood, 2021). An absence of a cohesive and systematic integration of trauma-informed practice, that is prioritised and supported at every level of the organisation, leads to a fragmented and inconsistent approach to care. This serves to perpetuate anxiety and insecurity at all levels of the system, and can lead to harmful, re-traumatising practices.

To implement trauma-informed care, there has to be an understanding of the structure of the current system and observations of how the people in the system function to stay safe and survive. For patients, safety is an act of self-preservation to predict the intentions and motivations of others, based on previous harmful relationships, and replaying actions that result in survival.

For staff, their intent is a moral endeavour to care (Seedhouse, 1994) and make people better. However, they are often caught up in the pressures of the role which are beset by policy and procedures that are challenges in the organisation; the ward, peers, and manifest and latent traumas in the patient group soon become a task beyond clinical teaching. This complex interrelationship frequently leads to high levels of anxiety and expressed emotion. In organisations or systems that lack an understanding of this, the default management position follows an organising principle of control of others in order to achieve outcomes (Carlisle & McGuire, 2020).

For patients, entering a therapeutic relationship with staff operating within a highly controlled environment serves to replay the very family/social care system they may be used to, which results in re-traumatising experiences. Events that are projected as "care interactions", oscillating between compliance (perceived as "progress") and independence (risking "breakdown"), can represent a misalignment of goals. Stability for both patients and staff is rarely achieved, particularly in the early stage of treatment. This represents a consuming existential risk. Great harm has occurred to them in relationships, sufficient to crystalise their mental maps of human interaction. They often find it psychologically excruciating to contemplate the prospect of other adults having control and authority over them. They do not have an expectation of kindness, compassion, and benevolent care. Rather the opposite is true; the expectation is that the intent of people in positions of power is to harm them even though they initially may disguise this.

The features aligned to an abusive system can be observed in examples of failed care such as Wharton Hall and Winterbourne View.[1] The organising principle of control of others holds within it actions of secrecy and silencing, invalidation, coercive control, violence, violation of boundaries, exclusion, and isolation. In few circumstances is this purposeful and planned. It is more a gradual and inexorable slip into unacceptable practice. Poorly led and ill-governed systems become self-organising. They form and shape to meet the needs of the decision-makers at every level with a combination of human and organisational factors (Carlisle & McGuire, 2020).

To some degree, most staff and patients in secure care are likely to have experienced some features of control in relationships and organisations. Whilst all have significant consequences to the recovery of complex trauma, developing therapeutic and healing relationships whilst navigating systemic philosophies that counter this will have insidious and damaging consequences to all involved. Boundaries become unclear, violations are increasingly likely, invalidation is common, and the trauma transmits, erodes, and erupts in all parties. A trauma-informed system not only focuses on adapting the environment, but also invests in care of the staff, understanding that they come with their own adversity and are sensitive to the transference of trauma of others.

The mental health difficulties of patients in secure services are predominantly viewed through the prism of *sickness*. This is an understandable position and, to a degree, is valid. Yet if we consider trauma in the context of its literal translation to mean "wound", then the paradigm shifts. The perspective turns to people who have sustained multiple and repeated psychological wounds over many years. These are reopened time and time again in an attempt to cure or at least manage symptoms, rather than a focus on providing an environment and relationships that heal. The misalignment arises when "trauma-focused interventions" attempt to address past experiences while the patients' energies are spent avoiding current and future harm. Trauma-informed care therefore must start in the here and now. Psychological and physical safety is the prerequisite (see Figure 20.1). This is not just the position of the organisation, it is the therapy. A therapeutic milieu is cultivated from the first contact, the building, the relationships with all staff involved in care.

A progressive trauma-informed system aims to develop a healing environment based on the organising principles of autonomy and fairness – something that has been compromised in those with complex trauma histories. It involves ensuring that relationships are based on safety, trustworthiness, choice, empowerment, collaboration, and respecting individuality with respect to culture, history, religion, and gender (SAMSHA, 2014).

Implementing a Trauma-Informed Model of Care in a Secure Hospital

Readers may expect the focus of this chapter to be on the trauma of patients or perhaps the secondary impact on staff of repeated exposure to traumatic narratives

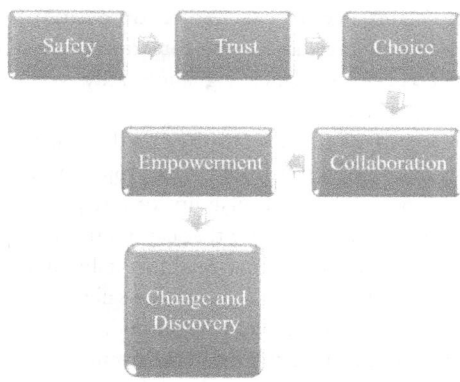

Figure 20.1   Principles of trauma-informed care (adapted from SAMHSA, 2014)

and material. In essence, though, it is only possible to arrive at a genuinely trauma-informed system through the exploration and active management of two other critical sources of organisational trauma, namely the impacts of the life histories of staff and of any trauma-genic practices, processes, or interpersonal patterns. Unaddressed, these factors are the touchpaper for re-traumatisation of patients and staff, and usually result in an over-reliance on long-established approaches that are often the only available defences against anxiety. Implementing this strategy at a women's medium secure care ward is the focus of this chapter and is presented in a series of vignettes.

A trauma-informed administration will acknowledge the reverberations of the individual and systemic traumas of not only all the people but the organisation itself. When an organisation has endured a threat to its existence, this becomes a psychic component and is played out in staff who were not even there. The historical and social context of the service is critical to understanding the development of systems and processes and the psychological makeup of staff and patients.

The reality for staff is that the recognition of what is happening in the traumatised organisation is often hidden in rigid policies and procedures. In order to generate a sustainable recognition of stress there needs to be a series of emotionally contained conversations about how staff function in work amongst distressing circumstances, acknowledging how the organisation chooses to operate to manage the risk in the framework of its heritage. In secure care, with high rates of self-harm and restraint, high rates of staff injury and sickness, and a quick turnover of temporary staffing, a women's ward can be a place many staff state active resistance to working into for their own concerns about managing distress; staff fight/flight/freeze is activated before they have taken on the shift.

Often a ward in crisis results in a change of clinical priorities. This can be seen as flight from intolerable anxiety. Relief is in short supply and space to safely reflect is extinguished. Yet there is an attempt to impose order on chaos, often at the expense of meaning. This is bound to fail and eventually will exacerbate the issues. In an environment where there is a sustained exposure to adversity and removal of protective factors, prolonged stress and anxiety can lead to dissociation in the team and the system functions in an automatic state, losing direction or coherence. This can look like absenteeism, presenteeism, avoidance, vigilance, tardy work, or any acts that conserve the self from being overwhelmed.

When asked, staff can articulate the stress they hold emanating from direct patient care with relative ease. In addition to this they can project limitations to the recovery from the stress into the system – the availability of rest periods, formal or informal reflection or reviews. An unhelpful culture that can focus on responsibility can make staff take steps to avoid experiencing blame. Staff inevitably not only become anxious about their physical and psychological safety, and the safety of colleagues and patients, but also concerned to their profession and livelihood. It is not uncommon to hear staff talk about their professional registration in the event that something goes wrong.

When traditional models of reflective practice are available to help navigate individual and collective experiences of a stressful or risky nature, it tends to locate all of the experience within the single situation or setting, and in teams where the staffing is (by mechanism of shifts or organisational pressure) irregular, there are few opportunities for the development of psychological safety, cohesion, and growth.

To counter this, there must be a broader psychological understanding of the multiplicity of the trauma systems everyone is involved in, and the relative contribution of each. Yet staff do not routinely have access to a systemic framework to inculcate and maintain this level of awareness. Without an active framework which privileges the emotional containment and psychological safety of staff, individuals and teams will struggle to over time to maintain a reflective and compassionate understanding of the fluid dynamics of the network of attachment relationships across the system.

A team that is functioning under threat or in fear can remain silenced – no one wants to be the weakest link. They can invalidate their own experiences and that of others in the team. Boundary violations which feel like support and comfort, or exclusion and isolation are inevitable. The organising principle of controlling the self, controlling other, and ensuring compliance to the wider system of the ward and organisation are maintained. Articulating the true impact of events is avoided. The team is primed to experience dissociation. To this end, the care believed to be on offer is fragmented as a sequence of events which are poorly aligned to meet the needs of the patient group and can lead to an impoverished employment experience which reverberates outside of the workplace.

Left unaddressed a traumatised and dissociated team cannot navigate relationships with patients safely; the barometer for risk shifts towards either hypervigilant or avoidant. The attunement and psychological safety of all members of the ward (staff and patients) remains under threat.

Delivering such a cultural and operational change is a complex and challenging task. This model of intervention requires an integrative and reflective space. There is an emphasis on prioritising space and time for thinking and reflection and a primary objective of building a culture of compassion, support, and reflection between staff. With persistent trauma-informed reflective practice and supervision, staff can be receptive and attuned, reflect and respond in ways that are coherent to the demands of needing to respond to the trauma in others.

The objective of developing a trauma-informed model of care is to move towards a system organised around autonomy and fairness, upholding the principles of safety, trustworthiness, choice, collaboration, empowerment, and respecting individual differences (adapted from SAMHSA, 2014). In doing this, acknowledging and validating various levels of traumatic material in the team is an important task. Working with trauma is evocative and yet most of what it evokes remains enshrined in the daily hassles of working with complexity. It can remain hidden or invalidated. Staff bring with them their own history of adversity and to a large degree believe it to be resolved or managed. In effecting a cultural shift in the emotional management of a service in a trauma-informed way, interventions that *realise* the trauma is there, *recognise* its signs, *respond* by providing intervention, and actively *resist re-traumatising* are integral to the model and are supported via a circle of containment in validating relationships and developing relational security for all (*Four Rs*: SAMSHA, 2014).

Context to the Vignettes: The Women's Ward

All patients are cis-female with some identifying as male. The patients present as a risk of harm to self or others at a level that requires enhanced physical and procedural security along with robust relational security. These terms appear to be formal – the essence of the environment is a model of care that aspires to autonomy and fairness; however, this is difficult to achieve in an institution where care and control are intertwined, and where, for patients, restriction is the critical component of perceived unfairness – patients are of a mindset before care starts that they are being unfairly treated and controlled as their freedom is removed. Where the organising principle is one of control, the conditions of the care relationships can all too easily involve coercive practices, invite silencing, invalidation, exclusion and isolation, and have a lack of cultural respect.

Most harmful experiences for the patients have occurred within their family of origin or in the care system. The chronic and consistent exposure to neglect and abuse shape their personalities, functioning and, importantly, their expectations about treatment from others, particularly those people who are in positions of power over them. Coming into a secure care environment is likely to replicate the conditions of harmful relationship dynamics and re-traumatise.

On the ward, the patients are at differing levels of acuity of distress or recovery. The service has no place to move patients on within its own unit: you arrive, you recover amongst your peers, you move on. This presents a critical dilemma to service providers and to supporting a systemic model of care; the environment is likely perpetually entrenched in trauma responses amongst all of the people on the ward. In becoming trauma-informed, the task is to recognise this and respond accordingly reducing the risk of re-traumatising experiences.

The staffing on the ward is a complement of qualified nurses, nurses in training, and nursing assistants. This is augmented by a multidisciplinary team consisting of a consultant psychiatrist, psychologist, social worker, occupational therapist, and other allied therapists all of whom have a clearly defined and regular role on the ward in relation to the team and the patients. Staffing is a problem for services; with sickness and injury there can be a high turnover of staff, and the women's ward is no exception. A basic premise for psychologically safe service provision is a workforce that is equipped to provide a safe base and safe haven: one where the team are regular/familiar and can observe the three tenets of secure care (physical, procedural, relational security) in consistent ways (Department of Health, 2010).

In order to make conditions conducive to a healing environment, it is critical to have a truly systemic investment in trauma-informed care through the structure of the Trust and across the lifecycle of the employees. In a secure care environment, there are inherent problems in any attempt to shift away from dominance and control towards an organising principle of autonomy and fairness. It is important to raise awareness of the impact of trauma corporately and clinically, and to develop explicit and implicit ways of collaborating and empowering, validating people, providing choice along with respecting and upholding the cultural values and needs of all.

The following series of continuous vignettes are fictional characters and will outline an example of common scenarios, and the implications will be discussed throughout.

Vignette 1: The Patient, Karen

Karen was admitted to the unit after setting fire to her room in the hostel where she lived. Information from hostel staff indicated this followed a dispute which a man with whom she had a romantic relationship. Karen has a history of violence using weapons, with reports of numerous assaults on men. Her medical records revealed long-term mental health difficulties with frequent and severe self-harm, and substance misuse. She is often referred to as a "complex individual".

Recognising the intensity of these difficulties, Karen's clinical team focused on allowing her to settle into the ward and were responsive to her requests. However, despite their care and concern, she would become oppositional and aggressive, and staff developed a plan to "not reward acting out". Often her behaviour escalated, and she was placed in seclusion.

Multi-disciplinary assessment revealed extreme childhood adversity. Karen was adopted aged two. Her adoptive mother was psychologically and physically unavailable, having developed a dependence on benzodiazepines and alcohol. From the age of six Karen was regularly sexually assaulted by her adoptive father. School was an unhappy place for her, and she was lonely, teased, and bullied. She suffered from enuresis throughout her childhood. As an adolescent she relied on alcohol and drugs to cope emotionally and was groomed and sexually assaulted by men after being befriended and introduced to them by girls older than her. She was pregnant at 14 and her parents arranged a termination. Shortly after she was placed in residential care where she was sexually exploited and subjected to repeated violence. She is known to have engaged in sex work and petty crime. Karen has three children all of whom were removed and placed in care.

Karen did not settle on the ward and appeared hypervigilant. She was often accused of getting involved in issues between staff and other patients and was seen to be interfering in matters that did not concern her. Her mood was deemed unstable and her interpersonal difficulties were attributed to her undiagnosed "personality disorder". Staff adopted greater vigilance in maintaining boundaries. Karen experienced this as psychological unavailability, provoking intense attachment behaviour.

Attempts to discuss her early adversity resulted in withdrawal and disengagement (dissociation). She would often engage in aggressive behaviour or self-harm the next day. She continued to feel unsafe and was constantly vigilant to indicators of threat, evaluating staff interaction with other patients as evidence of an abusive environment. This frequently led to emotive confrontation and seclusion.

Karen experienced overwhelming and intolerable feelings of shame about her past. This led to internally and externally directed rage which seemed inappropriate and incongruent to circumstances the next day. Staff perceived her anger and aggression as unjustifiable and without a trigger. It became clear that the impact of the past was not about the events themselves, which generally led to dissociation. Rather, it was the meaning of these events to her. She was terrified every day that therapists and nursing staff would want to talk about these things.

Staff with Complex Lives

It should be clear by now that a significant contribution to the trauma load in any organisation, particularly, in health and social care comes from the lived experiences and circumstances, past and present, of staff. Trauma and trauma-genic environments are pervasive and permeate the lives of people from all backgrounds and socio-economic groups. If trauma is considered merely as a matter of personal history, there is a fundamental and far-reaching error of logic, yet one which is common in organisational responses.

In a period of elevated anxiety on the ward, managing behaviour or illness can become the overriding objective at the expense of acknowledging of the complex lives of staff. Chronic stressors such as domestic violence or relationship problems, living with sick or disabled family members and having care responsibilities, poverty, substandard housing, house moves, divorce, and bereavement are common amongst the workforce. Still staff turn up to work, and to a significant degree such life stressors undoubtedly influence their capacity to build healing relationship with patients. Helping others heal is a difficult process, doing it when you are continually hurt is often a burden which may on occasion be unbearable.

Human Resourcing can only go so far. It is indisputable that Trusts employ staff with complex lives, with unresolved or cumulative traumas of their own, or with on-going life events which serve to distract from the task at hand (Carlisle & McGuire, 2020). These issues are a challenge to systemic working: Who notices what is happening to staff? How do they navigate their emotions and not over-identify or get overwhelmed with the emotions of others? Outsourcing these tasks to Human resources or occupational health is only a partial solution. A systemic approach to care treatment and culture which fails to integrate these elements will see interpersonal connections characterised by uncertainty, withdrawal, isolation, and negativity. This is often the context from which attributions of the patient emerge.

Vignette 2: The Staff Member, Maria

Maria has worked as a Nursing Assistant for eight years. She is of dual heritage. Her father is White British and her Mother is from Zimbabwe, although they separated when she was young. She has spoken to colleagues about her father's excessive use of violence and his temper.

Maria likes her job although it can be stressful at times, she works on the women's ward mostly. She regularly takes extra shifts on different wards but feels anxious and uncomfortable. She experiences racism at work but does not complain because other people do not see it. Maria feels lucky that she has good friends on the women's ward and they look after her if she's had a bad day or if she is faced with a risky patient.

Maria went through a contentious divorce a few years ago. Her relationship was characterised by violence and coercive control. Her husband denied these allegations and many of her friends stopped contact with her. She has three children at school but receives only inconsistent financial support from their father. She worries about them when she is at work. Often her salary is spent before the end of the month, she may have a week or so without money and she relies on pay-day loans.

The Meaning-Making of Trauma

If we are to accept then that the trauma load comes from multiple sources, then we must also accept that there are many different meanings given to trauma-genic experiences. These are individual, collective, and systemic, and often across the levels of the organisation, poorly aligned. Consequently, the needs of a person who has experienced chronic trauma (perhaps survival and managing shame) is at odds with both staff perceptions of their task and the objectives of the organisation.

The objectives of secure care are centred around the recovery model. Commonly this can mean recovery to how someone was before they were sick or recovery from a defined illness. This often lacks meaning and therefore trauma-informed approaches remain fragile and perhaps out of reach. It is important to guard against linearity of thought (sickness or recovery model). A focus on the number of ACES as individual "ticks" will lead only to partial and perhaps off-centre interpretations of a person's experiences and functioning. This is a key component in the emergence of re-traumatising environments. In the absence of routine enquiry (Felitti, 2010) there are few mechanisms to share meaning-making and plan for the environment.

Like many patients, for Karen, the devastating chronic impact was not merely what happened to her, terrible as this was. Far more powerful was the psychological adaptations she had to make to survive in a hostile and withholding environment. Psychological chaos, borne from rejection, exclusion, threat, and malice coalesced in a self-concept characterised by shame, guilt, self-hatred, worthlessness, interspersed with threads of unbearable rage and anger. Emotionally Karen believes she was at fault, she is flawed and at times deserves maltreatment. Revisiting her experiences is to contemplate her reality, a person alone and shameful who is to be hidden from others.

Maria takes pride in her resilience in the face of adversity. She states that nothing gets her down because she has seen everything in life. She would complain about the racism, but it is useless because she believes she will be ostracised further, so works hard to fit in. She recalls that, at first, she did not like working with the women because they were "draining" but now likes working with them because she understands where they came from and nothing can affect her.

Understanding the meaning each makes of their experiences is fundamental to being trauma-informed.

Vignette 3: Working with Patients with Complex Trauma

Maria spends a lot of time supporting Karen on the ward. She can feel sorry for her having no family, and she feels sad that she has had her children removed. There are times when Karen is distressed and Maria "feels her heart sink" as she is put on her observations. Karen wants to talk about her distress, Maria thinks she should be over this by now and feels "stuck" with Karen's story.

Karen used to like Maria but finds her dismissing when Maria is under stress. Karen would like to be able to talk about her children; she worries that what happened to her will happen to them. Maria says that Karen should count herself lucky because her own children are "nothing but trouble and great expense", but she "loves them really". Karen can feel the rage in her stomach and chest. She wants to punch Maria. Instead, she cuts herself for being so inept.

Maria is frustrated with Karen. She says she's there for Karen to talk to and is annoyed with Karen's self-harm. Maria attempts to cover up her annoyance, but suspects it leaks out a little. She thinks it doesn't matter to Karen as Karen ignores her anyway. Maria returns to the staff office after observation and hands over that Karen is moody and has cut herself. Maria shows her annoyance to her colleagues who agree that Karen is "hard work when she is like that". Maria feels validated by her colleagues.

The Challenges to Emotional Containment

Left alone to consider trauma-related presentations, in non-trauma-informed environments, practitioners are likely to feel overwhelmed and may even become traumatised themselves. The phenomenon of secondary trauma is a genuine risk to the health and wellbeing of practitioners. The concept of secondary stress is well defined, established, and evidenced (Choi, 2011; Craig & Sprang, 2010). The evidence base reveals this vulnerability to secondary trauma responses in staff occurs across the spectrum of caring professions and is particularly pronounced in those organisations that work with trauma (Cohen & Collens, 2013).

The meaning of trauma is misaligned between Maria and Karen. Maria struggles to consider Karen outside of her own frame of reference. Indeed, any current life stressors Maria has only served to irritate her that Karen is given opportunity to "get better" but fails to do so even when she is in a place of safety. When Karen self-harms, Maria's sense of helplessness leads to her re-framing Karen's behaviour as attention-seeking and Karen is rejected by Maria.

In the care team, the discussion of the sense of helplessness could be a useful transaction – however they lose the context of this and view the event as Karen failing to respond to the care offered. Karen is blamed for poor responsiveness to treatment. Maria's understanding is confirmed.

Thus, inevitably the misalignment in the dyad extends to the whole clinical team who are unable to detect the different perspectives of the staff and patient. Systemically the care delivered by the service does not attend sensitively to Karen's trauma, and instead attends to the risk of her self-harm or disengagement in a way that renders Karen helpless (i.e., expectation of concordance, threat of seclusion if she is distressed): the staff feel stressed and helpless. The risk of re-traumatising Karen is elevated as the team move towards coercive methods or exclusion and isolation to manage the care objectives.

Thus, without reflection, the trajectory of sickness/problem behaviour is located solely in the patient. Without context or a space for all of the people involved in Karen's care to consider their own responses and where that might come from, the discussions about care focus on the need for restraint or seclusion, rather than a psychological understanding of Karen's experiences: control is perpetuated and the risk of re-traumatisation continues.

Safe Space to Reflect and Grow

This chapter has set out the importance of a socially aware and responsive organisation with strong and sustained investment in trauma-informed policy, practice, and procedures. At ward level there was a programme of trauma awareness training which incorporated a bio-psycho-social understanding of attachment, developmental trauma, and adverse childhood conditions. The training emphasised the role of reflection on transference and the impact of working with the traumatic material and resultant difficult relational dynamics that commonly occur. This became the foundation for consistent reappraisal in the work environment between the ward psychologist, ward-based staff, and the wider care team.

Prior to the introduction of a trauma-informed model of care, the supervision strategies for nursing staff were often based on management targets and performance indicators ahead of clinical issues. The recording of supervision was variable. Senior staff ensuring supervision occurred were provided with support to make their supervision trauma-informed. The framework for this was based on the "Four Rs". This holds key assumptions that people *realise* that trauma and stress exist and are likely to be experienced by everyone; that the people can *recognise* the signs and symptoms of stress and trauma; can *respond* in a timely trauma-informed or trauma sensitive way; and make efforts to know about and *resist* re-traumatisation (SAMHSA 2014). Supervisors and senior staff became comfortable with enquiring about supervisee's psychological well-being and developing psychologically safe clinical relationships that supported reflection.

An additional intervention to the ward was weekly trauma-informed reflective practice. This joint thinking space was facilitated by the ward psychologist. Creating a safe space to explore and validate staff experiences working with the traumatic material and difficult relational dynamics of the patients, staff became accustomed to reflecting on their own bodily responses and thought processes and behaviour that were elicited.

Vignette 4: Maria's Participation in Reflective Practice

Maria is scheduled into the reflective practice session each week. In general, she likes these sessions as she can learn a bit more about the patients and also at least when she is in the session she's not "on obs" and is grateful for the time away from ward-based tasks.

In the session, the discussion turns to supporting Karen. The team are asked to consider what they understand about Karen and how they experience her. Maria reports that she likes Karen but expects that Karen should be better behaved and then she would be easier to manage. Curiosity and openness are fostered in the group and Maria's notion is explored in tandem with a psychological understanding of Karen's developmental trauma and life experiences. Maria reframes this and believes that Karen's self-harm is "just behaviour" which is a common label for a non-thinking approach to dismiss distress.

The team is asked, if behaviour is communication, what might Karen be communicating? The team start to volunteer their reflections not only on Karen, but other patients they see self-harming. Maria thinks Karen is communicating stress. Other staff remember that Karen has felt invalidated and powerless in her relationships and begin to wonder if that was happening prior to the last episode of self-harm. Maria at first reflects her frustration that most women are powerless in their relationship with their parents or men but just get on with it. She reflects that she gets on with it when she feels invalidated because of her heritage. As she makes this reflection, she feels a burning sensation in her face and stomach. Maria becomes aware that she has betrayed her pain to her colleagues – the very people who invalidate her. She feels vulnerable. The psychologist picks up on this instantly and offers Maria validation and support. The colleagues in the room also acknowledge their lack of awareness of this. It is agreed that this issue will be followed up safely in another forum.

Maria reflects that Karen has had very few experiences of being in control or having a say. Maria says "it must have been awful to have her children removed. She must be scared about what is happening to them too". Maria identifies feeling a "heart sink" when she is on Karen's observations. She suspects that this is linked to not being able to help Karen; Maria says she is frustrated and feels powerless. The team begin to reflect on the potential fear, powerlessness, and possible anger in Karen, knowing that she will likely be silenced by invalidating reactions from others, including eye rolling, sighing, or abruptly exiting the care dynamic. In considering this, the team reflect on how they can collaborate to develop a validating and soothing relationship with Karen where she is empowered to voice her concerns, Maria starts to have thoughts of hope for her working relationship with Karen.

Reflective spaces, whether they are in a group or a more intimate forum like one-to-one supervision, are important barometers for the impact of the care dynamics, monitoring risk, and supporting the health of the individuals in the team. There are inherent difficulties in the practitioner–patient relationship with power and control; however, cultivating and nurturing the team is about an authentic understanding of all participants and is critical to responding to trauma (wherever that trauma lies, in staff or patients) and preventing re-traumatisation. This should not stand alone, or be part of a project around a patient, it is a long-term investment in a trauma-informed model of care that should build consistency and have a regular reappraisal of the team's wellbeing.

Vignette 5: Safe, Collaborative, Empowering Practice

It is the week of Karen's eldest child's 10th birthday. She ruminates upon the birth and the precious time she had with her. She believes she can smell her daughter and feels an overwhelming surge of grief coupled with anger and distress. The loss feels like it happened yesterday. Karen cannot distract herself from the fear that her daughter is being harmed. Her urge to self-harm is strong and she loses her appetite. She wants to die.

At the initial assessment, alongside her developmental history, the care team sought to understand when significant anniversaries or trigger factors/emotional detonators were likely to occur. They discuss the upcoming birthday and predicted the impact upon Karen and prepare to provide extra support. The team prepare with a reflective space taking a compassionate focus on Karen's experiences. They make plans to draw up advanced decisions and a detailed care plan designed by Karen to help her through the week. Maria is looking forward to supporting Karen and hopes she will engage with the preparation.

Maria takes time to consider Karen's experiences and believes that they are developing a psychologically safe and trustworthy relationship. Karen appears to respond warmly nowadays, and she has learned from Karen that when she does not feel safe, she will withdraw. Maria has developed confidence in the way she speaks to Karen when she is like that.

Karen does not like to share her private thoughts; she has been invalidated too often. She worries that people will think she is a bad person for losing custody of her children, although she reflects that Maria seems more tuned in to what it is like to be a mother. Karen thinks she might be able to let Maria help her with the care plan once she has begun to set out what she might need to get through the next few days. Maria offers Karen some choices in terms of company, activities, therapeutic tasks that will offer comfort. Maria acknowledges that the week will be difficult for Karen, and Karen believes that she will be able to be upset without being told off or intensely scrutinised and gets through the week safely without feeling abject loneliness.

Summary

The vignettes have their limitations. However, they are designed to illuminate some of the intricacies that exist in trying to develop trauma-informed practices in systems that hold onto historical trauma, and in services that are ill equipped to consider multiplicity of trauma in staff and patients, particularly where the focus on outcomes is based on vague recovery models.

The Department of Health (in press) defines trauma-informed care as

> a whole system approach that adopts a lifespan perspective informed by the person's history and actively seeks to understand the impact of previous trauma and adversity on current functioning, emotional experiences and relationships. The model of care is structured to identify and eliminate process and practices which inadvertently recreate or reinforce the traumatic experiences of service uses and staff.

This chapter has reflected upon the implications of the multiplicity of trauma in navigating the implementation of a trauma-informed model of care. Service developers should consider the context of the lives of both staff and patients in the communities they come from and return to. It is incumbent upon them to ensure that there are adequate resources with time to think, and that safe reflective space and trauma sensitive supervision are in place. These are fundamental expectations ahead of services delivering trauma-informed systemic interventions or direct trauma interventions/therapy.

Note

1 The response to the whistleblowing of Winterbourne view set off a process of transforming care for people with Learning Disability that was a fundamental shift for practitioners and legislators (Department of Health, 2012).

References

Bloom, S.L. (2010). Trauma-organized systems and parallel process. In N. Tehrani (Ed.), *Managing trauma in the workplace: Supporting workers and organizations* (pp. 139–153). Routledge.

Bloom, S.L. (2012). Trauma organised systems. In C.R. Figley (Ed.), *Encyclopaedia of trauma. An interdisciplinary guide* (pp741–743). Sage Publications Inc.

Carlisle, J., & McGuire, F. (2020). *Systemic factors and trauma-informed care: Cultural change and managing trauma.* Presentation at Trauma-Informed Care in Forensic Settings Conference, 30–31 January 2020.

Choi, G.Y. (2011). Organizational impacts on the secondary traumatic stress of social workers assisting family violence or sexual assault survivors. *Administration in Social Work. 35*(3), 225–242. doi:10.1080/03643107.2011.575333

Cohen, K., & Collens, P. (2013). The impact of trauma work on trauma workers: A metasynthesis on vicarious trauma and vicarious posttraumatic growth. *Psychological Trauma: Theory, Research, Practice, and Policy, 5*(6), 570–580. doi:10.1037/a0030388

Craig, C.D., & Sprang, G. (2010). Compassion satisfaction, compassion fatigue, and burnout in a national sample of trauma treatment therapists. *Anxiety Stress Coping, 23*(3), 319–339. doi:10.1080/10615800903085818

Department of Health. (2010). *See think act.* Department of Health.

Department of Health. (2012). *Transforming care: A national response to Winterbourne View Hospital.* Department of Health.

Department of Health. (In press). *Reducing the psychological emotional impact on staff in high secure services.* Department of Health.

Facer-Irwin, E., Karatzias, T., Bird, A., & Blackwood, N. (2021). PTSD and complex PTSD in sentenced male prisoners in the UK: Prevalence, trauma antecedents, and psychiatric comorbidities. *Psychological Medicine*, online first view. doi:10.1017/S0033291720004936

Felitti, V. (2010). *The relationship of adverse childhood experiences to adult health status.* Retrieved from www.youtube.com/watch?v=Me07G3Erbw8

Karatzias, T., Shevlin, M., Pitcairn, J., & Thomson, L. (2019). Childhood adversity and psychosis in detained inpatients from medium to high secured units: Results from the Scottish census survey. *Child Abuse and Neglect, 96*, 104094. doi:10.1016/j.chiabu.2019.104094

NHS Strategy Unit. (2020). *Estimating the impacts of COVID-19 on mental health services in England.* Retrieved from www.strategyunitwm.nhs.uk/sites/default/files/2020-11/Modelling%20covid-19%20%20MH%20services%20in%20England_20201109_v2.pdf

SAMHSA. (2014). *SAMHSA's concept of trauma and guidance for a trauma-informed approach.* Retrieved from https://ncsacw.samhsa.gov/userfiles/files/SAMHSA_Trauma.pdf

Seedhouse, D. (1994). *Ethics. The heart of healthcare* (2nd Edition). Wiley. UK Parliament. (2021). *Domestic abuse and Covid-19: A year into the pandemic.* Retrieved from https://commonslibrary.parliament.uk/domestic-abuse-and-covid-19-a-year-into-the-pandemic/

21
THE IMPACT ON STAFF OF TRAUMA-INFORMED WORK IN FORENSIC SETTINGS

Michelle Smith

Introduction

When considering a trauma-informed approach to working within forensic ser-vices, focus generally centres on how we can shape services for the benefit of our service users. This is undoubtedly of paramount importance, but what is often less considered is the notion that to do this effectively we need to ensure that support systems for staff and organisations operate along the same trauma-informed principles. There has been a wealth of knowledge developed over the last few decades regarding trauma and its overarching impact. Notable contributions have been made from neuroscience, which have helped us to understand the intricacies of the impact of trauma on developing brain processes and the long-lasting impact it can have across generations. An understanding of the triune brain system and associated bottom-up approach to trauma described by van der Kolk (2014) helps us understand that addressing embodied impacts of trauma is crucial alongside the effects on disrupted emotional processing and cognitive connections. It is suggested that the process is no different when considering the impact of trauma in forensic staff populations.

This chapter will focus specifically on the impact of trauma-informed working on staff within the critical occupation of forensic services. It will firstly aim to review what we mean by the terms *critical occupation* and *trauma*, and explore the specific traumatic impacts reported when working within forensic services, summarising the literature in this area. It will seek to describe and clarify the variety of terms used within the literature to describe traumatic impacts within critical occupations (sec-ondary traumatic stress, compassion fatigue, vicarious trauma, burnout). It will con-clude by suggesting an approach to addressing traumatic impact which is framed

DOI: 10.4324/9781003120766-27

by well-evidenced trauma-informed stages – creating safety, facilitating emotional processing, and maintaining cognitive connections. This is based on the principle that we need to model as practitioners what we intend to offer to our service users. It will include an integration of applied models of boundary management, resilience, and psychological formulation as well as offering suggestions for a trauma-informed service model. It will also describe an approach to the management of human public services, which attends to integral trauma processes at individual, organisational, and public policy levels.

Critical Occupations

Critical occupations have traditionally been defined as those involving the performance of a critical role in the protection of society, combined with an exposure to incidents that may have a critical impact on physical and mental health (Parrish Meadows, Shreffler, & Mullins-Sweatt, 2011; Paton & Violanti, 1996). This has often included roles within the military and emergency services such as police, fire and rescue, emergency medical services. While these roles clearly include aspects of public protection and exposure to trauma, wider definitions include a range of other public service roles such as prison officers, healthcare staff, and social workers. It should be noted, however, that decisions about inclusion as a critical occupation are often guided by historical and social contexts. What may be considered a vital occupation at one point in time with in a given social context may not be included at later time points. The Covid-19 pandemic has demonstrated this very clearly, with critical occupations being extensively widened to include a greater range of key public services – education, food production, sale and distribution, transport and border staff and utilities, communication and financial services (Department of Education, 2021).

The definition of critical occupations currently extends to include work roles within the forensic arena such as prison officers, probation officers, forensic psychologists, forensic psychiatrists, and mental health professionals (Clarke, 2004). Forensic professionals have a core focus on public protection in their role of forensic risk assessment and in the discharge of this, often face constant and relentless exposure to events that can cause psychological and physical health-related issues and burnout (Clarke, 2004; Paton & Violanti, 1996). Examples include direct involvement with individuals who either demonstrate verbal and physical violence towards others, or to themselves; exposure to the use of illicit substances or contaminated equipment for such misuse; exposure to traumatic material from the life history of individuals within the criminal justice system; working in secure and often intimidating and dangerous environments; managing pressures on reduced staff to client ratios and the resulting impact on risk and safety; fear of the risk and magnitude of making mistakes and associated stress levels. This inexhaustive list of direct and indirect events can have a detrimental effect not only for individuals but also for the development and maintenance of services (Elliot & Daley, 2013; Wright, Powell, & Ridge, 2006).

Trauma

Definitions of trauma have expanded over years with the developing insight gained from a wealth of research in the area. Times of adversity and challenge in life are commonplace and can often cause temporary distress for individuals. When we refer to trauma in this chapter, we define this as a response to "an inescapably stressful event" (van der Kolk & Fisler, 1995; p.505) or series of events, which overwhelms individual or systemic mechanisms of care which usually offer "a sense of control, connection, and meaning" (Herman, 1992; p.33). Research has demonstrated the cumulative and long-term impact of developmental trauma in terms of childhood adversity (Felitti et al., 1998) and adverse childhood experiences (ACEs) are highly prevalent within the population of individuals who commit offences (Bellis et al., 2015; Farrington, 2003; Levenson, Willis, & Prescott, 2016; Scottish Government, 2018). It is also clear that trauma-informed principles have been integrated across a range of health, social, and educational services to date and are now starting to be considered across forensic services (British Psychological Society, 2019). This is creating a paradigm shift which more visibly acknowledges the difficult dialectic between accepted functions of forensic roles – risk management and compassionate care. Traditionally, forensic professionals have considered trauma in terms of its integration within psychological formulations of service users, to better understand their offending behaviour as a response to their traumatic experiences. Johnstone and Boyle et al. (2018) widened this idea with the introduction of the Power Threat Meaning Framework and enabled it to be applied to professionals and service users alike. The framework was originally developed to challenge the notion that emotional distress and mental health problems are illnesses to be treated within a purely medical model. However, the principles are specifically noted as applicable to those within the criminal justice system. The framework considers that negative power experiences occur for *everyone*, on an individual and systemic level, and can create both threats and interpretations which result in a range of behaviours, some of which can be viewed as survival strategies or threat responses. This allows us to consider that trauma experience and emotional distress are not exclusive to individuals accessing forensic services. Indeed, if we consider wider, collective definitions of trauma that include racial trauma, poverty, and social deprivation that create pervasive, lifelong cross-generational impact, how can we possibly conclude that staff working in forensic services are immune to this in a different way to that of our clients? These are undoubtedly universal experiences. Following this argument, it is entirely possible that the undeniable tensions experienced by forensic staff in the constant juggling of responsibilities in their role may be associated with the deleterious impacts noted in the literature.

Trauma Impact in Forensic Professionals

Terminology

The research literature notes a range of impacts on staff of working in forensic services, and different concepts have been proposed over the last few decades to describe these. One of the notable issues with this impact literature is the interchangeable use of terms across studies such as *secondary traumatic stress, compassion fatigue, vicarious trauma*, and *burnout*. These describe related yet distinctly different impacts, leading to difficulties in achieving an overarching understanding and creating confusion. It is important to create clear and distinct understandings of the definitions of these terms before looking at what studies can tell us about how forensic staff are affected by their work.

Secondary Traumatic Stress (STS) and Compassion Fatigue (CF). Originally introduced by Figley (1995), these terms have been used interchangeably in the literature and reshaped over time to describe professionals' sense of being psychologically overwhelmed by their observations of trauma, the depth of suffering experienced in working with this, and their perceived need to support individuals experiencing trauma (Barros et al., 2020). It is suggested that these terms are not only applicable to professionals but can include others such as carers, lay people, and loved ones (Branson, 2019). Both STS and CF are considered to result in psychological distress including avoidance, unwanted mental images, and over sensitivity to trauma-related stimuli, and can be akin to PTSD presentations (Devilly et al., 2009). It is suggested that STS and CF are acute phenomena and that they may result from shorter term or even a single exposure to trauma (Branson, 2019).

Vicarious Trauma (VT). Vicarious trauma describes the longer-term impact on the cognitive schemas, beliefs, expectations, and assumptions of the self and others that are internalised by professionals working with traumatised individuals. It has been described as a transfer of traumatic stress from survivor to therapist following the process of bearing witness to their stories (Hernandez, Ganggsei, & Engstrom, 2007) and has a distinct cumulative process (Pearlman & Saakvitne, 1995). It was introduced by McCann and Pearlman (1990) as part of their constructivist self-development theory, which sees the effects on therapists as an interaction between the characteristics of the situation, the individual's psychological needs and cognitive schemas. Branson (2019) reports that it presents as similar to the symptoms of primary trauma and has impacts across four areas: intrusive imagery, arousal, avoidance behaviours, and negative cognitions. It has been related to ethical professional practice impacts in terms of decision-making, emotional containment, and managing professional boundaries (Branson, 2019).

Burnout. Burnout is a much wider concept which applies across a range of occupations and results from the demands of the work role with limited access to supportive resources (Maslach, Schaufeli, & Leiter, 2001). In forensic services we can understand this more clearly as the long-term psychological strain of undertaking supportive work with individuals or groups with complex problems. Maslach and Leiter (2016) describe this as a prolonged response to chronic interpersonal stressors on the job and note the factors which distinguish burnout as (a) overwhelming exhaustion; (b) feelings of cynicism and detachment from the job; and (c) a sense of ineffectiveness and lack of accomplishment. Branson (2019) notes the similarity between burnout and VT, due to them both developing through a process of accumulation of experiences. There has been a greater focus in occupational psychology literature on the dialectic of *burnout* and the more positive conceptualisation of *engagement* using conceptual models of job stress such as the *Areas of Work Life model*. This focuses on the six areas of workload – workload, control, reward, community, fairness, and values – to understand the adaptations required to increase engagement and reduce burnout (Leiter & Maslach, 1999; Leiter & Shaughnessy, 2006).

Impact Studies

The impact of working with individuals across forensic settings, both secure and in the community, is widely accepted as complex across the forensic practitioner community and this is reflected in the literature. However, there is a paucity of empirical studies specifically focused on forensic professionals when compared to those of other critical occupations (Gil-Monte, Figueiredo-Ferraz, & Valdez-Bonilla, 2013).

Studies of non-forensic critical occupations such as mental health workers indicate that exposure to traumatic material associated with work-related stressors can result in negative outcomes in terms of psychological distress but the literature is divided in terms of the specific prevalence and weight of specific contributions to resulting STS, CF, VT, and burnout (Devilly, Wright, & Varker, 2009; Lee, Lim, Yang, & Lee, 2011; van Minnen & Keijsers, 2000).

Critical occupation studies with emergency service personnel such as fire and ambulance workers, some of which also include forensic staff such as police personnel, highlight increased levels of psychological strain in these roles. Organisational and traumatic stress reactions have been found to predict levels of strain similarly for police and fire personnel, but overall, organisational stressors are noted to offer a better predictor of job satisfaction than trauma symptomology for fire, ambulance, and police personnel (Brough, 2004). Furthermore, it has been found that longer serving police officers working with victims of sexual trauma showed greater levels of CF, STS, and burnout, indicating that greater exposure to traumatic material increases negative impact (Turgoose et al., 2017).

Staff working within community forensic services in forensic interviewing or support roles (child exploitation, child abuse, or sexual assault centres) have been found to display increased levels of STS, VT, and burnout. Impacts are felt within direct contact, outside of the professional role and also personally (Burns et al., 2008; Middleton et al., 2021), with experiences of intrusive images and thoughts outside of work, protective feelings towards children, dissociation, and an inability to discuss traumatic material (Burns et al., 2008). Organisational factors are reported to contribute to these experiences with job support, funding pressures, and increased caseloads being crucial factors (Starcher & Stolzenberg, 2000). A combination of personal and organisational factors has been cited to ameliorate these impacts, including supervision, training, peer support, and shadowing (Horvath et al., 2020), as well as humour and a combination of organisational, psychological, and social support (Burns et al., 2008).

Studies involving forensic staff in mainly secure environments include a range of professional groups such as prison officers, forensic psychiatrists, forensic psychologists, nurses, mental health workers, and therapists. Overall, they suggest a clear risk of increased levels of STS, CF, VT, and burnout, at mild, moderate, and severe levels, depending on the focus of study and methods used. However, their presence in staff is dependent upon a complex interplay including individual characteristics, organisational factors, and personal events outside the work context (Clarke, 2013). A range of contributing factors have been identified to explain the variation in findings in the literature. These include amount of exposure to traumatic events (van der Ploeg, Dorresteijn, & Kleber, 2003); gender and length of experience (Gould et al., 2013); levels of demand, control, and support within role (Dollard & Winefield, 1998); levels of role conflict and negative experience of work (Gallavan & Newman, 2013); levels of compassion satisfaction (Munger, Savage, & Panosky, 2015); levels of avoidance, intrusion, and hyperarousal in individuals (Cramer et al., 2020; Newman, Eason, & Kinghorn, 2019); personal trauma (Adams & Riggs, 2008; Knight, 2010); workplace stress other than specific traumatic exposure (Pirelli, Formon, & Maloney, 2020); maladaptive coping strategies (Barros et al., 2020); and difficulties in self-identifying issues and managing these (Johnson et al., 2011). Comparison studies across forensic and non-forensic critical occupations have demonstrated similar findings with a clear presence of STS, CF, VT, and burnout across both in comparison to the general population (Carleton et al., 2019), significant impact on job satisfaction and personal life (Bourke & Craun, 2014), and reductions in role performance dependent upon individual, organisational, and social factors (Bakker & Heuven, 2006).

It is clear that with such a mixed and complex picture regarding the impact of working in forensic roles, more research is required (Bradford & de Amorim Levin, 2020). Existing literature highlights the impact of forensic role conflict between risk management and compassionate care. Holding the idea of an individual as both a victim of and perpetrator of trauma can often create cognitive dissonance for the practitioner which is difficult to tolerate for prolonged periods of time. The impact on professional competence has been highlighted (Johnson et al., 2011), including the maintenance of interpersonal boundaries (Rocchio, 2020), varying interpersonal styles (Lambert, Chu, & Turner, 2019), and the importance of personally managing self-awareness, reactions to shame, and fear over rejection from others (Johnson et al., 2011). However, it is not an insurmountable task and despite the wealth of evidence for negative impact, there is growing evidence for positive impact. Cramer et al. (2020) identified the good health of mental health staff in their recent study of a forensic psychiatric setting and Gould et al. (2013) reported use of mostly adaptive coping skills in correctional officers despite the presence of burnout within this population. Brovko and Foote (2011) demonstrated a potential resiliency effect in their reported study of forensic professionals, and Silveira & Boyer (2015) has noted the presence of increased hope and optimism when working with victims of interpersonal trauma. The concept of vicarious resilience may help to explain this. Engstrom, Hernandez, & Gangsei (2008) introduced the idea that there could be positive experiences which arise from work undertaken with survivors of trauma. Hernandez, Ganggsei, and Engstrom (2007) identified it as a natural process which has not been previously defined or described and which requires further exploration. They propose that, with the correct environment, vicarious resilience offers the chance for staff to learn together with their clients and strengthen the conscious attention to positive effects, creating transformation in a strengths based manner (Hernandez, Ganggsei, & Engstrom, 2007).

Clearly there is an argument for increased focus on the impact for staff in forensic environments. Across different forensic settings, staff are holding an important critical role, within very challenging environments, with an often traumatised service user population. They are also carrying a range of personal, professional, organisational traumatic experiences themselves and can experience role conflict within their work. Research evidence suggests that their ongoing attempts to manage such role conflict and balance the complex risk versus treatment dialectic in an ethical/profession-ally boundaried way can have a profound impact on decision-making and ethical judgement and yet many have significant resources which can aid their resilience and lead to positive job satisfaction and outcomes.

Trauma-Informed Service Development

With clear traumatic impact for staff in forensic settings evidenced over time and the need to support them to manage this impact positively, an obvious question arises: why has this not been wholeheartedly integrated across forensic services before now? One contributing factor could be the parallel process dynamic which is referred to in the Sanctuary Model (described in detail below). This references the collective transference and counter-transference process of emotions, cognitions, and behaviours that can occur between service users and professionals and shape the way organisations operate at the most senior levels in terms of decision-making. Forensic systems are often set up to take a blame-focused approach to service users and staff who struggle with boundary management and resilience, and this seems to be founded on a long-standing culture where provoking shame is embraced over the safe, supported expression of vulnerability, within a holistic understanding of the person in the system. Recent developments in shame literature generally have indicated that shame responses which incorporate blaming tend to be less effective than clear boundary setting and accountability (Brown, 2010), and limit compas-sionate leadership of services (Brown, 2018). Another factor could relate to the fact that the forensic psychology discipline and wider correctional policy has been led by a paradigm that views forensic professionals as collective experts in terms of risk assessment and treatment, dominated by the Risk Need Responsivity model (Bonta & Andrews, 2016). Within this paradigm, "experts" are presumed not to have the same vulnerabilities as service users and thereby the system operates on a version of power that is defined by "power over" rather than "power with" or "power to". With the advent of wider frameworks integrating health and well-being perspectives such as the Good Lives Model (Ward, 2002), where power is collaboratively shared with service users and their experiences, this is being challenged in terms of equality and diversity. It seems clear then, that this shield of expertise is an illusion and protects individuals, organisations, and policy makers from truly integrating the vulnerability of physical, emotional, and cognitive impacts of exposure to trauma in forensic settings. The danger is that this is not a tenable long-term strategy and transform-ation is required.

The following approach, I propose, draws together suggestions for individual staff across three integral areas of trauma processing by using established applied models evidenced within forensic services. It addresses physical and emotional safety (creating safety bubbles) through use of an applied boundary management model; provides a tool for understanding and managing the emotional impact of forensic work (emotional processing) using a well-evidenced resilience model; and facilitates cognitive processes and risk-related decision-making (cognitive connection) using a trauma-informed formulation framework. All of these can be facilitated easily through existing established supervision networks and training systems. It additionally considers two approaches for the systemic development of organisations and public policy at both a micro and macro level: the *Sanctuary Model* (Bloom & Farragher, 2010; Bloom, 2013; Bloom & Farragher, 2013) and the *Human Learning Systems Approach* (Lowe et al., 2021). While a comprehensive evaluation of each approach is beyond the scope of the current chapter, an overview and introduction of each will be offered with recommendations for further reading.

Professional Boundaries (Creating Safety Bubbles)

Professional boundaries can be described as the limit or edge of appropriate practice (Gutheil & Gabbard, 1998). They can be considered across three main areas, often referred to as the *security triad* in forensic settings. They include environmental or physical boundaries (e.g., walls or gates in a prison), procedural boundaries (e.g., policies and operational processes), and relational boundaries (e.g., interpersonal relationships between staff and service users). The complex interplay between physical, procedural, and relational boundaries in balancing the dialectic between risk management and compassionate care in forensic settings is clear in the literature and can create risks and significant consequences (Davies & Nagi, 2017). These can include boundary inattention (forgetting forensic context), boundary crossings (minor lapses in judgement), and boundary violations (breach of policy/code of conduct) (Love & Herber, 2001). Applied models of boundary management such as the *Boundary Seesaw Model* (Hamilton, 2010) have been developed as a way to understand and manage such boundary risks and could usefully be incorporated as part of trauma-informed service design and delivery.

The Boundary Seesaw Model (Hamilton, 2010) was developed by drawing from cognitive analytic therapy (CAT; Ryle & Kerr, 2002), and dialectical behaviour therapy (DBT; Linehan, 1993) and the continuum of professional behaviour related to regulatory codes to understand observed boundary behaviour demonstrated by staff in a service for those diagnosed with severe personality disorder. The concept of a seesaw is used to describe a continuum of care and control with over-involved behaviours (*Pacifier* role) or under-involved behaviours (*Security Guard* role) at either end of the seesaw and care with explicit limits (*Negotiator* role) in the middle. Hamilton (2010) suggests that staff are likely to move along the seesaw with their professional interactions through safe, risky, and danger zones at some point. However, the key to effective boundary management is knowing the non-negotiable limits at the ends of the seesaw and being aware of these smaller boundary shifts so that they do not progress to larger boundary crossings or clear boundary violations, and balance is maintained at the pivot point of the seesaw. There is a recognition within this model that forensic staff are, because of the nature of their role and the population with which they work, operating more often at the edge of these boundary zones. It is important that boundary shifts and crossings are well attended to, documented, and reflected upon within services and, as Davies and Nagi (2017) highlight, supervision is vital to this collaborative observation process. Hamilton (2010) describes equally valuable systemic processes which, if implemented, can help to manage boundaries effectively at an organisational level. These include the development and communication of clear organisational values and procedures related to boundaries; an ethos of shared responsibility for boundary management; staff training, processes for boundary management reviews; monitored meaningful activity schedules for staff-service user interactions.

Resilience (Emotional Processing)

Definitions of resilience in the academic literature focus around two core themes; *recovery*, or the ability to bounce back after adverse experiences and *sustainability*, or a continued journey of recovery and growth (Reich, Zautra, & Hall, 2010). Conceptual models of resilience appear to take one of three different approaches: *compensatory*, *protective*, and *challenge*. Compensatory approaches view resilience as having a neutralising effect on the exposure to risk, where risk and compensatory factors equally contribute to the eventual outcome. Protective approaches see risk and protective factors interacting together to mediate negative outcome and moderating the exposure to risk. The challenge approach considers that the presence of risk factors (as long as they are not too extreme) can help with adaptation (a notion similar to the idea of herd immunity). Concepts of *survival*, *recovery*, and *thriving* are interlinked when considering resilience and also need to be examined. Survival relates to the idea that a person or system will continue to function; recovery indicates a return to baseline operation while thriving indicates the potential for transformation and cognitive shift with a stronger sense of self (O'Leary, 1998). Survival, recovery, and thriving concepts may indicate the stage of resilience response for an individual or organisation (Ledesma, 2014).

One process-based model of resilience, taking a protective approach, which has been developed specifically from research with intervention facilitators in secure prison settings, is the *Model of Dynamic Adaptation* (MDA; Clarke, 2004). The MDA highlights a range of factors which interact to result in either positive or negative psychological outcomes. These include factors relating to the person, the critical occupation, and additional dynamic factors. Person-specific *static* factors tend to be fixed or change in expected ways such as age, whereas person-specific *stable* factors demonstrate limited change or do so over time, experience or with support, such as coping style or emotional sensitivity. *Critical occupation* factors focus on organisational components such as the physical environment, risk of exposure to critical incidents, policies and procedures, and organisational support. *Dynamic* factors are unpredictable and can quickly change – the events that sometimes occur without any control such as a bereavement or a change in team members. Clarke (2013) suggests that this model of resilience can be applied functionally to any critical occupation and encourages ongoing research to explore the contributing value of all the differing factors – some may be unique to a particular setting while others may be common across critical occupations. It is suggested here, that if applied systematically within forensic services, alongside the boundary seesaw model, this could offer support for emotional processing of traumatic events at an individual and organisational level.

Power Threat Meaning Framework (Cognitive Processing and Decision-Making)

Psychological formulation is a tool for practitioners to work together with service users to make sense of the distress and difficulties with which they present (Johnstone & Dallos, 2013). While previous chapters have applied aspects of this in detail, the current chapter will provide a brief overview and offer reasoning for its inclusion as part of the trauma-informed approach for forensic professionals and organisations. The publication of the Power Threat Meaning Framework (PTMF) as an approach to formulation has offered a meta framework drawing from a variety of theoretical approaches and evidence to integrate more a social and contextual lens to the understanding of psychological distress than has previously been available (Johnstone & Boyle et al., 2018). It approaches formulation by asking a series of questions related to exploring the following areas:

- Power: What has happened to you? This includes power experiences across many areas – biological/embodied, interpersonal, coercive, legal, economic, social/cultural, ideological.
- Threat: How did it affect you? This includes core threats, needs, and power within relationships, within the body, emotional, economic, social/community, environmental, across knowledge, and meaning construction and within the development or maintenance of identity.
- Meaning: What sense did you make of it?
- Threat Response: What did you have to do to survive?
- Power Resources: What are your strengths?

This is designed to facilitate a collaborative and empowering overarching formulation by asking "What is your story?". The benefits of integrating the PTMF within trauma-informed forensic service development alongside the Boundary Seesaw Model and Model of Dynamic Adaptation is that it has application to service users, individual practitioners, teams, services, organisations, and public services at the widest strategic level. The model's theoretical basis and philosophical approach takes a radically different view, to traditional medical models, of how our current society and culture understands distress. If formulation is undertaken at each level using this framework, it may allow for more collective responsibility for transformational change at the cognitive processing level and works towards shifting culture change towards compassionate risk management within forensic settings.

The Sanctuary Model

The Sanctuary Model provides a scaffolded structure to aid the development of trauma-informed organisations which provide safe moral climates (Bloom & Farragher, 2010). It recognises that everyone has vulnerability to trauma, includes system-wide interventions for adversity and stress across all levels of an organisation, and provides ways to shape services in a more trauma-informed way (Bloom, 2013; Bloom & Farragher, 2013). It incorporates clear understandings regarding the significant effects of trauma exposure on individuals and systemically to organisations that become traumatically overwhelmed. Bloom (2010) posits that there is a parallel process dynamic which, due to the significant inter-relationship of individuals, groups, and organisations, means they develop similar emotional, cognitive, and behavioural ways of operating. In forensic services, the complex interplay between service users managing their traumatic experiences through the use of violence to others and/or self, and the inherent pressures on staff holding both risk management and care, while already balancing their own traumatic lived experience, mean that trauma responses bounce backwards and forwards between them. Place this within a wider system which is operating itself within an environment loaded with social and economic strain and the trauma responding becomes more complex. The Sanctuary Model suggests that these parallel processes must be addressed fully if organisations are to remain healthy and effective in their delivery of trauma-informed services to those who access them. It recognises the process of traumatisation and re-traumatisation especially when services have more authoritarian approaches and indicates the moral injury inherent in this. It suggests that if the correct moral climate can be created, then a parallel process of recovery can be achieved for all.

The model is founded on what is referred to as the four pillars. The first of these is *theory* which refers to the extensive empirical and theoretical evidence which underpins the model. Its theoretical basis is drawn from trauma theory, but also integrates business theory, systems theory, and empirical work from the development of UK Therapeutic Communities. The second pillar refers to the *Sanctuary commitments* which are akin to a moral compass which guides the operation of decision-making and problem solving. All members of a community adopting the Sanctuary Model adopt these values and they shape the operational guidance of norms in the culture which is created. The third pillar refers to a shared language which is adopted to refer to four key domains of recovery: Safety, Emotions, Loss, and Future. The final pillar refers to the Sanctuary toolkit which is a range of practical tools and skills designed to help the community to build a more effective practice of the Sanctuary commitments and to create community connection and potential for new behavioural habits.

If forensic settings wish to introduce changes to existing systems and services in line with a more trauma-informed approach, the Sanctuary Model offers a clear, robust, well evidenced and tightly structured template. Its value structure is in line with all previous components (Boundary Seesaw Model, Model of Dynamic Adaptation, Power Threat Meaning Framework) in that it stresses collaborative, shared responsibility with a view of working in an empowered manner with individual service users, staff, and with the organisational culture.

Future Directions

Working within forensic settings offers both challenges and opportunities and it is clear from the impact literature and the experiential knowledge of practitioners that staff and organisational well-being depend upon culture, climate, and the development of individual strengths. There is a building evidence base over time for the significant negative effect for staff of working in such challenging environments but also much potential for working with this in a positive, strengths-based manner. It has been suggested that a public health framework would be the most useful approach to take. Molnar et al. (2017) has outlined four stages to undertake this:

1. Define the problem and measure its scope
2. Identify the risk and protective factors for negative outcomes
3. Develop interventions and policies
4. Monitor and evaluate interventions and policies over time

Molnar et al. (2017) offers this caveat:"Without a concerted response from researchers, policymakers, and organization leaders, these professional groups are left vulnerable to the shared burden of trauma, accrued from chronic or acute hardship, known as VT or STS" (p.138).

The development of clearer trauma-informed models of working with forensic clients and supporting staff and organisations in the process have been outlined as a suggested way forward within this chapter. There needs to be a radical shift in systemic culture at the macro, public management level in order to integrate trauma-focused perspectives and processes. Human Learning Systems (Lowe et al., 2021) is a relational, systems-focused way of addressing the complexity of public services and offers the potential for such transformation.

Many forensic service users have also accessed a range of other human public services during the process of living with and processing aspects of their experienced trauma, for example social services, NHS, voluntary and charitable organisations. The Human Learning Systems approach includes all of these within its scope and defines public service activity as all those purposeful activities that support human freedom and flourishing (Lowe et al., 2021). In this way the task of human public service management becomes more aligned to previously mentioned notions of "power to" and "power with", which are clearly more trauma-informed than traditional approaches. It takes the position that New Public Management (NPM), an approach implemented in the 1980s with a focus on markets, managers, and metrics (referred to as the 3Ms), fundamentally does not fit with the operation of public service and can be dehumanising. It has a theoretical basis in complexity theory and offers a paradigm shift to the way public services are managed at the macro level, based on continuous learning and adaptation with a shared responsibility for the health of the system which is developed. It posits that three core shifts are required to achieve this:

- Motivation – staff need help and support within their practice rather than incentivisation and targets.
- Learning and adaptation – learning is the mechanism for improved function, adaptation, and improvement in a system.
- System health – this focuses on the quality of relationships since service users interact with the whole system not just individuals within it.

It offers opportunities to think about how we strategically develop forensic services at a wider system level including public policy structures which, despite attempts at integration, often remain very divided. It could also offer a shared opportunity for learning, experimentation, responsibility and accountability to the transformation of public sector management which could bring together the variety of services across health and social care, criminal justice, education and employment in a meaningful way for the benefit of the service user.

Further Reading

Further information on the Sanctuary Model is detailed in the following three texts for those looking to implement structured trauma-informed approaches in forensic services:

Bloom, S.L. (2013). *Creating sanctuary: Toward the evolution of sane societies* (2nd ed.). Routledge.

Bloom, S.L., & Farragher, B. (2010). *Destroying sanctuary: The crisis in human service delivery systems.* Oxford University Press.

Bloom, S.L., & Farragher, B. (2013) *Restoring sanctuary: A new operating system for trauma-informed systems of care.* Oxford University Press.

References

Adams, S.A., & Riggs, S.A. (2008). An exploratory study of vicarious trauma among therapist trainees. *Training and Education in Professional Psychology, 2*(1), 26–34. https://doi.org/10.1037/1931-3918.2.1.26

Bakker, A.B., & Heuven, E. (2006). Emotional dissonance, burnout, and in-role performance among nurses and police officers. *International Journal of Stress Management, 13*(4), 423–440. doi:10.1037/1072-5245.13.4.423

Barros, A.J.S., Teche, S.P., Padoan, C., Laskoski, P., Hauck, S., & Eizirik, C.L. (2020). Countertransference, defense mechanisms, and vicarious trauma in work with sexual offenders. *The Journal of the American Academy of Psychiatry and the Law, 48*(3), 302–314. doi:10.29158/JAAPL.003925-20

Bellis, M.A., Hughes, K., Leckenby, N., Hardcastle, K.A., Perkins, C., & Lowey, H. (2015). Measuring mortality and the burden of adult disease associated with adverse childhood experiences in England: A national survey. *Journal of Public Health, 37*(3), 445–454. doi:10.1093/pubmed/fdu065

Bloom, S.L. (2010). Organizational stress as a barrier to trauma-informed service delivery. In N. Tehrani (Ed.). (2010), *Managing trauma in the workplace: Supporting workers and organisations* (1st ed.) (pp.139–153). Routledge. doi:10.4324/9780203841068

Bloom, S.L. (2013). *Creating sanctuary: Toward the evolution of sane societies* (2nd ed.). Routledge. doi:10.4324/9780203569146

Bloom, S.L., & Farragher, B. (2010). *Destroying sanctuary: The crisis in human service delivery systems*. Oxford University Press.

Bloom, S.L., & Farragher, B. (2013) *Restoring sanctuary: A new operating system for trauma-informed systems of care*. Oxford University Press. doi:10.1093/acprof:oso/9780199796366.001.0001

Bonta, J., & Andrews, D.A. (2016). *The psychology of criminal conduct*. Routledge. doi:10.4324/9781315677187

Bourke, M.L., & Craun, S.W. (2014). Coping with secondary traumatic stress: Differences between U.K. and U.S. child exploitation personnel. *Traumatology, 20*(1), 57–64. doi:10.1037/h0099381

Bradford, J., & de Amorim Levin, G.V. (2020). Vicarious trauma and PTSD in forensic mental health professionals. *Journal of the American Academy of Psychiatry and the Law, 48*(3), 315–318. doi:10.29158/JAAPL.200025-20

Branson, D.C. (2019). Vicarious trauma, themes in research, and terminology: A review of literature. *Traumatology, 25*(1), 2–10. doi:10.1037/trm0000161

British Psychological Society. (2019). *The complexity of 'complex' trauma*. British Psychological Society.

Brough, P. (2004). Comparing the influence of traumatic and organizational stressors on the psychological health of police, fire, and ambulance officers. *International Journal of Stress Management, 11*(3), 227–244. doi:10.1037/1072-5245.11.3.227

Brovko, J.M., & Foote, W.E. (2011, March). Vicarious traumatization: Are forensic psychologists vulnerable to trauma exposure? Presented at the 42nd Annual American Psychology-Law Society Conference, Miami, FL.

Brown, B. (2010). *The gifts of imperfection: Let go of who you think you're supposed to be and embrace who you are*. Hazelden.

Brown, B. (2018). *Dare to lead: Brave work, tough conversations, whole hearts*. Random House.

Burns, C.M., Morley, J., Bradshaw, R., & Domene, J. (2008). The emotional impact on and coping strategies employed by police teams investigating internet child exploitation. *Traumatology, 14*(2), 20–31. doi:10.1177/1534765608319082

Carleton, R.N., Afifi, T.O., Taillieu, T., Turner, S., Krakauer, R., Anderson, G.S., … & McCreary, D.R. (2019). Exposures to potentially traumatic events among public safety personnel in Canada. *Canadian Journal of Behavioural Science, 51*(1), 37–52. doi:10.1037/cbs0000115

Clarke, J. (2004). *The psychosocial impact on facilitators of working therapeutically with sex offenders: An experimental study* (Unpublished doctoral thesis). University of York.

Clarke, J. (2013). The resilient practitioner. In J. Clarke & P. Wilson (Eds), *Forensic psychology in practice: A practitioners handbook* (pp.220–239). Palgrave MacMillan.

Cramer, R.J., Ireland, J.L., Hartley, V., Long, M.M., Ireland, C.A., & Wilkins, T. (2020). Coping, mental health, and subjective well-being among mental health staff working in secure forensic psychiatric settings: Results from a workplace health assessment. *Psychological Services, 17*(2), 160–169. doi:10.1037/ser0000354

Davies, J., & Nagi, C. (2017). Supervising the therapists. In J. Davies & C. Nagi (Eds), *Individual Psychological Therapies in Forensic Settings: Research and Practice* (pp.228–242). Routledge.

Department for Education. (2021). *Critical workers and vulnerable children who can access schools or educational settings*. Department for Education.

Devilly, G.J., Wright, R., & Varker, T. (2009). Vicarious trauma, secondary traumatic stress or simply burnout? Effect of trauma therapy on mental health professionals. *Australian and New Zealand Journal of Psychiatry, 43*(4), 373–385. doi:10.1080/00048670902721079

Dollard, M.F., & Winefield, A.H. (1998). A test of the demand–control/support model of work stress in correctional officers. *Journal of Occupational Health Psychology, 3*(3), 243–264. doi:10.1037/1076-8998.3.3.243

Elliott, K.A., & Daley, D. (2013). Stress, coping, and psychological well-being among forensic health care professionals. *Legal and Criminological Psychology, 18*, 187–204. doi:10.1111/j.2044-8333.2012.02045.x

Engstrom, D., Hernandez, P., & Gangsei, D. (2008). Vicarious resilience: A qualitative investigation into its description. *Traumatology. 14*(3), 13–21. doi:10.1177%2F1534765608319323

Farrington, D.P. (2003). Developmental and life-course criminology: Key theoretical and empirical issues:The 2002 Sutherland Award address. *Criminology, 41,*221–225. doi10.1111/j.1745-9125.2003.tb00987.x

Felitti,V.J.,Anda, R.F., Nordenberg, D.,Williamson, D.F., Spitz,A.M., Edwards,V., … & Marks, J.S. (1998). Relationship of childhood abuse and household dysfunction to many of the leading causes of death in adults:The adverse childhood experiences (ACE) study. *American Journal of Preventive Medicine, 14*(4), 245–258. doi:10.1016/S0749-3797(98)00017-8

Figley, C.R. (1995). *Compassion fatigue: Coping with secondary traumatic stress disorder in those who treat the traumatised.* Bruner/Mazel.

Gallavan, D.B., & Newman, J.L. (2013). Predictors of burnout among correctional mental health professionals. *Psychological Services, 10*(1), 115–122. doi:10.1037/a0031341

Gil-Monte, P.R., Figueiredo-Ferraz, H., & Valdez-Bonilla, H. (2013). Factor analysis of the Spanish burnout inventory among Mexican prison employees. *Canadian Journal of Behavioural Science, 45*(2), 96–104. doi:10.1037/a0027883

Gould, D.D.,Watson, S.L., Price, S.R., &Valliant, P.M. (2013).The relationship between burnout and coping in adult and young offender center correctional officers:An exploratory investigation. *Psychological services, 10*(1), 37–47. doi:10.1037/a0029655

Gutheil, G., & Gabbard, G.O. (1998). Misuses and misunderstandings of boundary theory in clinical and regulatory settings. *American Journal of Psychiatry, 155*(3), 409–414. doi:10.1176/ajp.155.3.409

Hamilton, L. (2010).The boundary seesaw model: Good fences make for good neighbours. In A. Tennant & K. Howells (Eds), *Using time not doing time* (pp.181–194). Wiley-Blackwell. doi:10.1002/9780470710647.ch13

Herman, J. (1992). *Trauma and recovery:The aftermath of violence from domestic abuse to political terror.* Basic Books.

Hernandez, P., Ganggsei, D., & Engstrom, D. (2007). Vicarious resilience: A new concept in work with those who survive trauma. *Family Process, 46*(2), 229–241. doi:10.1111/j.1545-5300.2007.00206.x

Horvath, M.A.H., Massey, K., Essafi, S., & Majeed-Ariss, R. (2020). Minimising trauma in staff at a sexual assault referral centre:What and who is needed? *Journal of Forensic and Legal Medicine, 74,* 102029. doi:10.1016/j.jflm.2020.102029

Johnson,W.B., Johnson, S.J., Sullivan, G.R., Bongar, B., Miller, L., & Sammons, M.T. (2011). Psychology in extremis: Preventing problems of professional competence in dangerous practice settings. *Professional Psychology: Research and Practice, 42*(1), 94–104. doi:10.1037/a0022365

Johnstone, L. & Boyle, M. with Cromby, J., Dillon, J., Harper, D., Kinderman, P., Longden, E., Pilgrim, D., & Read, J. (2018). *The power threat meaning framework:Towards the identification of patterns in emotional distress, unusual experiences and troubled or troubling behaviour, as an alternative to functional psychiatric diagnosis.* British Psychological Society.

Johnstone, L., & Dallos, R. (2013). *Formulation in psychology and psychotherapy: Making sense of people's problems.* Routledge.

Knight, C. (2010). Indirect trauma in the field practicum: Secondary traumatic stress, vicarious trauma, and compassion fatigue among social work students and their field instructors. *Journal of Baccalaureate Social Work, 15*(1), 31–52. https://doi.org/10.18084/basw.15.1.l568283x21397357

Lambert, K., Chu, S., & Turner, P. (2019). Professional boundaries of nursing staff in secure mental health services: Impact of interpersonal style and attitude toward coercion. *Journal of Psychosocial Nursing and Mental Health Services, 57*(2), 16–24. https://doi.org/10.3928/02793695-20180920-05

Ledesma, J. (2014). Conceptual frameworks and research models on resilience in leadership. *SAGE Open, 4*(3), 1–8. doi:10.1177/2158244014545464

Lee, J., Lim, N.,Yang, E., & Lee, S.M. (2011).Antecedents and consequences of three dimensions of burnout in psychotherapists: A meta-analysis. *Professional Psychology: Research and Practice, 42*(3), 252–258. doi:10.1037/a0023319

Leiter, M.P., & Maslach, C. (1999). Six areas of worklife: A model of the organizational context of burnout. *Journal of Health and Human Services Administration, 21*(4), 472–489.

Leiter, M.P., & Shaughnessy, K. (2006). The areas of worklife model of burnout: Tests of mediation relationships. *Ergonomia: An International Journal, 28*, 327–341.

Levenson, J.S., Willis, G.M., & Prescott, D.S. (2016). Adverse childhood experiences in the lives of male sex offenders: Implications for trauma-informed care. *Sexual Abuse, 28*(4), 340–359. doi:10.1177/1079063214535819

Linehan, M.M. (1993). *Cognitive-behavioural treatment of borderline personality disorder.* New York: Guilford Press.

Love, C.C., & Heber, S.A. (2001). Staff-patient erotic boundary violations. *Journal of Psychosocial Nursing, 7*, 4–7.

Lowe, T., French, M., Hawkins, M., Hesselgreaves, H., & Wilson, R. (2021). *New development: Responding to complexity in public services: The human learning systems approach.* Routledge. doi:10.1080/09540962.2020.1832738

Maslach, C., & Leiter, M.P. (2016). Understanding the burnout experience: Recent research and its implications for psychiatry. *World Psychiatry, 15*(2), 103–111. doi:10.1002/wps.20311

Maslach, C., Schaufeli, W.B., & Leiter, M.P. (2001). Job burnout. *Annual Review of Psychology, 52*(1), 397–422. doi:10.1146/annurev.psych.52.1.397

McCann, I.L., & Pearlman, L.A. (1990). Vicarious traumatization: A framework for understanding the psychological effects of working with victims. *Journal of Traumatic Stress, 3*(1), 131–149. doi:10.1002/jts.2490030110

Middleton, J., Harris, L.M., Matera Bassett, D., & Nicotera, N. (2021). "Your soul feels a little bruised": Forensic interviewers' experiences of vicarious trauma. *Traumatology.* Advance online publication. doi:10.1037/trm0000297

Molnar, B.E., Sprang, G., Killian, K.D., Gottfried, R., Emery, V., & Bride, B.E. (2017). Advancing science and practice for vicarious traumatization/secondary traumatic stress: A research agenda. *Traumatology, 23*(2), 129–142. doi:10.1037/trm0000122

Munger, T., Savage, T., & Panosky, D.M. (2015). When caring for perpetrators becomes a sentence: Recognizing vicarious trauma. *Journal of Correctional Health Care, 21*(4), 365–374. doi:10.1177/1078345815599976

Newman, C., Eason, M., & Kinghorn, G. (2019). Incidence of vicarious trauma in correctional health and forensic mental health staff in New South Wales, Australia. *Journal of Forensic Nursing, 15*(3), 183–192. doi:10.1097/JFN.0000000000000245

O'Leary, V.E. (1998). Strength in the face of adversity: Individual and social thriving. *Journal of Social Issues, 54*(2), 425–446. doi:10.1111/0022-4537.751998075

Parrish Meadows, M., Shreffler, K.M., & Mullins-Sweatt, S.N. (2011). Occupational stressors and resilience in critical occupations: The role of personality. In Perrewé, P.L. & Ganster, D.C. (Eds), *The role of individual differences in occupational stress and well being (Research in Occupational Stress and Well Being, Vol. 9)* (pp.39–61). Emerald Group Publishing Limited. doi:10.1108/S1479-3555(2011)0000009006

Paton, D., & Violanti, J.M. (Eds). (1996). *Traumatic stress in critical occupations: Recognition, consequences and treatment.* Charles C Thomas.

Pearlman, L.A., & Saakvitne, K. (1995). *Trauma and the therapist: Countertransference and vicarious traumatization in psychotherapy with incest survivors.* W.W. Norton.

Pirelli, G., Formon, D.L., & Maloney, K. (2020). Preventing vicarious trauma (VT), compassion fatigue (CF), and burnout (BO) in forensic mental health: Forensic psychology as exemplar. *Professional Psychology: Research and Practice, 51*(5), 454–466. doi:org/10.1037/pro0000293

Reich, J.W., Zautra, A.J., & Hall, J.S.E. (2010). *Handbook of adult resilience.* Guilford Press.

Rocchio, L.M. (2020). Ethical and professional considerations in the forensic assessment of complex trauma and dissociation. *Psychological Injury and Law 13*, 124–134. doi:10.1007/s12207-020-09384-9

Ryle, A., & Kerr, I.B. (2002). *Introducing cognitive analytic therapy: Principles and practice.* John Wiley & Sons Ltd. doi:10.1002/9780470713587

Scottish Government. (2018). *Understanding childhood adversity, resilience and crime.* Retrieved from www.gov.scot/publications/understanding-childhood-adversity-resilience-crime/

Silveira, F.S., & Boyer, W. (2015). Vicarious resilience in counselors of child and youth victims of interpersonal trauma. *Qualitative Health Research, 25*(4), 513–526. doi:10.1177/1049732314552284

Starcher, D., & Stolzenberg, S.N. (2020). Burnout and secondary trauma among forensic interviewers. *Child & Family Social Work, 25*(4), 924–934. doi:10.1111/cfs.12777

Turgoose, D., Glover, N., Barker, C., & Maddox, L. (2017). Empathy, compassion fatigue, and burnout in police officers working with rape victims. *Traumatology, 23*(2), 205–213. doi:10.1037/trm0000118

van der Kolk, B.A. (2014). *The body keeps the score: Mind, brain and body in the transformation of trauma.* Penguin Books.

van der Kolk, B.A., & Fisler, R. (1995). Dissociation and the fragmentary nature of traumatic memories: Overview and exploratory study. *Journal of Traumatic Stress, 8*(4), 505–525. doi:10.1002/jts.2490080402

van der Ploeg, E., Dorresteijn, S.M., & Kleber, R.J. (2003). Critical incidents and chronic stressors at work: Their impact on forensic doctors. *Journal of Occupational Health Psychology. 8*(2), 157–166. doi:10.1037/1076-8998.8.2.157

van Minnen, A., & Keijsers, G.P. (2000). A controlled study into the (cognitive) effects of exposure treatment on trauma therapists. *Journal of Behaviour Therapy and Experimental Psychiatry. 31*(3-4), 189–200. doi:10.1016/s0005-7916(01)00005-2

Ward, T. (2002). Good lives and the rehabilitation of offenders: Promises and problems. *Aggression and Violent Behavior, 7*, 513–528. doi:10.1016/S1359-1789(01)00076-3

Wright, R., Powell, M.B., & Ridge, D. (2006). Child abuse investigation: An in-depth analysis of how police officers perceive and cope with daily work challenges. *Policing: An International Journal of Police Strategies & Management, 29*(3), 498–512. doi:10.1108/13639510610684728

22

TRAUMA-INFORMED CARE AND CULTURE CHANGE IN AN NHS FORENSIC SERVICE

Victoria Hiett-Davies

A trauma-informed approach to forensic mental health involves re-examining and changing many of our assumptions and the way we work with and think about colleagues, service users, and the organisation. This chapter describes the development and implementation of a trauma strategy within Forensics in a large UK mental health trust, building on existing good practice around trauma-informed care (TIC). This involved a process of drawing these practices together, learning from each other and developing further through a common trauma-informed framework, changing habits and routines, embedding core trauma-informed practices and foundation values in our services, education and development, and an organisational commitment to promote resilience in our staff. The strategy equally intended to promote our service-users feeling of safety and being supported, with increased engagement with staff who understand trauma reactions and responses, having care experiences that do not add to previous trauma or re-traumatise, with improved outcomes.

For TIC to truly become a part of our everyday working and thinking, there are key elements that are crucial. TIC does not occur via application of an isolated set of practical interventions and approaches; instead, a shift in the culture of the organisation is paramount. An agenda to change practice to be more trauma-informed needs to use processes that, in themselves, reflect the principles of TIC to support that shift. Moving away from "What's wrong with you?" towards "What has happened to you?" based practice, and applying compassionate thinking thereafter, requires an all-systems culture change from *blame* to *just*.

TIC is an organisational response to meet the needs of traumatised people within the organisation. It understands that so many of the people working and living in our services have had traumatic events in their lives. We already recognise that people have had and do have difficulties and past trauma, and we have processes to capture that

DOI: 10.4324/9781003120766-28

information and ensure that it is documented. But what do we do with this information then? How does it relate to people's everyday experiences of being in our services and how is it translated into the approach and care that is provided to both our staff and service users? There is a tendency to acknowledge the trauma and view it as a silo event, one that happened years ago which renders it somewhat irrelevant to current experiences and behaviours. As a case in point, a colleague once asked, "people have had worse trauma than him, so why does he behave so badly now?" Trauma-informed services recognise that our past experiences can and do impact on how we experience day-to-day events. For our service users, there must be an awareness that being in our services can be traumatising; seeing others frightened or angry, loss of agency and empowerment, diagnosis and loss of family contact are a few of many potentially traumatising and re-traumatising examples. For our staff, we must remember that they too can have past experiences of trauma in their personal and working lives, and that they too can be traumatised or re-traumatised by their work. With so much of the work within forensic services revolving around individual trauma and adverse experiences, both within the service user group *and* in our staff, developing and embedding a trauma-informed agenda is both highly relevant and paramount.

A trauma-informed and formulation-driven whole system approach to care is indicated. Furthermore, it is not sufficient to think that we can transform our service users' experiences of care without transforming the experiences of the people who work with them. Change is needed at all levels of our system to enable wider trauma-informed principles to become embedded within our forensic culture. A willingness within our systems to consider and reflect upon the impact of trauma on one another is a key element. It is essential to be curious and less assumptive that we know what is going on for the person, and to have compassionate and open conversations with the people who know themselves and their histories best. Historically, the traditional medical model of care has led and dominated our services; however, the determination of a diagnosis and application of medically orientated interventions is increasingly viewed as too narrow and limiting to address the spectrum of service users' experiences and needs. Simultaneously, the evidence base for understanding and adopting trauma-informed principles, not only at service user level but also at an organisational level, has grown significantly (Bloom, 2013; Harris & Fallot, 2001; SAMSHA, 2014).

Any shift towards such understanding and change must be underpinned by investment and commitment at every level of an organisation. The efficacy of TIC requires full integration of knowledge about trauma into policies, procedures, and practises to help reduce re-traumatisation, enhance recovery, and promote staff well-being. Embedding core trauma-informed approaches into everyday practice, to shape the foundation values in our services, provide education and development, and to drive organisational commitment to create the conditions that promote resilience in our staff and service users, constitutes some of the necessary changes. Promoting such work within services via a multi-model approach provides permission to be curious and ask questions; thus, fostering relationships within the leadership teams to support such a broad agenda is crucial.

The move towards trauma-informed services is evident within the United Kingdom and beyond, and the calls for such approaches from those living and working within our services are becoming louder. The drive towards this agenda is clear across many organisations and consequently there are more and more data and narratives relating to service user and staff experience to inform strategy and practice. Broadly, TIC views training, development, supervision, and support for staff as essential. This attention to staff needs has the potential to reduce burnout and staff turnover, improve staff resilience, staff sickness, and reduce re-traumatisation (Sweeney, Clement, Filson, & Kennedy, 2016). In addition, there is good evidence that TIC can influence a reduction in restrictive practises such as seclusion, long-term segregation, physical and mechanical restraint, and enforced medication (LeBel & Goldstein, 2005).

Background

To establish trauma-informed principles and responses within an organisation, it is important to consider what that might look like to the people who use and work within our service. Garnering the interest and passion of the larger group of people already working toward TIC in their own areas and creating a "community of interest" with those people who want to influence and engender this agenda is key. A narrative of wanting change and being curious about what that could look like was becoming clear within services dominated by disenfranchised staff tired of a culture of "That's just how we always do it". To consolidate and link these interested parties, two separate conferences were held: the first for interested staff and a second for service users and carers. Facilitated by the two trauma agenda leads, the conferences acknowledged existing good practice, as well as gaps in our service, and captured the hearts and minds of those people involved. Establishing best practice and asking the question "what is possible?" opened an avenue in the trauma-informed arena for curiosity and change. Involving service users and carers provided rich information about how it felt to be on the other end of an organisation. Hearing the voices of our service users disrupted some of the pre-sumptive narrative around "what we do and how we do it" and allowed for a more thoughtful approach informed by all stakeholders. Following the conferences, a working group (LEEP: Lived Experience Expert Panel) was established from the Peer Support Development team to ensure the continued involvement of people with lived experience.

The trauma conferences aimed to shine a light on and demonstrate the import-ance of TIC within our forensic services. To undertake the work and embed TIC into clinical practice, the conferences started the conversation about where this strategy could be piloted. Ultimately, it was agreed that nine teams would be put forward from within the forensic services in the initial phase. From these discussions, came five key arms that were deemed vital to the strategy by the community of interest. Agreed collaboratively, the key arms were: staff health and well-being, education and develop-ment, clinical scoping, a TIC framework, and an internet-based virtual hub to bring together staff, their knowledge, expertise, and shared experiences.

Staff Health and Well-being

Stress and unaddressed trauma in staff can have a significant impact on healthcare culture and the ability to respond effectively to the needs of service users. The impact this has on staff burnout, sickness, and retention are well known (Health and Safety Executive (2001), and processes in place within the organisation, such as exit questionnaires, staff sickness returns, and staff surveys, capture this information. Within this arm of the strategy, there was to be a focus on how we could ensure the impact of the work was viewed as equally important to clinical outcomes. To achieve this, the trauma agenda highlighted two elements: to create a culture and provision to support and educate staff about good and effective trauma-informed clinical supervision, and to assert the role of trauma-informed reflective practice as a key structure to be invested in within our service. Furthermore, a separate 'reflective practice' agenda aligned with TIC has been developed to ensure that these elements are equitable for all, with recognised standards and acknowledged and invested in by the leadership team.

In 2017, a post-incident peer support (PIPS) framework was rolled out across the Forensic directorate (Hiett-Davies, Milburn, & Regal, 2017). This framework was developed in response to National Institute for Health and Care Excellence (2015) which recommended the general, practical, and social support and guidance to anyone following a traumatic incident, whilst the government commissioned report on *Thriving at Work* (Stevenson & Farmer, 2017) recommended the establishment of a framework to coordinate support for those employees at higher risk of stress or trauma. The framework encompasses three elements of support following defined types of significant incidents which have a structure of providing social and organisational support, normalisation and signposting. Staff were trained to facilitate *defusion* for staff involved (immediately post-incident), *peer support de-brief* for staff within two weeks of an incident, and *service user review* for service users following an incident. The framework's purpose is to provide time for staff to begin to process the incident and gain immediate support from their peers, facilitated by trained staff and designed to support coping in the immediate term. The service user review ensures that the views of the individual involved are gathered and discussed, and that a plan to further support the person is generated collaboratively. The PIPS framework and the associated training needs are promoted within the trauma agenda.

Development and Education

Developing a trauma-informed training package is integral to a trauma-informed service. Providing staff with the understanding and tools needed to respond with compassion, care, and curiosity is vital. To engender a narrative around what has happened for the individual provides a space in which colleagues can think and work proactively with the person, rather than simply rely upon reactive responses in difficult moments. Compassion for the other can be difficult to maintain when staff stay only in the moment and encounter a set of behaviours and presentations which in turn may generate fear, stress, or dismissive responses. Creating a training set, through which the thread of compassion runs, pays attention to the phenomena evident in many staff, namely compassion fatigue, over-reliance upon restrictive practices, disrupted boundaries, and disengagement. Consequently, a two-day trauma awareness training package was developed and delivered to each of the nine "seeded" teams. The team training approach was important to ensure that the whole team, rather than individuals or an individual discipline, committed to the trauma-informed agenda. This whole system approach was adopted for the purpose of bringing together and training all staff involved in service user care to enable the embedding of a trauma-informed culture across the clinical environment. Provision was made to deliver two sets of this two-day training to each team to ensure that all staff from every discipline could attend and engage, and in total 206 staff were trained from our forensic services.

The training included an understanding of the impact of trauma on the individual and how it might have affected them. This encouraged thinking about some of the presentations our staff experience, how these behaviours may have developed over time, and how these might constitute forms of protection throughout that person's life. Attachments and how these are formed and the impact that difficult and chaotic attachments might have on the person we see now were also discussed. Throughout the training, emphasis was placed on how our staff might feel and respond to someone in distress, and honest conversations about how it is to be on the end of that distress were encouraged. It was interesting to note that, pre-training, from the evaluation feedback from the teams, staff consistently reported that they did not feel that they had the skill set required to work with trauma and felt that their role consisted of the reactive containment and management of service user behaviours. Staff narratives around loss of compassion, seeing a person as "difficult and risky" and forgetting the person's own story and what has happened to them, were also regular themes. Indeed, a clear sense of guilt, anger, and a loss of self-worth, empathy and motivation permeated the commencement of training sessions. However, such dialogue invariably changed over the course of the two days as staff became more energised and motivated towards change. The training provided interventions and approaches that can help in moments of distress, and tools such as grounding, sensory techniques, and distress care plans to address the person's own experience were taught. Use of formulations and the concept of the *window of tolerance* (Ogden, Minton, & Pain, 2006) and how these should inform distress care planning were introduced to the groups for them to better understand and cater for the individual's whole life, experiences, and presentations.

Clinical Scoping

From the initial conferences, a scoping exercise highlighted the breadth and range of interventions and approaches already being offered across forensic services, and we now have a comprehensive map of local provision and expertise. This provided a foundation for exploration of where best practice occurs and where the gaps in provision were. Future provision and possible developments were also derived from this work. The act of drawing together the knowledge and expertise within forensic services and developing a community of interested people allowed for that expertise to be shared, and diluted traditional silo working. Links can now be made across the services to people with specific areas of expertise and information disseminated through the virtual hub. New possibilities around the use of video training and video conferencing have come to the fore, and although this may reduce face-to-face contact, it has broadened the training arena and made this agenda more accessible for more people.

Virtual Hub

The virtual internet hub was developed to provide a portal for organisational engagement and communication, providing links for the community of interest and beyond. Having a central place for staff to link to, share good practice and learn from others, and to export good practice from one service to another is seen to be key. Educational and training needs can be addressed through the hub, with all playing an important role in sharing expertise and providing learning opportunities for others. The hub is accessible to all staff and has links to and from other relevant sites, such as staff health and well-being, clinical practices, and suicide prevention. It is essential that "being trauma informed" is not a stand-alone practice and does not sit in isolation across a system. Creating a truly trauma-informed service ensures that trauma and trauma-informed practices and thinking constitute a thread that runs through and touches all aspects of the organisation. The production of the hub pays attention to this and has generated unity through promotion of the agenda and instilling the idea that being trauma aware and responsive is everyone's business.

Trauma-Informed Framework

Identifying what we mean by TIC, what it looks and feels like, the core practices and foundation values that are embedded in our services and how this links to personal recovery and staff health and well-being are a central part of the work. To establish this, we need to ensure that we have the knowledge, skills, and impetus to develop and maintain TIC, and to create a culture in the organisation to enable this to flourish. Achieving this supports the goal of good recovery and ameliorates the impact of vicarious trauma and re-traumatisation for both staff and service users. Using a trauma framework allows staff to work with a structure that enables them to plan their trauma-informed service. They can view and action plan against each element as separate entities in a practical way, whilst working towards bringing them together as a whole. The purpose of this approach was to ensure that attention to trauma became less additive and more integrative.

The Five Pillars of Trauma-Informed Care

The framework is comprised of the behaviours and processes that reflect each of the five pillars of trauma-informed care outlined by Covington (2016): Safety, Collaboration, Trustworthiness, Choice, and Empowerment. These pillars formed part of the staff and service-user evaluation and from these a benchmarking tool was developed. In addition, a set of standards for the teams to work towards was created.

Safety: Environmental and Psychological

Environmental safety involves working towards ensuring that people within our services feel safe in their environment. This requires staff to take a step back and really look at their service, *what does it look and feel like?* Many teams recognised that their services were built around a risk-orientated formula: chairs that were too heavy to move, tables bolted down, rooms that were bare, restrictions on many items, staff using toilets to get away from work in order to cry because they had nowhere else to go, and little attention paid to the sensory ambiance, as the usual smell, look, and sounds were no longer noticed. Environments could be modified to be conducive to feelings of safety, and the positive impact this might have on the traumatised individual was not considered.

TIC is underpinned by psychological safety. This is a critical factor in collaboration and learning. When people feel psychologically safe, learning and positive change can take place. Rather than focusing on self and self-protection, we can work and learn together and focus on joint goals once we feel safe expressing opinions and offering solutions without fear of judgement or criticism. There is a clear relationship between psychological safety and engagement, and consequently this is a crucial element when working collaboratively with our service users who struggle to trust and engage with others, who often do not feel that they have a voice or that it will be heard. Developing a psychologically safe service works on the premise that the individual's views and thoughts will be respected and paid attention to, and that this is understood and felt by the individual. From a learning perspective, opinions and questions are viewed as constructive, and not knowing or understanding is acceptable. Generally, our services expressed a view that they felt psychologically safe. However, closer examination revealed examples where staff and service users did not feel safe. Ward rounds were one such example; traditionally hierarchical, consisting of a mixture of disciplines who carry authority, nursing staff reflected at the conference that at times they felt intimidated in this arena or felt that they were there to simply advocate for their service users without having a voice themselves. A direct consequence of this was that the views of the service users were not heard adequately either. Staff were less likely to ask for help, give feedback, share innovative ideas, or discuss problems, leading to a much less cohesive and collaborative discussion with shared goals and outcomes at its heart. This lack of psychological safety (and therefore, inclusion) was also felt by service users. Fears around reporting mistakes, questioning practices, and querying decisions were shared by staff and service users, with such fears often as a direct result of previous negative experiences. More generally, service users reported that they did not feel part of the decision-making process, and some felt that their views were never listened to or even considered. In such instances, there was little opportunity for shared learning or collaborative working as a team.

Collaboration

It is important that people are given the opportunity to make a meaningful contribution to their care and work, providing a sense of agency, empowerment, and choice.

A cohesive approach to helping people feel safe is informed by a shared understanding of what works best for individuals and works towards reducing the intensity and frequency of moments of overwhelm and distress. There must be a consistent process of engagement to access people's views and inclinations, and an understanding and recognition of the centrality of this. Within our services, there was a willingness to work collaboratively with service users; however, staff reflected within the conference that the nature of our forensic care stymied their capability to truly work in this way. Examples of "having to manage and respond" to difficult and risky behaviours appeared to negate staff ability to collaborate with the person. In those moments, the culture of "doing to" came to the fore, apparently at the expense of utilising the opportunities for collaborative crisis-planning (outside of episodes of overwhelming distress). Environments were created based on staff assessment of risk rather than working collaboratively to create an environment which felt safe to the people who stayed there. Assumptive thinking based on "what we have done before works" formed a basis for managing risk, and a pre-set activity timetable excluded those who were not interested in what was on offer or felt threatened within groups. Teams worked in collaboration with service users to develop care plans but recognised that, ultimately, the multi-disciplinary team would decide on the course of treatment for the individual. Meanwhile, plans to manage violence and aggression, self-harm, security, and other forensically relevant risk areas tended to be developed and held by ward staff.

Trustworthiness

Trust is the foundation to developing meaningful relationships and delivering TIC. It creates the conditions necessary for care to be received and to flourish in a meaningful way. There must be clear and concise expectations of all, with transparent communication upheld. There was a recognition from those at both the conferences that services are often unpredictable and in flux. From these forums it was reported that it was commonly perceived that there were no clear pathways of care and no expectations of behaviours or expected responses. Service users reported that they were not routinely kept informed of changes to their care timetable, and were not informed of changes to their routine. Furthermore, staff reported that communication between management and staff was not always clear or well circulated, and there was a feeling that decisions were made by senior figures that were not in the best interests of staff. Naturally, this impacted on staff ability and willingness to trust that their leaders were open and transparent and held their staff in mind when making decisions that impacted on them. In some areas this had created a *them and us* culture, with a loss of cohesiveness and increase in suspiciousness and cynicism around the motives of each party. This dynamic within the staff team was paralleled within the service user and staff dynamic.

Choice

People's preferences must be sought and prioritised. There needs to be an awareness that people who are distressed and overwhelmed may have difficulty in processing information and then making good, adaptive choices. Equally, it must be recognised that at times they may believe that their voice has been denied, invalidated, or not been heard, and that their past experiences may shape this belief. We need, therefore, to create different ways to provide the same information, with good choices, and that this is available as required in a non-shaming and non-threatening way. From the conferences, our services recognised that often there was no such information available for people, and what information there was, was in a "one size fits all" format. There was also an acknowledgement of a "doing to, not doing with" culture that was underpinned by a power imbalance apparent to all. Routines and regimes that gave people little space for choice were reported to dominate our forensic services. Simple, everyday staff practices like knocking on service user doors and walking in before receiving a response, assuming that service users consented to be subjected to rubdown searches without asking them, set seating plans for meals and rotas to use the laundry were just some of the opportunities to provide choice that were often missed. These regimes enable systems to run smoothly and basic interventions and activities to be attended to. However, we can forget that, for our service users, these day-to-day interventions are the basis for many of their interactions with others, and that providing them with choice can provide a sense of safety, worth, agency, and empowerment.

Empowerment

Every person should be seen as an individual with unique experiences and a personal history. By recognising people's strengths and building skills, we can maximise their empowerment. It is clear within our forensic services that there is a power imbalance between staff and service users. Service users are not free to leave, see their family as they wish, or choose how they eat their own meals. They cannot decorate or design their rooms as they want them to be. Equally, there are many examples where loss of empowerment for staff is evident. Inflexible working, processes and procedures to adhere to, decision-making not always at "ground level" can leave a staff team feeling disempowered. Rules, regimes, and restrictions are important to any organisation because they provide boundaries, containment, consistency, and safety for all. However, within this element of the strategy we look at ways in which we can increase a sense of empowerment for our staff and service users. We want to create a culture where identifying and developing skills is a priority. We can empower people by collaboratively looking at where they have strengths and how we capitalise on those; creating activity timetables that are person-centred and strengths based; and having conversations about what the person enjoys rather than what we have to offer. We can ensure that staff have access to training that is relevant to their skill set and interests, and put processes in place to make sure that clinical supervision provides a safe space for discussion and ensures that identified goals are acted upon.

Implementation of Process into Practice

The initial phase of engagement for the strategy encapsulated both the conferences and fostering relationships with senior leaders via various forums and written communications. This resulted in nine forensic inpatient teams being nominated as leads for the trauma-informed agenda, forming a starting point to embedding the work across all forensic services. These teams were based across the forensic directorate within high, medium, low secure settings and prison in-reach. They covered a cross section of the service user population, including Women's Services, Male Mental Health Admission/Acute Services, Personality Disorder Services, and Intellectual Disability Services. Each team appointed two staff "champions" with whom the trauma agenda leads would work closely with, having secured a commitment for protected time for those champions from their respective service leads.

A pre-intervention evaluation of TIC was co-developed by the agenda leads and undertaken by Lawday & Lawday (2019) to establish current areas of need across the identified teams in relation to TIC. The measures were selected following a review of published literature relating to milieu rating scales/ward atmosphere, as well as validated measures of trauma-informed practice, and a "walk through" of each service. Every team staff member was asked to complete anonymous, pre-evaluation assessments relating to ward atmosphere:

- *The Essen Climate Evaluation Schema* (Schalast & Tonkin, 2016) a 17-item questionnaire corresponding to 1 of 3 subscales: patient cohesion, experienced safety, and therapeutic hold/support.
- *Attitudes Related to Trauma-Informed Care* (ARTIC: Baker, Brown, Wilcox, Overstreet, & Arora, 2016), with 7 subscales consisting of underlying causes of problem behaviour and symptoms, responses to problem behaviour and symptoms, on-the-job behaviour, self-efficacy at work, reactions to the work, personal support of TIC, and system-wide support of TIC.
- *Professional Quality of Life Scale* (ProQOL: Stamm, 2009) comprising of 3 subscales: compassion satisfaction, burnout, and secondary traumatic stress.
- *Bespoke benchmarking tool* measuring staff and service users' experience of safety, collaboration, trust, choice, and empowerment (Covington, 2016).
- *Trauma awareness training questionnaire* immediately post-training consisting of 16 questions based around the training they had received and its impact on themselves, their team, and their service users and repeated 18 months later at post-evaluation.

The walk-through of services was conducted by the agenda leads and a member of the LEEP team and occurred from the admission point for service users. This provided an insight into how the service felt from an environmental and psychological perspective, aiming to highlight good practice as well as barriers to promoting safety.

The next phase of the strategy was to introduce the champions to the information from the pre-intervention assessments and benchmarking tool. These were used by the teams to create an action plan, based on highlighted areas around the five pillars, where each team wanted to improve. The action plan called for the teams to evidence their trauma-informed practices against the trauma strategy standards, as developed by the agenda leads (adapted from McGuire & Carlisle, 2018; Mersey-care NHS Foundation Trust). Based on the five key pillars (separating "safety" into two elements of psychological and environmental), the set of nine standards also incorporated staff well-being, staff development, and crisis planning. By employing this set of trauma-informed standards, each team was empowered to work towards establishing and then providing evidence of the shifts and changes that they had made. Further areas for development were then identified and planned for by the teams.

Trauma Awareness Training Evaluation

Each delegate was provided with a questionnaire immediately post-trauma awareness training to capture staff's initial thoughts and impressions. This questionnaire was designed to capture both the practical aspects of the training as well as the content. Each delegate was asked if they were willing to participate and all returns were anonymous. A further post-training questionnaire was included in the service evaluation format six months later. Every member of staff from the teams was asked to complete this. From this information a thematic analysis was completed to provide a snapshot of the impact of the training. Of the staff group, responders to the follow-up training questionnaire, 33% had received the training. This reflects the reported high turnover of staff due to natural progression and movement across services and trusts and reinforces the importance of training for trainers to ensure sustainability.

Evaluation

Details of the evaluation are reported by Lawday and Lawday (2019; 2020). Both the pre- and post-intervention evaluation was sent out to staff via trust email and all data received was managed and analysed by the principle researcher. Overall, there were 113 staff respondents at pre-intervention, 51 staff respondents at post-intervention. (There was a notable reduction in responses compared to the baseline period. Possible reasons include demands of the role during the Covid-19 pandemic response, staff absence or turnover, acuity of clinical need.) Service users received their evaluations via the post to their wards and were supported by staff or agenda leads and LEEP members, and were requested to complete the questionnaire which focused on their views of the service based on the five pillars. Pre-intervention there were 47 service user respondents and 47 service user respondents post-intervention.

All measures were repeated in the post-intervention evaluation which occurred 18 months later. The benchmarking tool asked questions relevant to the five pillars of TIC, at pre- and post-intervention. At post, all questions saw an improvement on average, in particular the Choice and Collaboration questions. Statistically significant improvement for all five pillars of TIC was found. There was also significant positive change on six of the seven subscales of the ARCTIC measuring attitudes to trauma amongst staff. On the Professional Quality of Life Scale, average staff ratings of compassion satisfaction had increased, while reported levels of burnout and secondary traumatic stress had reduced.

Service user responses post-intervention saw a slight deterioration in average scores, in particular on the trust, choice, and empowerment benchmarking survey scales. Unfortunately, the measures were taken during lockdown due to Covid-19, which is likely to have significantly affected the sense of choice and empowerment that service users felt at the time. The positive changes in other areas were tested for statistical significance. There was a statistically significant difference in the scores for pre-responses compared with post-responses.

Focus groups with employees from each of the nine seeded teams were also arranged following the intervention. In each session facilitators sought the opinions of participants in relation to their experiences of being part of the introduction of TIC in their service. These were designed to gather the narrative of the staff teams with a standard set of questions to each and were facilitated by the agenda leads. A series of seven prompt questions were used and the outputs of every discussion were recorded in written format and then thematically analysed to give a snapshot of how TIC has impacted within those sites.

The focus groups highlighted increased compassion for each other and their service users as a priority and an important shift in their working, being able to consider what has happened for the other and responding with compassion rather than blame. There was an overwhelming focus on better team cohesion, psychological safety, a shared language, and better service user outcomes. Staff reflected that there was an increase in curiosity and desire to understand the drivers behind the person's behaviour or trauma response, with a willingness to ask questions and discuss different approaches to care without fear of criticism. Working towards ensuring that care for all in our service is sensitive to needs and is experienced as safe, predictable, and consistent was a running theme throughout. Within the focus groups, staff identified being able to recognise the impact of traumatic events on colleagues and themselves. Staff described being more empathetic towards their colleagues, being able to approach each other to offer support more readily. Having a shared language and enhanced understanding promoted better communication and contributed to a change in culture.

Teams had shifted their practices around staff and service user well-being, giving consideration to their environment. Staff reflected within the focus groups that they had not previously considered the environment as having an impact on our service users or themselves. Stepping back and viewing their environment through "fresh" eyes influenced and altered their perception. Several teams considered the entrance to their ward area and the route new admissions are taken on to arrive there. One team reflected on a new admission who had arrived distressed having been driven past the main entrance and round the back of the hospital to arrive at the side door to the ward, believing he was being taken to a concentration camp.

Other teams focused on the immediate surroundings within the ward environment, re-configuring rooms that could be used as a sensory or a quiet room. Putting up curtains that had otherwise been viewed as potential for being used in "risky" ways and reconsidering service users' experience of mealtimes, bedroom spaces, and lounge areas. Several teams turned their attention to mealtimes and redesigned the eating area to make meals a more pleasurable experience rather than simply a process of eating.

Many teams changed previous pathways of care to develop a trauma-informed pathway, adopting interventions and approaches from pre-admission to transition and discharge with a focus on safety, engagement, and feeling contained as opposed to risk, ward activity timetables and restrictions. Teams rethought the process of engagement and the views they held of service users who were "dis-engaged". These teams created more flexible timetables which allowed service users to have choice in activities and whether these were with groups or individual. These were tailored to the service user needs and built entirely around staff understanding of the individual's capacity and ability to engage with others.

The analysis from both training evaluations was equally positive, with staff reporting a sense of being heard and invested in. Post-training, all teams reported that trauma training significantly impacted on service user care and outcomes while 54% of staff felt that their practice would improve following the training. With the knowledge and understanding around the presentations and behaviours that staff work with every day, good use of clinical interventions such as formulation, distress signature, collaborative care planning, sensory work, creation of pathways through service, and being with and listening to were given as some examples of change to practice. Staff reflected within the training evaluation that they had re-thought risk assessments and risk management plans through the lens of distress rather than risk alone, having a positive impact on restrictive practices. All teams shared examples of this shift of focus and described better outcomes for both the staff and service user. Several teams had changed their risk management plans to incorporate trauma and ensure that the service user experiences were understood in the context of how they might present. Staff reflected that changing the focus of risk to a more balanced view of both *risk* and *distress* enabled a reduction of re-traumatising responses from staff. This shift in focus promoted service user empowerment where they could tell their story, be understood, and supported in a way that was helpful to them. Teams were embedding the use of formulations to develop collaborative care plans which truly address the persons' difficulties and how they want to be supported. Following the training staff reported a re-framing of their role and understanding the importance of day-to-day containment and engagement in the persons' recovery which had a positive impact on their feelings of empowerment and being valued within the team. Staff reported feeling that they had a purpose and motivation to change, were skilled with something to offer and empowered to make change, and were confident in their own ability and willingness to share and receive good practice ideas.

The focus groups, trauma-informed standards, training and evaluations enabled our forensic services to achieve genuine TIC that demonstrated measurable positive differences to the lives of the people they work with as well as to their own working lives. It is evident that these trauma-informed areas are the beacons of our forensic service and stand as evidence of the positive impact of TIC. They have demonstrated positive change to their culture, a culture that had previously been underpinned by the ethos that "this is how we have always done it"; those practices and approaches have been re-thought and reconsidered through the trauma-informed lens.

Next Steps

There remains much work to do to better establish TIC across an organisation. There are more changes that need to happen to ensure that being trauma informed is not seen as a "silo" but as an approach and way of thinking that spans and influences all areas. A full commitment from organisation leads to support the trauma agenda is vital, with their visible investment to communicate the trauma strategy both internally and externally as a core part of business. Much thought and investment are needed to ensure that training packages are both sustainable and relevant to staff teams. A "train the trainers" programme is in place and all champions of the TIC teams will be trained to ensure sustainability within their service. Equally, we will see our champions working closely with other teams within their services, supporting them through the benchmarking tool to action planning and achieving the standards. The author continues to work closely with and align trauma-informed work with all other relevant areas of the organisation such as staff health and well-being, just and restorative culture, influencing policies and procedures, training department, suicide prevention, Quality Improvement, as well as our Positive and Safe Violence Reduction department to name a few. Instilling trauma awareness and knowledge within our interdependencies ensures that trauma and its impact is not seen in silo, or something "other" and not connected to other areas and agendas. Embedding an understanding of trauma and compassion as the foundations to all areas of the work is imperative. The continued work with our Positive and Safe Violence Reduction leads within the trust is especially important because of their influence "setting the tone" for all staff and training and developing them to work with and support our service users before, during, and after crisis. In recent years, Violence Reduction training has broadened its focus to include *preventative* strategies as well as *management* strategies. Therefore, prioritising "primary strategies" to avoid conflict in the first place, having effective "secondary strategies" to intervene and de-escalate risk-indicating situations, and being able to deliver safe "tertiary strategies" to manage crisis continues to be influenced by the trauma agenda. However, equally important in this area is the consideration we must give to our staff in relation to the impact those crises can have on them.

From a global, national, and local level, research, papers, other Trusts, evaluations, and trauma-informed pilots all demonstrate the necessity of a trauma-informed agenda which should be built on. The NHS long-term plan (NHS, 2019) is clear with regards to trauma-informed services and it is likely that organisations will need to demonstrate a robust and working trauma-informed agenda in the future. TIC and its place within healthcare is growing and there is a spotlight on those organisations with this agenda at the heart of its work. Becoming a trauma-informed service does not only relate to the work that we do with our service users but transcends this to an all systems approach, where all have a shared language of compassion and understanding. It is the development of a service which understands that we all react and respond in different ways when under duress, when the nature of our work is difficult, stressful, and traumatising at times. That TI service responds to our staff and service users with the understanding – we are all doing the best that we can with what we have.

With acknowledgements to the steering group: Lawrence Jones, Andrea Cockram, Maureen Tomeny, Julien Eve, Emma Watson, and Mary Di Lustro, as well as Tom Harris (Positive and Safe Violence Reduction manager) and Christine Milburn (co-agenda lead).

Further Reading

Dana, D. (2020). *Polyvagal exercises for safety and connection: 50 client centred practices.* Norton. This book provides the reader with a "grab-bag" of polyvagal-informed exercises with understandable explanations of the ways the autonomic nervous system directs daily living.

Harris, M., & Fallot, R. D. (Eds). (2001). *Using trauma theory to design service systems.* Jossey-Bass. A useful read for anyone wanting to establish trauma-informed services, taking the reader through developing TIC from system to service level.

Kurtz, A. (2020). *How to run reflective practice groups: A guide for healthcare professionals.* Routledge. For readers wanting to develop reflective practice within their service, this is very relevant as a step by guide.

References

Baker, C. N., Brown, S. M., Wilcox, P. D., Overstreet, S., & Arora, P. (2016). *Development and psychometric evaluation of the attitudes related to Trauma-Informed Care* (ARTIC) scale. *School Mental Health, 8*(1), 61–76. doi:10.1007/s12310-015-9161-0

Bloom, S. (2013). The sanctuary model: Changing habits and transforming the organizational operating system. In J. D. Ford, & C. A. Courtois (Eds), *Treating complex traumatic stress disorders in children and adolescents: Scientific foundations and therapeutic models* (pp.277–293). Guilford Press.

Covington, S. (2016). *Becoming trauma informed tool kit for women's community service providers.* Centre for Crime and Justice Studies.

Harris, M., & Fallot, R.D. (Eds). (2001). *Using trauma theory to design service systems.* Jossey-Bass.

Health and Safety Executive. (2001). *Tackling work-related stress: A manager's guide to improving and maintaining employee health and wellbeing.* The Stationery Office.

Hiett-Davies, V., Milburn, C., & Regal, S. (2017). *Post incident peer support framework.* Unpublished Report, Nottinghamshire Healthcare NHS Foundation Trust. Available on request.

Lawday, R. E, & Lawday, D. R. (2019). *Evaluating the implementation of trauma-informed care improvements across Nottinghamshire Healthcare NHS Foundation Trust: Establishing a baseline of service and staff measures in seeded sites.* Unpublished Report, Nottinghamshire Healthcare NHS Foundation Trust. Available on request.

Lawday, R. E., & Lawday, D. R. (2020). *Evaluating the implementation of trauma-informed care (TICE) improvements across Nottinghamshire Healthcare NHS Foundation Trust: 2020 follow up comparison to 2019 baseline of service user and staff measures in TICE strategy seeded sites.* Unpublished Report, Nottinghamshire Healthcare NHS Foundation Trust. Available on request.

LeBel, J., & Goldstein, R. (2005). Special section on seclusion and restraint: The economic cost of using restraint and the value added by restraint reduction or elimination. *Psychiatric Services, 56*(9), 1109–1114. doi:10.1176/appi.ps.56.9.1109

McGuire, F., & Carlisle, J. (Eds). (2018) *Standards for trauma informed care.* Mersey Care NHS Foundation Trust. Unpublished report.

National Institute for Health and Care Excellence. (2015). *Violence and aggression: Short-term management in mental health, health and community setting* (NICE Guidelines NG10).

NHS. (2019). *The NHS long term plan.* NHS.

Ogden, P., Minton, K., & Pain, C. (2006). *Trauma and the body: A sensorimotor approach to psychotherapy.* Norton.

SAMHSA. (2014). *SAMHSA's concept of trauma and guidance for a trauma-informed approach.* US Department of Health and Human Services.

Schalast, N., & Tonkin, M. (Eds). (2016). *The Essen climate evaluation schema—EssenCES: A manual and more.* Hogrefe Publishing.

Stamm, B. H. (2009). *Professional quality of life: Compassion satisfaction and fatigue version 5* (ProQOL). Retrieved from https://proqol.org/proqol-measure

Stevenson, D., & Farmer, P. (2017). *Thriving at work: The Stevenson/Farmer review of mental health and employers.* Department for Work and Pensions and Department of Health.

Sweeney, A., Clement, S., Filson, B., & Kennedy, A. (2016). Trauma-informed mental healthcare in the UK: What is it and how can we further its development? *Mental Health Review Journal, 21*(3), 174–192. doi:10.1108/MHRJ-01-2015-0006

23

TRAUMA AND RESTORATIVE JUSTICE

Estelle Moore

Justice is not some abstract thing. It's a force that sits at the very centre of who [we] are ... do we have the capacity to shatter denial ... and allow suffering to speak ... allow every voice to be lifted?

Cornel West (2015) NACRJ Conference, USA

The word "justice" can be highly emotive, especially if you have experienced or been responsible for traumatic harm. Annually, millions of survivors of harm and their relatives enter criminal justice buildings, their architecture symbolically representative of the processes (typically experienced as "cold, imposing and distant") that occur following harm (Toews, 2018). Justice conveys the idea that somewhere there is concern for fairness, possibly for peace, and for the well-being of others. These ethics are so fundamental in many societies that these principles are often embodied in roles undertaken by senior legal adjudicators, leaders, and elders in communities worldwide. Coupled with the notion of "restoration" (the act of returning something to a former owner, or place, or condition), in the context of harm, restorative justice (RJ) sounds important and promising of hope in the wake of tragedy or trauma. Important aspirations indeed – how might they translate into practice within services where harm is the *reason for referral* and often a recurrence within the walls of hospitals that are positioned to promote safe treatment for people who have typically lived under threat and struggled thereafter to live safely alongside others.

In her review of the history of RJ as a field of practice, Liebmann (2007) refers to RJ as "the most ancient and prevalent approach in the world to resolve harm and conflict" (p.37). Since the majority of the people who come into contact with prison and mental health services have experienced a personal history of multiple traumas (Dandurand & Vogt, 2020; Fox, Perez, Cass, Baglivio, & Epps, 2015), the historical focus on *punishment* following harm has left our systems ill-equipped to deal with the legacy of trauma, and therefore with comparatively limited options to date for trauma–informed healing. Retributive (penal) systems have a set of aims (Wenzel, Okimoto, Feather, & Platow, 2007) that may unhelpfully compound the harms that

DOI: 10.4324/9781003120766-29

brought residents to the doors of the units in the first place. It has been argued that our failure to "get at these root causes" remains characteristic of our response to offending actions (Oudshoorn, 2016; p.122). We might ask, why would a young person be expected to be willing to take responsibility for their actions when no one is accountable for the harm done to them (Oudshoorn, 2015)?

Justice (of the kind that you either get or you don't) can easily become politicised by campaigners of all persuasions, with the unwanted consequence that the person(s) who define it are rarely the victim-survivors (Goodmark, 2015). People described as mentally disordered offender patients often find themselves treated as both victims *and* perpetrators (McKenna, Jackson, & Browne, 2019). We all have the potential to be made the "other": the appeased or the aggressor. How might the benefits of RJ as an element of a trauma-informed forensic healthcare system best be represented and maximised?

Following Braithwaite's seminal work (2002), RJ is defined as a process that includes a response to offending. This chapter explores how RJ, and more widely restorative *practices*, can be operationalised within mental health settings with the potential to possibly repair some of the harms of trauma with a view to future accountability for not repeating it. The subject of RJ commands a wide and diverse literature today and there is much that this chapter cannot address. The focus here is on the rationale for emboldening the voice of the harmed and including victim-survivor perspectives within and beyond the offender-patient population. If conflict is handled well, this can resonate with the "felt sense" (embodied) experience in mental health settings of containment and safety, and this has the potential to increase trauma awareness and compassion throughout the system, reaching both harmed and harmer identities.

What Is Restorative Justice?

Restorative Justice is an approach to offending which invites victims, offenders, and relevant others to *engage with influence* over the way the consequences of crime are addressed to meet (some of) the needs of the victim(s) and offenders (van Denderen, Verstegen, de Vogel, & Feringa, 2020). The key to RJ is the reparation of harm (Dandurand & Vogt, 2020). With a greater focus on broken relationships than broken laws, the spectrum of RJ practices seeks to achieve moral and social repair with positive psychological consequences (Latimer, Dowden, & Muise, 2005; Lloyd & Borrill, 2020; Braithwaite, 2003; 2006).

The wide definition of what constitutes restorative practice has led some to argue that the term RJ has become too diffuse (Wood & Suzuki, 2016), covering not only criminal but also transitional justice (that is, truth and reconciliation commissions) informed by RJ principles. For simplicity here, the basic model of RJ via its *three pillars* is set out in Table 23.1.

Fundamentally, RJ involves engaging safely in facilitated dialogue with the hope of arriving at shared understanding and/or agreement (Dandurand & Vogt, 2020). Formats for RJ practice might include preparatory meetings, review with supporters, conferencing (face-to-face meetings that tend to follow a scripted schedule), other forms of mediation (where facilitators go between potential participants until there

Table 23.1 Three pillars of restorative justice (Zehr, 2020): addressing the aftermath of crime, encouraging the repair of harm

---

Harms and needs: crime causes harm and justice requires active repair
• Who was harmed? What was the harm? How can it be repaired?

Obligations: the parties encounter one another and set out how they will repair together
• Who is responsible and accountable and how can he/she repair the harm?

Engagement of stakeholders in the direction of transformation of the relationship
• Victims and offenders have active roles in the justice process.

---

is sufficient common ground for a meeting), and in some cases letter writing or review that shifts perspectives but may not bring participants into the same room at the same time. Opportunities to participate in what happens next after an offence and to draft agreements post-harm (e.g., plans that will support future safety, tolerance, or well-being, or that more fundamentally set out a recognition of the impact of the wrongdoing) can generate feelings of connection for participants distanced or, worse, damaged by the harm. These are some of the reliable features of restorative justice from the perspective of the harmed who are in a position to engage (Liebmann, 2007).

There is evidence that these features can also be outcomes when the harm directed against the victim has been very serious (Umbreit, Vos, & Coates, 2006) or sustained (Pico-Alfonso et al., 2006). The severity of the impact of an incident is not necessarily a predictor of the interest in, or potential power of, RJ. A critical factor is likely to be a readiness on the part of the survivor to seek healing or perhaps simply acknowledgement of the harm they suffered. Until recently this was not a "formal" option for victims of the harm perpetrated by those with a diagnosis of mental disorder because access to these resources was not on offer (Drennan, Cook, & Kiernan, 2015; Power, 2017). Some of the reasons for this are explored below.

Restorative practices have a range of different goals in different contexts – from offender rehabilitation in the prison system (Calkin, 2021) and diversion from it (Bonta, Wallace-Capretta, Rooney, & McAnoy, 2002) to reintegration, to making amends in communities, neighbourhoods (Ward, Fox, & Garber, 2014; Willis & Hoyle, 2019), and in domestic contexts (Burkemper & Balsam, 2007). Restorative practices generally involve scaffolding ways in which those involved in a crime (as survivors, witnesses, and/or perpetrators) can make a contribution to how the impact of the offending is handled. There is international variability with regard to public perception of the degree of culpability for crimes committed *when unwell*, and by extension, knowledge of the relationship between mental disorder and risk (Whiting, Ryland, & Fazel, 2020). Views as to what extent the person is considered responsible for causing harm inevitably permeate the offer of restorative practices in mental health settings, but have not entirely constrained it. Paying attention to the context and what has happened to people, as well as their mental state at the time of their offending, can offer a way forward: combining healing with/through accountability.

Although hopeful that present barriers to the success of RJ in prisons can be over-come, Dhami and colleagues have argued that RJ has not found the same "significant utility" inside prison settings as it has outside (Dhami, Mantle, & Fox 2009). Some prison systems have an RJ philosophy (Latimer et al., 2005). Many offer victim-offender mediation, community service work, offending behaviour and victim awareness programmes, whereby RJ operates in conjunction with traditional crim-inal justice, not as an alternative (Miers, 2001). RJ features at different stages of the process: pre-charge, post-charge and pre-conviction, pre-sentence, post-sentence, and pre-vocation. Is has been found to help prisoners achieve the goals of facing up to crimes and repairing damage in preparation for community return (Van Ness, 2007).

What Is the Value of Victim-Survivor Inclusion in Harm Repair?

Situating the experience of people who have been harmed (*victim-survivors*) as piv-otal in this chapter, evidence for the value of RJ *for victims* is shared here. On the basis of their findings from a major review of research on RJ in the UK, in which 36 comparisons were made between RJ and conventional criminal justice, Sherman and Strang (2007) report that RJ significantly reduced crime victims' symptoms of post-traumatic stress disorder (PTSD). It also reduced the desire for revenge, improved their satisfaction with the outcomes, and reduced crime-related costs (such as the cost of repeat offending). These outcomes resonate with earlier work in the United States. Informed by 30 years of evaluation research of restorative justice programmes, McCold (2003) analysed 98 such interventions, noting public support for RJ, for victims of offending, and for the process of reparation as key findings. He reported that participation rates in restorative practices were very high and were typically associated with the recommendation to others of the process, and shared support for the value of mediation.

Detailed examination of attempts through RJ to reduce PTSD following victim-isation (or secondary victimisation in the case of family members) has since produced some strong (Angel et al., 2014) and other more modest support for RJ over cus-tomary justice procedures (Lloyd & Borrill, 2020). Post-trauma symptoms including arousal and reactivity, re-experiencing of the harm, avoidance of cues related to the scene of the harm, anger, negative beliefs, and self-blame have reportedly been lowered by engagement in restorative meetings, particularly if questions (such as "why me, why then?") are met with satisfactory explanations.

Walters (2015) has demonstrated the positive impact of an apology (not offered in all exchanges) for secondary victims, and others who were processing the possibility of forgiveness. Restorative processes foster empowerment because sensitively addressing harm builds strength in the longer term. The following example encapsulates the pos-sibility that something can come from harm, which means that the suffering/loss of another was "not for nothing".

This mother (Paula, whose son was killed by Lawrence) reflects:

> I stood up at the end of the meeting and held my hand out to Lawrence –
> he took my hands in his and kept saying over and over again how sorry he

was. Going home in the car I felt as though every bit of energy had been drained from me. Around three days later I felt that, after four long years, I had received some closure on what had happened that night. I would urge anyone who is in similar circumstances to do what I have done.

Paula – quoted in Liebmann, 2007; p.226

The Risks of Victim Exclusion in Mental Health Settings

Offender-oriented RJ (which might involve a perpetrator in a potentially positive, albeit one-sided, process), even where the outcome includes accountability, has attracted critique for its failure to really involve victim input or redress in the process (Wood & Suzuki, 2016). There are many useful programmes in prison and health services e.g., Life Minus Violence (Ireland, 2007) and Aggression Replacement Training (Brännström, Kaunitz, Andershed, South, & Smedslund, 2016) that support offenders to learn the skills (self-control, moral development, etc.) in order to reduce the likelihood of offending behaviour. Nonetheless, it might be possible to complete such courses with limited engagement as to the impact of offending on those who are deeply harmed by violence. As people, we tend to be reluctant to talk about interpersonal violence and traumatisation; shame can play a central role in avoidance of further exposure or harm and the apparent safety of silence (Nathanson, 1994). However, paying *too little* attention to victimisation, such that a person who had been victimised would not see the value in participation in a restorative process, risks the loss of this viewpoint in recovery, and the opportunity for those harmed to experience repair. This somewhat inaudible exclusion is one of the barriers to restorative practices becoming embedded in hospital culture, as treatment has a tendency to do *for* or *to* patients, rather than working *with or alongside* them.

Organisational failures, poor communication, inflexible practice, and struggles with power as they are played out in teams (Stevens, Hulme, & Salmon, 2021) will also impact on the embedding of quality restorative practice (Liebmann, 2007). Discrimination that excludes those with mental disorder from a restorative process on the basis of the additional presence of mental health needs, is another (Drennan et al., 2015). There are of course situations in which people simply do not want communication with a person who has harmed them, or whose position with regard to accountability is inevitably fragile but not impossible to resource with a suitable infrastructure.

Mercer (2006) asked victim-survivors why they preferred *not* to meet their offenders, and heard that too much time had passed since the offence, I prefer to forget it, I was too angry, my mother was too angry, I have support, and I have other priorities. In mental health settings, the fear of not being taken seriously, or of repeat attack by the same/other perpetrator(s) in some form, has also been articulated. The latter may be a particular pressure in institutions where patients/inmates are resident for years, and trauma histories circulate. Dominance and control are often maintained via implicit threat in the stories of incidents told by peers and staff, often with reputational impact (Edgar, O'Donnell, & Martin, 2003).

There are many voices in the arena of recovery from harm that have historically been under-acknowledged for a multiplicity of reasons. The Violence Abuse and Mental Health Network (VAMHN) have poignantly asked: "why is it that victims invariably report shame, in a way that their abusers do not?"; and "how might we work with people who have personal experience of violence, abuse and mental health problems to generate research questions that actually illustrate pathways to resilience?". Julich's (2006) research highlights a common desire amongst victim-survivors of child sexual abuse to be able to tell their story in a safe forum, and certainly to ensure that there are consequences for the offender, but not necessarily punishment. There are individuals with very specific needs (such as those who have both experienced sexual abuse and also perpetrated it, and may experience exclusion as a consequence of both). Adaptive responses to shame-based beliefs can be fostered once (if) shame is expressed and acknowledged.

Judith Herman's work on justice from the victim's perspective (2005) articulates not only the impact of violence (in this study, against women), but also the impact of the legal proceedings that so often have to be endured to secure a conviction. Herman argues that whereas victims need social acknowledgement and support, the court requires them to endure credibility challenges. Whilst they need a chance to tell their stories safely, courts tend to dissect and decontextualise their accounts. The process inevitably over-exposes victims to re-livings of their experience, hence Herman's reference to court as the "theatre of shame". It is known that histories of trauma, sometimes of much depth, both individually and generationally, are likely to be disturbed by interactions with the justice system (Branson, Baetz, Horwitz, & Hoagwood, 2017). All injustices are intersectional: there is limited point in fair and legal process if poverty and racism have restricted the distribution of life and liberty (see Crenshaw, 1991).

Justice as "an Ever-Evolving, Nuanced, and Lived Experience"

In Western (liberal, democratic) culture, justice is sometimes used to equate the length of a prison sentence with recognition of the harm caused by the offending. However, viewing justice from a dichotomous position (the harmer is convicted or not; they are sentenced, or not; guilty or not; the harmed is a victim, or not) does not usefully include the full depth of the victim-survivor perspective. Researchers, who have listened to the survivors of domestic and sexual violence (e.g., Daly & Curtis-Fawley, 2006), highlight victim views that are neither restorative nor retributive, but carry a focus beyond the damage in the immediate relationship, towards repair between the victim and their community, in some cases. It is important to remember that the majority of interpersonal offences are committed by a person known to the victim: partners, lovers, siblings, friends, neighbours, teachers, carers, and religious leaders with whom (typically insecure) attachments have been further ruptured by the harm. No one approach, RJ included, could ever adequately address *all* the needs of victims of crime (Richards, 2009); equally the option for repair should be available to all.

Table 23.2 Different types of justice interests of victim-survivors (McGlynn & Westmarland, 2019; Toews, 2006)

- What are the consequences of offending for the perpetrator? Consequences as justice: let this not happen again (the significance of harm is highlighted)
- How is the harm recognised? Recognition as justice: more than being "believed" or taken seriously by others, recognition brings support and the experience of being acknowledged (there is some attempt to remedy the injury to self-respect)
- How is dignity embodied in the victim-survivor experience? Dignity as justice (dignity can be embodied in social standing and connectedness)
- How can victim-survivors "have a say; speak out"? Voice as justice (active participation in the decisions and directions of justice processes, bearing witness to harm)
- Can this harm be prevented from happening again? Individual justice may be less of a priority than a desire to address underlying causes of crime, Prevention as justice
- In the aftermath of trauma, can a shattered sense of belonging be met/rebuilt with empathy, support, and dignity? Connectedness as justice
- Relationships, safety, empowerment, information, venting, growing, accountability, and meaning are the "justice needs" of people affected by wrongdoing (Toews, 2006)

Based on an empirical investigation of the main justice interests of victim-survivors of a range of offences, including sexual offences, McGlynn and Westmarland (2019) offer a framework of themes that they observe to be "kaleidoscopic". That is, they define a form of justice that has evolved from the process of constant refraction through new experiences or understandings. The most frequently occurring justice interests of victim-survivors elicited in their study through the techniques of Positive Empowerment Approach (EPA) are set out in Table 23.2. Practice-based evidence from restorative practices in prison settings generated a comparable profile of justice needs (Toews, 2006).

From this commitment to justice from the perspective of survivors we can infer the importance of prevention and connectedness as critical in recovery. If these were features of the response to harm, this could begin to undermine the justice gap that failures of the criminal justice system readily generate (Daly, 2016).

Consequences of Injustice: How Can the Impact of Harm Be Addressed?

In the UK we have come a long way from early applications of RJ in the 1970–1980s through to government strategy and endorsement of RJ in youth legislation (Davey, 2005). Consideration is given here to the evidence available that RJ can play a part in current and future Trauma-Informed Forensic Mental Health services in the UK, a more recent strategic development (Drennan & Cooper, 2018; Public Health England, 2021). In both literatures (RJ with/without diagnoses of mental ill-health), there is an acknowledgement that "meaning-making" can be lost in conventional criminal justice systems where the focus is on internalising wrongdoing.

Do we understand why an offence occurred? (Yes; "because this offender is a bad person"?). What will be healing for those affected, even where outcomes include tragedy? ("Keep the risky person away from others, forever if necessary"?). There are many hidden costs in the justice system if such implications are drawn; retributive attitudes sometimes prevail in society (Pycroft & Christen-Schneider, in press) and can undermine access to RJ. In the Netherlands, Zebel and colleagues (2017) studied the seriousness (in terms of perceived wrongfulness, harmfulness, and duration of incarceration) of crimes perpetrated and whether this predicted the engagement in mediated contact between offenders and victims. They found that willingness to participate in victim-offender mediation after very harmful offences did increase over time, whereas it decreased with time where harm had been less impactful.

Sometimes victim-survivors and/or their families urgently require the punishment or safe disposal of an offender. In the UK, the Office of the Victims' Commissioner (2018) highlights the specific needs of families who have been subjected to terrifying offences by those whose judgement is impaired by mental illness, and who may endure the felt and real sense of a lack of ongoing safeguarding and equitable support for their situation. Frequently, victims also seek to understand *why* the offence occurred; why *to them*, and they do have hope that the perpetrator can take some steps towards making amends for all concerned (Donovan & Donovan, 2018).

Harm repair has therefore to be offered as a genuine process for the benefit of victims who suffer with the impact of the harm, with the potential (but no guarantee) for healing (Drennan, 2018). One of the complexities encountered in considering the role of RJ as part of a system of trauma-informed care and practices for mental health is that the majority of offender patients have inhabited both identities: harmed and harmer. Trauma, abuse, and mental health are inter-related (Jonas et al., 2011).

It is known that people with mental disorder are more likely than others to have experienced abuse and to be victimised (Heads, Taylor, & Leese, 1997; Kahlifeh et al., 2015). Those who had experienced psychological abuse suffer the same rates and severity of symptoms (including PTSD) as those who have experienced physical abuse, with a clear implication relating to mental harm and its impact over the lifespan (Pico-Alfonso et al., 2006), in some cases in relation to the harm they have themselves perpetrated (Harry & Resnick, 1986). Additionally, staff in forensic mental health services may be drawn to the work because of the lived experience of trauma in their lives, or then in relation to the impact of facing violence on a regular basis (Jacob & Holmes, 2011; Jacobowitz, 2013).

Not all restorative practices will decrease anger or distress; indeed, a small number of studies have shown the opposite (e.g., Wenmers & Cyr, 2005). As is known from the ever-increasing body of knowledge on trauma, even with the best of intentions, the trauma of harm can be magnified rather than resolved without due care, attention, thought, and preparation. A trauma-informed approach can at least acknowledge the prevalence of trauma on all sides and the importance of creating a sense of safety for those re-exposed through insensitive practices that parallel aspects of offending and re-play loss of control in the person's life (Moore, 2019).

An example from secure hospital practice: when an experienced member of staff was approached about RJ, he exploded with anger expressed at the failures of the system to support him in an impossible role. He had been punched in the face by an articulate patient who had a local frustration (a phone-call with a family member that he found unproductive and reminded him of exclusion and despair). There was no other external provocation for the assault. In turn, this reminded the member of staff of a number of other situations he had faced over a long career in mental health. To make matters worse, he had gone out of his way to assist this patient on that day. His family had been waiting for him to return home from the shift, and this was delayed even further by his having to go to the Accident and Emergency unit for treatment. The break to his nose remains as a visible reminder to this day. About 12 months later, after the patient had sought the opportunity to apologise and to meet, to give an account of his actions, the member of staff stated that he would not want to hear any words of regret about what happened; he would not find them credible. His preference was not to "play the game of RJ". Another six months on, he decided to engineer his own response. The patient and staff member eventually shared their contentment with a resolution fuelled at first by the mutual respect of temporary withdrawal of cooperation on both sides, and thereafter acknowledgement of the potential to harm and the value of genuine, rather than hurried and "false", connection. The member of staff preserved his belief in the importance of his job, a vocation he had committed his life to. The patient learnt that displacement of his anger was not likely to elicit support from those he actually respected, and this shifted his future accountability in a healthier direction. Is there a lack of RJ impact here? Certainly, the process took time and there was no facilitated restorative meeting. Rather, this might be considered a genuinely victim-led process, because the harmed person took control of the timing of his re-setting of the professional alliance – an example of justice with a dignity (Table 23.3) that was very important to both men.

The Application of RJ in Mental Health Settings: Individual and Group Possibilities

The role of the forensic psychiatric hospital is primarily to treat (that is, reduce the risk posed by) those who have committed an offence. Where this is a serious offence (e.g., homicide, assault, other violence), in the context of diagnosable of mental disorder, referral is likely to be a high secure hospital (NHS England, 2019). By virtue of their mental state presentations, cases involving mental illness would be designated as "complex and sensitive" in relation to RJ (van Denderen et al., 2020). Typically, the context in which offenders with mental disorder might reside can present both opportunities (access to RJ) and challenges (e.g., in light of risk, can a meeting progress safely?).

Developments in the South of England within medium secure services have illustrated the range of possibilities for introducing restorative practices, and more fully acknowledge the experience of victims within mental health services (Drennan, in press). In one of the UK's high secure hospitals, the journey towards more restorative

Table 23.3 Principles of RJ practices (after Braithwaite, 2003)

Restoration	Address and repair harm (focus on the future not the past)
Voluntary	Participate at own free will (minimising coercion), accessible
Neutral	Experience fairness and lack of bias
Safe	Non-blaming, non-labelling (very important in Mental Health services)
Trauma-informed	Not compounding of social injury (one on top of another)
Respectful	Maintaining of dignity for all parties
Additional adaptations in mental health settings/for "sensitive" case material: (see Cook et al., 2015; Wild, 2016; Drennan, 2018; Van Denderen et al., 2020; Power, 2017)	
Training	Required to appreciate complexity (i.e., understand trauma) and create the "safe and trusted" context for a restorative process
Preparation	To be more extensive and include review of the seriousness of the offending, the passage of time, mental state stability and risk assessment
Assessed resilience	Of harmers to cope with the experience of re-integrative shaming (ability to hear and accept the impact of harm)
Support	To be offered by the wider system for the process of repair
Co-facilitation	Of RJ meetings, including conferences between RJ facilitators and unit staff
Follow-up	To promote adherence to/review of plans to make adjustments/ allowance for mental state variations

practice started with review of the conflict situations that had led to patients being separated within and across the 210-bed site, and an offer to clinical teams to support restorative mediation to address this. Six years on, the teams can refer patients *and* staff (so frequently the victims of assault, Newman, Roche, & Elliott, 2021) for restorative justice. Some principles underpinning RJ practices and adaptations for complex cases, including cases where mental health/ill-health features, are illustrated in Table 23.3.

By way of example, a member of staff who had been assaulted twice by the same male patient (with an extensive trauma history including of being raised in a country with ongoing civil war, and suffered displacement, discrimination, and abuse) presented his feedback to the RJ team. The harmer (patient X) struggles with persistent paranoid ideas about younger male staff. Sadly, this mental state is enduring. Nevertheless, in spite of this, and after careful preparation, they participated in a restorative meeting, and this quote illustrates some of the gains of the process for the member of staff, the person harmed in this case:

> I wanted to say thank you all for helping me to recover from the incident six months ago. The meeting and support since has helped me to come to a point where me and X [patient] will be working together again; I hope to be able to realise my duty as a professional in helping him to move forwards.

The whole process has helped me to become a better member of staff and I hope to stay here rather than leaving, as I had considered doing at the start of the year.

The impacts on staff of constant exposure to the threat (Jacob & Holmes, 2011), risk, and reality of violence as a secondary traumatisation are more thoroughly addressed in Chapters 20 and 21 of this book.

The need is acknowledged for staff undertaking RJ in mental health settings to be supported by managers and multi-disciplinary teams, and to allow time for the organisation, training, and procedural plans to be operationalised. This way those most familiar with the patient's hopes and intentions can be involved and advocate where required. In the prison system, the benefit of strong resident/officer relationships is critical to the maintenance of stable prisons and building trust, a critical component in rehabilitation (Liebling, Arnold & Straub, 2015). Similarly, for restorative practices to take hold in any institutional setting, the constructive engagement of the wider context providing a network of support has seemed instrumental for RJ casework (Cook, Drennan, & Callanan, 2015; Moore & Dudley, 2016; Cook, 2019; Tapp, Moore, Stephenson, & Cull, 2020). The same is true for the development of restorative wards (Cooper & Whittingham, in press), where conflict resolution becomes part of community life for residents.

There are limitations here with a literature base in early development: more rigorous formal evaluation is required. It is possible that positive feedback about RJ may be the result of a reporting bias in these studies because "cases" are not randomly selected to participate in the process, but referred on the basis of the presence of need. At this time only qualitative data on referrals that do not take hold because one or other party dismisses them out of hand from the outset is available. However, we can draw on trauma-informed principles to make sense of the (sometimes necessary and protective) shield of avoidance and its origins in intolerable experiences (Tomkins, 1987). This perspective supports a compassionate working understanding of (otherwise) complex and often counter-intuitive responses.

The Application of RJ to Index Offence Referrals

Index offences are those that precede an admission to a mental health hospital or unit. Offending that occurs in the context of mental disorder can be very confusing and distressing for victims, their relatives, and the perpetrators and their relatives (Cook et al., 2015). To address the possible needs of the harmer and harmed in this situation requires a team-based approach and the structure of the RJ process to support and sponsor safety through potentially highly evocative encounters. In their research with offender patients in the Netherlands, van Denderen and colleagues (2020) found that mental stability (in the presence of a diagnosis of psychotic disorder) and realistic expectations about what victim-offender-contact would be likely to involve were associated with better outcomes for RJ conferences in which the harmed and harmers actually met face to face. The research team speculated that insight into the harm generated by offending (and forgiveness by victims) did not necessarily impact recidivism or treatment goals, but was associated with higher engagement (including in RJ) and demonstrable therapeutic change.

Category of mental disorder was not predictive of engagement in the process, but it was acknowledged that capacity for communication was helpful, as was the management of the victim-offender liaison. This is important, as Willis and Hoyle (2019) found that socioeconomically disadvantaged offenders appeared more likely to experience communication difficulties, and were less likely to be perceived by third parties as sincere or willing to desist from offending. In their research, social disadvantage and street cultural capital emerged as impactful in relation to participation in RJ processes (Willis & Hoyle, 2019).

Working on the index offence, if all (or possibly some) parties are willing, presents inter-agency challenges that can be addressed by partnership alliances. RJ interventions of this kind require that all those involved (staff, patients, participants, other stakeholders) are familiar with how the RJ process will interact with concurrent/future criminal justice processes. RJ is not an alternative to prosecution/conviction, but it can be an opportunity to potentially reduce the impact of high distress and the longstanding pain of unresolved harm and trauma.

From the perspective of both the perpetrator of harm and the harmed person/people, restorative work may assist in emboldening the narrative about the harm and its impact in a way that can address unanswered questions, rumination, and/or other preoccupations associated with it. Even if there cannot be a meeting (in some instances due to death), justice work can support the process of "closure" in situations where narratives are incomplete, unprocessed, and recur/re-appear in the form of nightmares, flashbacks, avoidance, and/or self-harm. Unmet "justice needs" (Daly, 2014) generate unfinished stories, and yet "meaning making" is a critical part of the journey in the direction of recovery from trauma and making meaning of life after loss (Ferrito, Needs, & Adshead, 2016).

The Application of RJ in Mental Health Settings: System-Wide Implications

Shifting the culture of the organisation towards fairness in responding to the risk of harm is a wider aim that is informed by the drive to prioritise safety in healthcare systems. Clear indications as to what are acceptable (safe) and unacceptable (risky) behaviours can be articulated for residents/patients and staff. So-called "just cultures" are fostered by mechanisms promoting awareness, not just an emphasis on liability, wherein contributors ideally learn and develop in an atmosphere of trust (Stretton, 2020). The focus on improvement is assumed to be helpful in raising performance rather than establishing causality (and blame). These principles have resonance in the wider literature on restoration. Just cultures highlight the humanity that trauma-informed practice draws attention to. Practitioners faced with daily encounters that will inevitably impact on their decision-making under pressure in the workplace, or foster omissions in care, are sometimes placed under unique occupational pressures. Repeatedly facing the threat of violence is a good example of such a challenge.

Restorative Foundations for Trauma-Informed Health Systems

Research repeatedly demonstrates the known association between trauma, a major risk factor for illness, and the development of mental ill-health and offending behaviour. Historically the criminal justice system has ignored the problem of unhealed trauma (Pycroft & Christen-Schneider, in press). Preliminary findings about the application of RJ principles in situation of harm of many kinds are promising. Where mental health services work restoratively they find that their relationships are stronger, there is a significant reduction in violence on wards, victims are engaged in the service more meaningfully, and elements of the service are able to engage with conflict and repair broken relationships in a hopeful way (Cook et al., 2015; Cooper & Whittingham, in press). The fostering of empathy between people with a history of harm enables everyone's gifts to contribute to the co-production of responses to harm.

Restorative practices create spaces for listening, for trust-building, reparation, and apology – places in which harming and harmed parties find a new strength to co-exist. Violence is (sometimes) what we do with suffering when we do not know what else to do (Russell, 2020). RJ offers the opportunity to reintegrate *both/all sides* (staff and patients, patients and patient peers, staff and staff peers, the organisation and its stakeholders) into communities that might be able to consider (historical and transgenerational) root causes, and the possibility of a valued life thereafter, in spite of the path of destruction that trauma has engraved. Along with other principles of empowerment, RJ invites us to ask of the harmed and harmer, not "what's wrong?", but "what's strong?", and to support institutions to avoid sustaining the very problems they believe they are solving (Russell, 2020).

Further Reading

Wallis, J. (2014). *Understanding restorative justice: How empathy can close the gap created by crime.* Policy Press. For readers interested in the relationship between empathy, responsibility, shame, forgiveness, and closure. This text explores the journey from harm to healing with compassion and provides a summary for those new to restorative practices.

References

Angel, C. M., Sherman, L. W., Strang, H., Ariel, B., Bennett, S., Inkpen, N., ... & Richmond, T. (2014). Short-term effects of restorative justice conferences on post-traumatic stress symptoms among twelve experiments in restorative justice: The Jerry Lee program 535 robbery and burglary victims: A randomised, controlled trial. *Journal of Experimental Criminology, 10,* 291–307. doi:10.1037/t12199-000

Bonta, J., Wallace-Capretta, S., Rooney, J., & McAnoy, K. (2002). An outcome evaluation of a restorative justice alternative to incarceration. *Contemporary Justice Review, 5*(4), 319–338. doi:10.1080/10282580214772

Braithwaite, J. (2002). *Restorative justice & responsive regulation.* London: Oxford University Press.

Braithwaite, J. (2003). Reintegrative shaming. In P. Bean (Ed.), *Crime: Critical concepts in sociology* (pp. 345–361). Routledge.

Braithwaite, J. (2006). Accountability and responsibility through restorative justice. In M. Dowdle (Ed.), *Public accountability: Designs, dilemmas and experiences* (pp.33–51). Cambridge University Press.

Brännström, L., Kaunitz, C., Andershed, A. K., South, S., & Smedslund, G. (2016). Aggression replacement training (ART) for reducing antisocial behavior in adolescents and adults: A systematic review. *Aggression and Violent Behavior, 27*, 30–41. doi:10.1016/j.avb.2016.02.006

Branson, C. E., Baetz, C. L., Horwitz, S. M., & Hoagwood, K. E. (2017). Trauma-informed juvenile justice systems: A systematic review of definitions and core components. *Psychological Trauma: Theory, Research, Practice, and Policy, 9*(6), 635–646. doi:10.1037/tra0000255

Burkemper, B., & Balsam, N. (2007). Examining the use of restorative justice practices in domestic violence cases. *Saint Louis University Public Law Review, 27*, 121–134.

Calkin, C. (2021). An exploratory study of understanding and experiences of implementing restorative practice in three UK prisons. *British Journal of Community Justice, 17*(1), 92–111.

Cook, A. (2019). Restorative practice in a forensic mental health service: Three case studies. *Journal of Forensic Psychiatry & Psychology, 30* (5), 876–893. doi:10.1080/14789949.2019.1637919

Cook, A., Drennan, G., & Callanan, M. M. (2015). A qualitative exploration of the experience of restorative approaches in a forensic mental health setting. *The Journal of Forensic Psychiatry & Psychology, 26*(4), 510–531. doi:10.1080/14789949.2015.1034753

Cooper, S. L., & Whittingham, L. (In press). Victimisation experiences of individuals with autism spectrum disorders and restorative practice approaches to repairing harm. In N. Tyler & A. Sheeran (Eds), *People with autism in the criminal justice and forensic mental health system: A handbook for practitioners*. London: Routledge.

Crenshaw, K. (1991). Race, gender, and sexual harassment. *Southern California. Law Review, 65*, 1467–1476.

Daly, K. (2014). Reconceptualizing sexual victimization and justice. In I. Vanfraechem, A. Pemberton, & F. Ndahinda (Eds), *Justice for victims: Perspectives on rights, transition and Reconciliation* (pp.378–394). Routledge.

Daly, K. (2016). What is restorative justice? Fresh answers to a vexed question. *Victims & Offenders, 11*(1), 9–29. doi:10.1080/15564886.2015.1107777

Daly, K., & Curtis-Fawley, S. (2006). Restorative justice for victims of sexual assault. In K. Heimer & C. Kruttschnitt (Eds), *Gender and crime: Patterns of victimization and offending* (pp.231–265). New York University Press.

Dandurand, Y., & Vogt, A. (2020). *Handbook on restorative justice programmes. 2nd edition: Criminal justice handbook series*. United Nations Office on Drugs & Crime. United Nations.

Davey, L. (2005). The development of restorative justice in the UK: A personal perspective. Building a global alliance for restorative practices and family empowerment, part 3. IIRP's Sixth International Conference on Conferencing, Circles and other Restorative Practices, March 3-5, 2005, Penrith, New South Wales, Australia.

Dhami, M. K., Mantle, G., & Fox, D. (2009). Restorative justice in prisons. *Contemporary Justice Review, 12* (4), 433–448. doi:10.1080/10282580903343027

Donovan, R., & Donovan, V. (2018). *Restored and forgiven: The power of restorative justice*. Bridge-logos Inc.

Drennan, G. (2018). Restorative justice applications in mental health settings – Pathways to recovery and restitution. In J. Adlam, T. Kluttig, & X. B. Lee (Eds). *Violent states and creative states: From the global to the individual. Book II: Human violence and creative humanity* (pp.181–194). Jessica Kingsley Publishers.

Drennan, G. (In press). *Restorative justice practice in mental health settings: Minding the gap*.

Drennan, G., Cook, A., & Kiernan, H. (2015). The psychology of restorative practice in forensic mental health recovery. In T. Gavrielides (Ed.), *The psychology of restorative justice. Managing the power within* (pp. 105–120). Routledge. doi:10.4324/9781315553788

Drennan, G., & Cooper, S. (2018). Restorative practice in mental health – gathering momentum. *Restorative Justice Council, Resolution, 63*, 12–13.

Edgar, K., O'Donnell, I., & Martin, C. (2003). *Prison violence: The dynamics of conflict, fear and power.* Willan.

Ferrito, M., Needs, A., & Adshead, G. (2016). Unveiling the shadows of meaning: Meaning-making for perpetrators of homicide. *Aggression & Violent Behaviour, 34,* 263–272. doi:10.1016/j.avb.2016.11.009

Fox, B. H., Perez, N., Cass, E., Baglivio, M. T., & Epps, N. (2015). Trauma changes everything: Examining the relationship between adverse childhood experiences and serious, violent and chronic juvenile offenders. *Child Abuse & Neglect, 46,* 163–173. doi:10.1016/j.chiabu.2015.01.011

Goodmark, L. (2015). Law and justice are not always the same: Creating community-based justice forums for people subjected to intimate partner abuse. *Florida State University Law Review, 42,* 707.

Harry, B., & Resnick, P. J. (1986). Post-traumatic stress disorder in murderers. *Journal of Forensic Sciences, 31*(2), 609–613.

Heads, T., Taylor, P., & Leese, M. (1997). Childhood experiences of patients with schizophrenia and a history of violence: A special hospital sample. *Criminal Behavior & Mental Health, 7,* 117–130. doi:10.1002/cbm.157

Herman, J. (2005). Justice from the victim's perspective. *Violence Against Women, 11,* 571–602. doi:10.1177%2F1077801205274450

Ireland, J. L. (2007). Introducing a new violence treatment programme: Life Minus Violence. *Forensic Update, 90,* 50–56.

Jacob, J., & Holmes, D. (2011) Working under threat: Fear and nurse–patient interactions in a forensic psychiatric setting. *Journal of Forensic Nursing, 7*(2), 68–77. doi:10.1111/j.1939-3938.2011.01101.x

Jacobowitz, W. (2013). PTSD in psychiatric nurses and other mental health providers: A review of the literature. *Issues in Mental Health Nursing, 34*(11), 787–795. doi:10.3109/01612840.2013.824053

Jonas, S., Bebbington, P., McManus, S., Meltzer, H., Jenkins, R., Kuipers, E., ... & Brugha, T. (2011). Sexual abuse and psychiatric disorder in England: Results from the 2007 Adult Psychiatric Morbidity Survey. *Psychological Medicine, 41*(4), 709–719. doi:10.1017/S003329171000111X

Julich, S. (2006). View of justice among survivors of historical child sexual abuse. *Theoretical Criminology, 10,* 125–138. doi:10.1177%2F1362480606059988

Kahlifeh, H., Moran, P., Borschmann, R., Dean, K., Hart, C., Hogg, J., ... & Howard, L.M. (2015). Domestic and sexual violence against patients with severe mental illness. *Psychological Medicine, 45*(4), 875–886. doi:10.1017/s0033291714001962

Latimer, J., Dowden, C., & Muise, D. (2005). The effectiveness of restorative justice practices: A meta-analysis. *The Prison Journal, 85,* 127–144. doi:10.1177/0032885505276969

Liebling, A., Arnold, H., Straub, C. (2015). Prisons research beyond the conventional: Dialogue, 'creating miracles' and staying sane in a maximum-security prison. In D. H. Drake, R. Earle, & J. Sloan (Eds), *The Palgrave handbook of prison ethnography. Palgrave studies in prisons and penology* (pp.56–80). Palgrave Macmillan. doi:10.1057/9781137403889_4

Liebmann, M. (2007). *Restorative justice: How it works.* Jessica Kingsley Publishers.

Lloyd, A., & Borrill, J. (2020). Examining the effect of restorative justice in reducing victims' post-traumatic stress. *Psychological Injury & Law, 13,* 77–89. doi:10.1007/s12207-019-09363-9

McCold, P. (2003). A survey of assessment research on mediation and conferencing. In L. Walgrave (Ed). *Repositioning restorative justice* (pp.67–116). Willan.

McGlynn, C., & Westmarland, N. (2019). Kaleidoscopic justice: Sexual violence and victim-survivors' perceptions of justice. *Social & Legal Studies, 28*(2), 179–201. doi:10.1177%2F0964663918761200

McKenna, G., Jackson, N., & Browne, C. (2019). Trauma history in a high secure male forensic inpatient population. *International Journal of Law & Psychiatry, 66,* 101475. doi:10.1016/j.ijlp.2019.101475

Mercer, V. (2006). *The Manchester adult restorative justice project: Evaluation 2005-6.* Greater Manchester Youth Justice Trust.

Miers, D. (2001). *An international review of restorative justice.* London: Home Office.

Moore, E. (2019). *Treating trauma for public safety: The contribution of psychological support for patients in high security hospitals.* Retrieved from www.bacp.co.uk/bacp-journals/healthcare-counselling-and-psychotherapy-journal/october-2019/treating-trauma-for-public-safety/

Moore, E., & Dudley, A. (2016). Broadmoor Hospital's restorative journey. *Resolution, 57.*

Nathanson, D. L. (1994). *Shame and pride: Affect, sex, and the birth of the self.* WW Norton & Company.

Newman, C., Roche, M., & Elliott, D. (2021). Exposure to workplace trauma for forensic mental health nurses: A scoping review. *International Journal of Nursing Studies, 117,* 103897. doi:10.1016/j.ijnurstu.2021.103897

NHS England. (2019). *NHS long term plan implementation framework.* NHS England.

Office of the Victims' Commissioner. (2018). *Entitlements and experiences of victims of mentally disordered offenders.* Retrieved from https://s3-eu-west-2.amazonaws.com/victcomm2-prod-storage-119w3o4kq2z48/uploads/2018/10/VC-Victims-of-Mentally-Disordered-Offenders-Review-2018.pdf. Accessed 19 March, 2019.

Oudshoorn, J. (2015). Trauma-informed rehabilitation and restorative justice. In T. Gavrielides (Ed.), *The psychology of restorative justice. Managing the power within* (pp.181–204). Routledge.

Oudshoorn, J. (2016). *Trauma-informed juvenile justice in the United States.* CSPI.

Pico-Alfonso, M., Garcia-Linares, M., Celda-Navarro, N., Blasco-Ros, C., Echeburúa, E., & Martinez, M. (2006). The impact of physical, psychological, and sexual intimate male partner violence on women's mental health: Depressive symptoms, posttraumatic stress disorder, state anxiety, and suicide. *Journal of Women's Health, 15*(5), 599–611. doi:10.1089/jwh.2006.15.599

Power, M. (2017). *International innovations in restorative justice in mental health – next steps for Australia.* Retrieved from: www.griffith.ed.ac/_data/assets/pdf_file/0019/107443/Michael-Power-Churchil-Fellowship-Restorative-Approaches-in-Mental -Health-V2.pdf

Public Health England. (2021). *The effectiveness of trauma informed approaches to prevent adverse outcomes in mental health and wellbeing: A rapid review.* PHE Publications.

Pycroft, A., & Christen-Schneider, C. (In press). An exploration of trauma-informed practices in restorative justice: A phenomenological study. *International Journal of Restorative Justice.*

Richards, K. (2009). Taking victims seriously? The role of victims' rights movements in the emergence of restorative justice. *Current Issues in Criminal Justice, 21*(2), 302–320. doi:10.1080/10345329.2009.12035847

Russell, C. (2020). *Rekindling democracy: A professional's guide to working in citizen space.* Cascade Books.

Sherman, L.W., & Strang, H. (2007). *Restorative justice: The evidence.* London: Smith Institute.

Stevens, E.L., Hulme, A., & Salmon, P.M. (2021). The impact of power on health care team performance and patient safety: A review of the literature. *Ergonomics, 64*(8), 1072–1090. doi:10.1080/00140139.2021.1906454

Stretton, P. (2020) The 'just culture': Why it is not just, and how it could be. *British Journal of Healthcare Management.* doi:10.12968/bjhc.2020.0058

Tapp, J., Moore, E., Stephenson, M., & Cull, D. (2020). "The image has been changed in my mind": A case of restorative justice in a forensic mental health setting. *Journal of Forensic Practice, 22*(4), 213–222. doi:10.1108/JFP-05-2020-0023

Toews, B. (2006). *The little book of restorative justice for people in prison: Rebuilding the web of relationships.* Good Books.

Toews, B. (2018). 'It's a dead place: A qualitative exploration of violence survivors' perceptions of justice architecture. *Issues in Criminal, Social and Restorative Justice, 21* (2), 208–222. doi:10.1080/10282580.2018.1455511

Tomkins, S. (1987). Shame. In D. L. Nathanson (Ed.). *The many faces of shame* (pp. 133–161). Norton.

Umbreit, M. S.,Vos, B., & Coates, R. B. (2006). *Restorative justice dialogue: Evidence-based practice.* St. Paul, MN: Center for Restorative Justice and Peacemaking. Retrieved from http://rjp. umn.edu/img/assets/13522RJ_Dialogue_Evidence-based_Practice_1-06.pdf

van Denderen, M.,Verstegen, N., de Vogel,V., & Feringa, L. (2020). Contact between victims and offenders in forensic mental health settings:An exploratory study. *International Journal of Law and Psychiatry, 73,* 101630. doi:10.1016/j.ijlp.2020.101630

Van Ness, D.W. (2007). Prisons and restorative justice. In G. Johnstone & D.W.Van Ness D. (Eds), *Handbook of restorative justice* (pp.312–324).Willan Publishing.

Walters, M.A. (2015).'I Thought "He's a Monster"… [But] He Was Just… Normal' examining the therapeutic benefits of restorative justice for homicide. *British Journal of Criminology, 55*(6), 1207–1225. doi:10.1093/bjc/azv026

Ward, T., Fox, K. J., & Garber, M. (2014). Restorative justice, offender rehabilitation and desistance. *Restorative Justice, 2*(1), pp. 24–42. doi:10.5235/20504721.2.1.24

Wenmers, J., & Cyr, K. (2005). Can mediation be therapeutic for crime victims? An evaluation of victims' experiences in mediation with young offenders. *Canadian Journal of Criminology and Criminal Justice, 47,* 527–544. doi:10.3138/cjccj.47.3.527

Wenzel, M., Okimoto,T., Feather N.T., & Platow, M. (2007). Retributive and restorative justice. *Law & Human Behaviour, 32*(5), 275–389. doi:10.1007/s10979-007-9116-6

West, C. (2015). *Justice for the future.* Keynote speech:The 5th National Association of Community and Restorative Justice.

Whiting, D., Ryland, H., & Fazel, S. (2020). Forensic mental health treatment and recidivism. In F. Focquaert, E. Shaw, & B. N.Waller (Eds), *The Routledge handbook of the philosophy and science of punishment.* Routledge, 2021. doi:10.4324/9780429507212

Wild, C. (2016). *Can Restorative Justice be effective with victims and offenders with a mental disorder? A note on challenges, development and outcomes.* Unpublished manuscript.

Willis R., & Hoyle C. (2019). The good, the bad, and the street: Does 'street culture' affect offender communication and reception in restorative justice? *European Journal of Criminology.* November. doi:10.1177/1477370819887517

Wood, W. R., & Suzuki, M. (2016). Four challenges in the future of restorative justice. *Victims & Offenders, 11*(1), 149–172. doi:10.1080/15564886.2016.1145610

Zebel, S., Schreurs,W., & Ufkes, E. G. (2017). Crime seriousness and participation in restorative justice:The role of time elapsed since the offense. *Law and Human Behavior, 41*(4), 385–397. doi:10.1037/lhb0000242

Zehr, H. (2020). *The little book of Restorative Justice.* Goodbooks: USA ISBN: 978-1-56148-376-1

24

THE FUTURE OF TRAUMA-INFORMED FORENSIC PRACTICE

Lawrence Jones and Phil Willmot

In the introduction to this book, we wrote about trauma as a new paradigm in forensic practice. Many contributors to this book have pointed out that the idea that early trauma is an important precursor to many chronic physical and mental health problems has been around a long time. However, the idea that it might be important to consider trauma in forensic settings has yet to catch on widely. This book points at some of the systemic barriers that stand in its way: social attitudes and a criminal justice system that stigmatise offenders and prioritise retribution and punishment over rehabilitation or restoration; a penal system that is underfunded and unable to prioritise therapy when it is often desperately fighting to maintain order and control in prisons; a forensic mental health system that is built around a diagnostic framework that scarcely recognises the importance of trauma. To this list we might add managers, policy makers, academics, and clinicians may struggle to understand or empathise with the clients we serve because our lived experiences are so far removed from theirs.

This is not a new or a unique situation. In 1992, 359 years after Galileo was forced by the inquisition to recant his belief that the earth moved round the sun, Pope John Paul II issued a public apology for his treatment (Montalbano, 1992), though in fairness to the Catholic Church, they had removed the ban on Galileo's teaching as early as 1835 (Heilbron, 2005), 202 years after his trial. These facts perhaps illustrate an important truth about paradigm shifts – that the paradigms that individuals and groups choose are determined not only by the available data, but by their beliefs, values, vested interests, inertia and fear of change, and by unwillingness to admit being wrong.

Before condemning the Roman Catholic Church for their choices, we should perhaps all reflect on the factors that influence our adoption or rejection of a trauma-informed worldview. How much is it due to the weight of research evidence we have been exposed to, and how much to the fact that trauma-informed care fits or clashes

DOI: 10.4324/9781003120766-30

with our social and political worldview; or to professional or personal allegiances; or to the fact that it represents a radical new way of thinking about forensic practice, which may be either exciting or threatening? Reflecting on the factors that influence our own choice of paradigms can help us to consider what might influence the choices of those we wish to persuade. That is not to say that we should behave in a deceptive or manipulative manner, but rather that we should use arguments that connect with and matter to those we seek to persuade, rather than trying to beat them down with sheer weight of data. The areas of dissent we highlighted in the introduction relating to the possible negative perceptions of being seen as "traumatised", stigmatised, robbed of a valorised diagnosis, or of demeaning medics or mothers, all need to be appreciated and worked with. Had Galileo appreciated that, he would have seen that no amount of solid scientific data would have persuaded an organisation that believed the bible to be the inerrant word of God. So, what can we do if we are to avoid waiting centuries for the trauma paradigm to become mainstream?

Connect with Groups Who Share the Same Values and Goals

It is relatively easy to ignore or dismiss arguments for change when they come from a narrow group of individuals or professions who can easily be dismissed as unimportant or as trying to further their own agenda. It is much harder to ignore those arguments when they come from many different quarters. We should therefore build connections with people and groups who share the same goals.

Connect with Service Users

The voices of service users have rarely been heard in forensic research or policy making. Where we have been able to include them in this volume, we believe that they have provided an important and powerful illustration not only of the need for a trauma-informed approach to their care, but of the inadequacy and failure of approaches that have not been trauma-informed. Service users represent a vast, largely untapped, source of knowledge about the causes of offending and how to tackle it.

Forensic and mental health research have tended to privilege quantitative methods, especially large-scale, complex randomised control trials and meta-analyses that are beyond the means or expertise of most scientist practitioners, and which inadvertently perpetuate a notion of offenders as a faceless homogenous mass, rather than as unique individuals. However, small-scale qualitative studies or single case studies based on the lived experience of clients are far more achievable and help to give voice to the people we work with and to present them as real and human.

Case studies can take a range of different forms. Personal narratives of people who have been through an experience of change are a good example of this. If we look at the history of interventions that have ended up having a significant amount of evidence to support their efficacy, it is clear that many of these were developed by practitioners who were applying techniques that they were using to deal with their own problems. Linehan and Shapiro describe developing DBT and EMDR respectively, based on their own experiences and insights.

Case studies narrated by practitioners are also invaluable and can be seen as one means whereby service users lived experience of what works can be passed on from one service user to others. Looked at in this way it can be seen as a responsibility of practitioners to collate and pass on what works to the community of service users; in this respect they are in a privileged position of hearing multiple narratives of different people engaged in change processes.

Connect with Minorities and Advocacy Groups

Forensic psychology has previously had very little to say to marginalised groups who are over-represented in forensic systems, such as people of colour, veterans, or those with intellectual disabilities. As contributors to this book have demonstrated, a trauma-informed approach provides a framework for considering these and other aspects of diversity and individual difference. It should encourage us to work more closely with diverse groups and those who advocate for them, to better understand the particular impact that trauma has on them. This in turn should enable those groups to have more of a voice in shaping policy and practice.

Connect with Colleagues

While forensic services ought to provide a safe haven, all too often they can be dangerous, traumatising, and retraumatising, not just for service users, but also for colleagues. As contributors to this book have demonstrated, effective trauma-informed culture and practice should improve staff morale and job satisfaction, and reduce sickness and turnover, and that is something that service managers and trade unions should welcome.

Connect with Other Fields

When it comes to trauma-informed practice, forensic services are an outlier. Education, social care, and mental health services have all adopted trauma-informed practice. We do not need to "reinvent the wheel" where we can adopt what other agencies are already doing.

Look Beyond Scientific Data for Arguments

We write this as Europe and North America are, hopefully, emerging from the effects of the COVID pandemic. Reviewing public discourse over the last 18 months about the virus, the focus has perhaps shifted the science of virology and epidemiology to arguments about the economic and social impact of different policies and debates about the balance between personal responsibility and personal freedom. So it is with many areas of debate, and perhaps particularly in the areas of crime and justice; it is difficult to limit discussion to the scientific issues when economic, social, and moral arguments often carry more weight. We should be prepared for this and develop a wider range of arguments.

Develop the Economic Arguments

Even if there was not an overwhelming moral argument for investing in education and children's services to prevent childhood trauma, there is a powerful economic argument for investing in preventing abuse and maltreatment in children under ten, rather than trying to treat them once they reach prison or hospital. The current cost of keeping one person in prison for a year is over £40,000 (Ministry of Justice, 2020). The same amount would fund approximately 100 Sure Start places for children from the most deprived communities (Cattan, Conti, Farquarson, & Ginja, 2019).

Develop the Moral Arguments

There needs to be more discussion about the ethics of incarcerating trauma survivors in institutions that are retraumatising (Jones, 2015). The youth justice system has been dealing with this question for some time now and has made significant progress in reducing the number of incarcerated young people by identifying those young people it sees as vulnerable who can and should be diverted from the damaging effects of incarceration.

We also need to consider how best to communicate ideas of trauma-informed justice in wider society. It is perhaps easier to have that discussion in relation to some groups – young people, veterans, women – than others.

Develop a Research Agenda

We have argued that paradigm change requires more than empirical evidence to drive it. However, it very much also needs empirical evidence. A number of areas suggest themselves.

Perhaps one of the most pressing questions is to clarify what we mean by trauma, or by "criminogenic trauma" that increases the likelihood of a trajectory into offending. We know that childhood maltreatment is widespread, as is adversity in later life. Since persistent and serious offenders form a small minority of the population, it seems safe to conclude that not all adversity leads to criminality. This book has pointed to some of the features of "criminogenic trauma" – abuse or maltreatment that is chronic and pervasive, that seriously undermines the survivor's ability to feel safe or to trust the people or institutions around them. However, this is probably not a complete or final definition and it will be important to develop a more complete understanding of the factors that make trauma or adversity more likely to be criminogenic. Although not intended, the accounts of service users from a variety of backgrounds and services in this book are remarkably consistent in reflecting a pattern of chronic and pervasive threat and unpredictability that they link to their offending. Qualitative data reflecting the lived experiences of service users will provide a rich source of data that can help us to identify the features of criminogenic trauma.

To access these narratives, we need to develop more sophisticated ways of overcoming or working with the natural self-protective reluctance or denial of trauma narratives particularly among people who have not worked on these experiences as part of an intervention aimed at offsetting the impact of these experiences. Most of the narratives in this book were obtained by clinicians who had developed a trusting safe relationship and who had made an informed judgement about whether the process of disclosure and exploration would not trigger any response that could not be contained by the individual doing the disclosing.

While this book has highlighted some of the limitations of the current paradigm, that paradigm is based on a massive body of data and research. A trauma-informed approach is likely to add to the existing research rather than replacing it. As discussed in Chapter 1, clarifying the processes by which trauma contributes to established criminogenic needs should help to elucidate the features of criminogenic trauma and how to mitigate its effects.

Evaluation must be central to trauma-informed practice if we are to know whether it is effective. While it is more difficult in the short or medium term to evaluate the effectiveness of trauma-informed cultures on recidivism, it is easier to evaluate the impact on workforce outcomes such as job satisfaction or staff turnover.

Elaborating Our Understanding of Psychological Processes Linked with Trauma and Offending

The need for a more sophisticated approach to the ways in which people respond to different kinds of trauma is another area for growth in the future. As we have seen in this volume, a range of different ways of thinking about developmental processes in the backgrounds of people who have offended have been described. Future exploration might attempt to clarify the different kinds of adversity that people can experience and the processes that are linked with this. An interesting attempt to begin this kind of thinking is offered by Brown (1992) who – way ahead of her time – developed a typology of abusive and oppressive experiences (a typology of "what happens to people") and reactions to these as an alternative to diagnosis.

This work might usefully look at a wider range of difficult or traumatic experiences.

Racism

While in this volume a number of contributors have attended to issues around racism, this is an area that has been grossly neglected by those working with trauma historically (Quiros, Varghese, & Vanidestine, 2020) and is much in need of research, responsive changes in practice consciousness raising and exploration. Constructs like microaggressions (Sue, 2010) are a result of recent attempts to articulate the impacts of racism and need to be developed and explored clinically and academically. It feels as if this is an area that has only recently begun to attract attention and the more one looks at it, the more shocking the clinical and academic neglect of this area becomes. Why have we not been openly discussing and exploring ways of addressing systemic racism in the criminal justice system, and indeed in ourselves as practitioners? This is a challenging area for us and needs to be kept on the table going forward, not allowed to drift into the background and be conveniently ignored or denied. The tendency for ways of seeing to "come and go", much as fashions do, militates against changes in this area becoming embedded.

The fact that many of the statistical tests developed by psychologists were developed in the context of people working on eugenic agendas (Ellis, 2021) is a clarion call to psychologists to think carefully about what we mean by "norms" and how we apply the idea that a population can be characterised using norms. It is critical that as forensic practitioners we do not become complicit in perpetuating racism. Indeed, Ellis reminds us that the misuse of psychology in forensic contexts historically creates an imperative for us to look long and hard at our own practices across the board.

Sexism

The Power Threat Meaning Framework (Johnstone & Boyle et al., 2018) highlights a range of power-related processes that impact adversely on people. This work, along with feminist thinkers like Brown (1992, 2017), points towards the importance of developing a more nuanced understanding of the harmful impacts of patriarchy on women and – in a different and less harmful way, as men are also the beneficiaries of patriarchy – on men who get caught up in behaving in oppressive ways towards women and each other. Several contributions have explored some aspects of the harm caused by different ways of doing masculinity.

Homophobia

There is little literature on Lesbian, Gay, Bisexual, Trans-sexual, and Questioning – and the wider array of sexualities and identities being discussed in the literature – people who have offended, exploring the possible contributions of processes such as homophobia, biphobia, and transphobia on the developmental processes that resulted in them offending, as well as the ways in which these impact on their mental health. Graziano and Wagner (2016) bemoan the lack of research on trauma in this group among people who have been incarcerated. This, again, is a significant gap in the literature that needs to be addressed.

Ableism

Chapter 6 of this book highlights also the adverse impacts of trauma on people with intellectual disabilities. The adverse impacts of stigma and negative or patronising responses to people with intellectual disabilities has not been adequately researched. This is also true for people from the d/Deaf community, as Chapter 7 reminds us.

The Francis report (2013) highlighted the plight of many people with intellectual disabilities in institutional settings, pointing up their vulnerability to exploitation and systemic abuse. The under-recognised and under-reported abuse that can be systemic and culturally embedded in organisations of all kinds working with people without a voice, or for whom having a voice is problematic, means that huge amounts of abuse go unrecognised and are met with silence. This silence is as true of people who have offended in these contexts as it is of those who have not. This too is an area requiring attention going forward.

Trauma Among Older People Who Have Offended

The age profile of people in prisons includes a significant number of elderly people. The different ways in which trauma impacts on older people and the different kinds of experience associated with different historical epochs are ill understood. In addition, the ways in which trauma experiences accumulate over the life course and the changing trauma response in relation to this needs to be considered. Older people also offer the opportunity to explore the processes of desistance and turning points towards and away from offending, and this links with trauma.

Existential Trauma

It is not unusual for practitioners to explore difficult issues such as sexuality and violence with people caught up in forensic services. It is however much more unusual to hear about practitioners discussing mortality and people's beliefs about mortality and the ways in which these feelings and beliefs impact on the individual's lives and lifestyles. Mortality is a major theme in everybody's lives, and the way in which it is understood – or indeed avoided – can have a very significant impact on the ways in which an individual lives their life. Existential psychotherapies – e.g., Yalom (2011) – attempt to explore these issues, as do different cultural and religious approaches. There is much work to be done in exploring and understanding cultural and personal ways of living with mortality and how these can contribute to the development of offending and mental health difficulties. Kerig and Becker (2010) describe a process that they term *futurelessness*, whereby an individual who has experienced trauma begins to act as if they are not going to have a future and therefore "lives for the moment" and does not invest in a possible life in the future. This is one example of an existential position in relation to mortality linked with the intense experience of lack of safety associated with other kinds of trauma.

Other related existential traumas include the ways in which people do not choose a whole array of aspects of their lives, e.g., having a body, having feelings, being a particular gender, being born in particular circumstances. This experience of being thrown, as it were, into a world without any sense of choice is also troubling and difficult for people to cope with. This also can impact on an individual's decisions about what is important for them to prioritise in their lives.

Different Trauma Processes Evolving in the Context of Different Temperaments and Neurodiversity

The way in which an individual responds to a traumatic experience is unique to them. This unique response is shaped by other experiences (e.g., the protective impact of attachment and social capital) but also plays out differently for people of different personality traits or neurodiverse presentations such as autistic spectrum traits (e.g., Westphal, 2016). Dell'Osso et al. (2018), for example, found among patients with a diagnosis of borderline personality disorder that there was a higher incidence of subthreshold autistic spectrum traits and these were linked with a higher incidence of sexual and violent abuse. In addition, adults with an autistic spectrum neurodivergence are reported to find a much broader range of stimuli traumatic (Rumball, Happé, & Grey, 2020) and to be prone to abusive exploitative behaviour in the context of relationships, particularly those with people who do not have a similar neurodiversity to themselves, where there is a "double empathy problem" – each individual being susceptible to misunderstanding the other's point of view (e.g., Pearson et al., 2020). Both of these social processes are encountered clinically and are linked both with trauma and offending patterns.

As a construct, the double empathy problem is a useful concept for understanding relational misattunement due to a range of deep-seated differences between people, not just autistic spectrum disorder. It is played out between people who are not trauma-informed in relation to people who are traumatised; it is played out between people of different cultures, different genders, and all sorts of different beliefs, religions, and political orientations. These are all contexts where relational ruptures can result in significant trauma, particularly if it gets played out repetitively and systemically, without any support or opportunity to step back, make sense and act on it. This is an area that could be fruitfully researched and developed.

Culpability and Credulity

A strong theme in the American literature exploring links between trauma and offending is the question of culpability (e.g., Javier, Owen, & Maddux, 2020). If people do things in states of mind where they are thought to be "less capable of being responsible", then there are possible implications for their legal status. Consequently, much effort has been put into trying to understand what are seen as more traditional questions for forensic psychologists: how do we know if people are lying so that they can get a lesser sentence – or indeed, in some countries help to build a case against the death penalty? How do we assess trauma and its role in offending in the context of various vested interests? This kind of question, while raising a clinically important issue, if foregrounded too much can result in a harmful process of not believing people who are telling the truth about their abuse. The question is: what are the consequences of believing somebody who is lying and how does this contrast with the consequences of not believing somebody who is telling the truth? This kind of cost benefit analysis is one that practitioners need to use all the time. While often the solution to this dilemma is to go for a state of protected uncertainty where one holds on to both possibilities when we are working with people who have not been believed all their lives even this stance can be experienced as yet another episode of disbelief. Exploration of this clinical dilemma and its impacts on service users and possible perceptions of taking a credulous stance by others would be a useful area for further development.

Staff Trauma

Carlisle and McGuire (2020) reported that staff starting in jobs in a secure hospital had experienced more adverse childhood experiences than the average of community groups. Staff then are bringing with them a significant amount of trauma-related lived experience. It may be partly this that has led them to be attracted to a helping profession. While this is a much neglected strength in staff, it is also a neglected vulnerability. Trauma awareness and coping training is not only for the residents in forensic settings, it is critical for staff also. This is a neglected area and needs to be taken more seriously. Working in forensic settings can be immensely rewarding, but it can also be highly stressful and, indeed, traumatising if staff are exposed to serious violent or abusive behaviour. Having this kind of history can be an asset in these contexts but it can also result in the individual being vulnerable to being harmed by the work. In other kinds of employment there is an accepted idea of an *industrial injury*. Traumatic exposure of staff needs to be seen in this light. It is as serious and harmful for some people's lives. It should not be seen as "part of the job" and to be expected. It needs to be understood and anticipated. Staff need to develop a range of strategies to facilitate their capacity to respond positively to this kind of challenge or, if this is deemed to be needed, to be given the option to move into less challenging roles in the interests of their mental health.

If an organisation accept that staff are going to be "burnt out" and implicitly see this as "part of the job" without trying to offset this harm then it is being complicit with an iatrogenic culture.

Organisational Trauma

A number of contributors have discussed the ways in which organisations can add to the trauma an individual has experienced (e.g., Chapter 20). There is a growing literature on the ways in which organisations can be traumagenic. Bloom (e.g., 2014) argues that organisations can react in ways that are both similar to individuals experiencing trauma and that can have a traumatising impact on those living and working in and with them. For instance, she describes organisations becoming hypervigilant, preoccupied with things that went wrong in the past, anxious, suspicious, making decisions on the spur of the moment without thinking them through or, on the other hand, not reacting, becoming insensitive and non-responsive to the needs of those living and working in them. Both of these organisational reactions are seen as being responses to organisational trauma, serious incidents, for instance, that have resulted in staff becoming preoccupied with the possibility that it could happen again.

As a model this has heuristic value. However there has been little research looking at these kinds of dynamics. More work needs to be done to elucidate this kind of process. Other models, looking at a similar idea from a very different perspective, are offered by psychodynamic thinkers who see much of what can happen in staff teams as being influenced by unconscious reactions to trauma-derived processes in the service user group (e.g., Hinshelwood, 1987; Kurtz, 2020) or similar processes from higher management and political contingencies – for example the threats of budget cuts. Developing models and languages for talking about, understanding, and accomplishing reflective spaces that respond to this range of sources of unprocessed trauma is a critical task for the future; in doing this we need to find ways of valuing native and so-called "folk" epistemologies addressing trauma.

Traumatising or Iatrogenic Therapy

An under-researched area is the ways in which therapies can be traumatic. Working with trauma is a complex and challenging therapeutic task. In therapy focusing on trauma with people who have not offended, it is typically seen as important to do a significant amount of preparation to get the individual to a point where they can begin to explore the trauma without reacting by feeling retraumatised or dropping out and avoiding the therapy. Trauma work precipitates the kinds of difficulties and symptoms the individual is struggling to manage and if this happens then it is important that they and the therapist – or multidisciplinary team – are ready and prepared for a range of reactions to the work so that it can be supported and contained. With people who have offended, all these considerations need to be attended to in addition to looking at the possibility that the work could precipitate some kind of offending behaviour. People will sometimes respond to exposure or processing work by becoming angry or dissociating. Sometimes this behaviour emerges before or after sessions and has to be managed by staff. At worst, this can result in deterioration or people leaving or dropping out of therapy. If trauma is linked with offending, then work on trauma runs the risk of triggering offence-related trauma responses. This can be either direct, e.g., becoming aggressive in the session, or it can be indirect, e.g., behaving in a sexualised or a violent way outside the session, after exploring an experience of sexual abuse.

Jones (2007) highlighted a number of ways in which therapies can be potentially harmful. Not all therapies are harmful, and not all of the harms experienced are going to be traumatic however. The kinds of outcomes that are going to be more problematic are those that result in trauma reactions of different kinds. Therapists can become overly involved with their patients and sadly can also have abusive relationships with their patients. This is sometimes a parallel to what happened in the context of the individual's own abuse if, for example, they had been abused by an adult caregiver. This then can have an accumulative impact, not only do they have to deal with the trauma of the abuse, but they also have to deal with the loss of trust in those who are supposed to be helping them.

Post-Traumatic and Post-Release Adjustment Trajectories

A significant area to explore in the future is the differences in response to trauma and, related to this, post-release adjustment trajectories. Some people respond relatively well while others do not. Why is this? This is relevant to patterns of response to the task of building a life after release from prison – in itself a potentially traumatic experience. Layne and Hobfoll (2020) have explored this and identified a set of post-traumatic adjustment trajectories.

People experience kinds of adjustment that are responses to the actual availability of resources in their lives, or their anticipation based on past experience, and react in different ways to this in terms of a range of trauma responses aimed at both gaining resources and managing the emotions linked with not having resources. Layne and Hobfoll highlight different patterns of adjustment for trauma; these are equally relevant to thinking about safety (risk). In the lead up to offending there is a pattern of loss of offence resisting resources (protective factors) that is impacted on by the parallel trajectory of resource loss in trauma reactions.

Layne and Hobfoll describe a set of post-traumatic adjustment trajectories: *decline* gradual or delayed, *distress tolerance* (just about coping but not back to pre-trauma functioning), *phasic adjustment* (going through good phases and "bad" phases), *severe decline*, *chronic maladaptive functioning*, *stress resistance* (not being impacted significantly), *resilient recovery* (springing back after an initial deterioration), *prolonged recovery* (gradually getting back to "normal"), and *growth*. Anyone with experience working with ex-offenders will immediately recognise these patterns as also relevant to the post-release adjustment trajectories of ex-offenders. Conceptually then, these descriptions offer a framework for looking at the interaction between trauma as it is triggered and pre-offending patterns of change in people released from custodial settings. More work needs to be done exploring why different people follow different trajectories and the ways in which provision of psychological and material resources can possibly prevent some of the more precipitative patterns of deterioration.

In addition, the conservation of resources (COR) theory principles, developed for understanding trauma, need to be explored in relation to trauma-related return-to-crime processes:

> Basic COR theory tenet: Individuals (and groups) strive to obtain, retain, foster, and protect those things they centrally value.
>
> **Principle 1: Primacy of loss principle.** Resource loss is disproportionately more salient than resource gain.
>
> **Principle 2: Resource investment principle.** People must invest resources in order to protect against resource loss, recover from losses, and gain resources.
>
> **Principle 3: Gain paradox principle.** Resource gain increases in salience in the context of resource loss. That is, when resource loss circumstances are high, resource gains become more important—they gain in value.
>
> **Principle 4: Desperation principle.** When people's resources are outstretched or exhausted, they enter a defensive mode to preserve the self which is often defensive, aggressive, and may become irrational.
>
> *Hobfoll, Halbesleben, Neveu, & Westman, 2018; p. 106*

Interventions that Move Away from Simple Assumptions of Agency

Some contributors have suggested that interventions with trauma need to attend to a range of psychological processes other than/as well as those relying on the use of language. Assumptions of agency are central to much of the therapeutic literature historically. Recent developments have pointed trauma therapies away from language towards interventions focusing on the body or which acknowledge that trauma can be linked with a propensity to experience radical shifts in states of consciousness, some of which increase the possibility of offending (e.g., offence-related altered states of consciousness). This is an area that requires systematic investigation: how does dissociation work among people who offend? How do people make sense of their own experiences of dissociation? Are there trauma-related states that could be protective also?

Research into the Effects of Positive Developmental Experiences

The emphasis in a trauma-informed perspective is on *negative* or aversive experiences resulting in people being hurt, hurting themselves, or hurting other people. It is equally useful, however, to think about *positive* experiences. Most people who have worked with people who have significant trauma histories will have the experience of working with people on finding memories or experiences that were nurturing and valuable to them. The obvious examples of this are attachment experiences. Even if it is difficult, most people can generate a positive experience from their childhoods – feeling loved, achieving in education, or a loyal pet. Layne and Hobfoll (2020) describe positive resource cycles following trauma experiences; others describe a process of post-traumatic growth. The key area here is finding ways of describing what it is that happens when people experience post-traumatic growth. One observation Layne and Hobfoll have made is that having resources provided at an early stage post-trauma is critical to preventing deterioration. However, what is it that leads to post-traumatic resilience and flourishing? What would a list of good things that can happen to you look like? The opposite of a list of ACEs? What mechanisms then would be in play in this context that led to non-problematic growth?

Intervention and Change

One of the strongest themes of this book has been a refocusing of attention onto contexts and the environment, and, in particular, the ways in which those contexts can be harmful, oppressive, and unjust. In some ways the psychological perspective runs the risk of hiding the context. In order to bring about change, do we help people to accept deprived situations, think positively about oppressive conditions, accept the pain of being unloved, stifle the cries of outrage at society for allowing abuse to take place, or do we try and change that society and validate the pain and face its intensity and honour its integrity? The answer to this has to be both, it is a false dichotomy – especially if not accepting the injustice of deprivation, or thinking negatively about oppression, or fighting against the pain of being unloved, or the nature of the cries of outrage are harming people. Of course, we need to help people, but we need also to try to change society. Not to address the underlying causes of crime is to be complicit with it. This is a reality that we can no longer deny as forensic practitioners.

How do we do this? There are a range of ways in which this can be done. The work needs to start with ourselves, developing a critical stance towards our own practice. Asking questions like: to what extent am I being complicit with harmful organisational practices and or dynamics? In what ways am I being racist or sexist or homophobic explicitly or implicitly? How can I listen more effectively to voices that have been repressed or excluded? Working with the organisations we work in to increase trauma awareness and responsivity and awareness of harmful dynamics like racism in policies, procedures, cultures, and reflective practice. Indeed, trauma- and diversity-informed reflective practice – as suggested by McGuire, Carlisle, and Clark (Chapter 20) – is a critical process for shaping perspectives and offering an opportunity to step back from the work and identify complicity and ways forward. This requires an understanding of our own shifts in states of consciousness from thinking to unthinking and a containing framework to allow and nurture useful and constructive responses to emerge (see Kurtz, 2020). Without this kind of work the double empathy problem (DEP) and a range of avoidant responses will inevitably lead to an escalation in mutual misunderstandings resulting in different kinds of troubled or troubling behaviour. We need to understand the ways in which trauma narratives and narratives of racism and oppression repeatedly get swept under the carpet, avoided, denied, and overlooked. The psychology and sociology of this kind of process needs to be a core part of our training and research agendas.

We need also to be letting the world know about this. Forensic practitioners are perhaps the only group of people who get to hear these stories. The rest of society rarely hears them. In a meeting with the National Union of Journalists in 2017, exploring the ways in which journalists document crime, it was clear that journalists do not have access to the back-stories behind the crimes that they reported. They indicated that they were interested in them, but just did not have access to the information. Therapists cannot easily pass these stories on as they are confidential. What do we do with them then? Do they end up in a *cul de sac*? Surely, we have a responsibility to pass them on to inform politicians, journalists, educators, academics, and society at large about the extent to which crime and people involved with crime have been exposed to these processes. Surely, we have a responsibility to try to move society in the direction of being trauma-informed and responsive and, ultimately, less unjust. The fact that the people we work with have hurt people themselves should not exclude them from the right to be heard; two wrongs do not make a right. Indeed, it could be argued that it is primarily through taking an *active stance* in relation to addressing processes like privilege, racism, and sexism in society that we can develop better psychologies of power, abuse, oppression, and trauma. Who better than forensic practitioners to do this? Brown (2017) provides a useful account of the major and decisive impact of feminism on bringing the trauma perspective out into the open – a perspective that would never have emerged if it hadn't been struggled for actively.

Conclusion

Hopefully this book has challenged practitioners to revisit their practice and consider working in new ways. Hopefully also it has opened possibilities for new ways of assessing and intervening to try to change the impacts of trauma, oppression, and adversity on people's lives.

References

Bloom, S. (2014). Creating, destroying and restoring sanctuary within caregiving organizations. In A. Odgers (Ed.), *From broken attachments to earned security: The role of empathy in therapeutic change* (pp. 55–90). Karnac Books Ltd.

Brown, L. S. (1992). A feminist critique of the personality disorders. In L. S. Brown & M. Ballou (Eds), *Personality and psychopathology: Feminist reappraisals* (pp. 206–228). Guilford Press.

Brown, L. S. (2017). Contributions of feminist and critical psychologies to trauma psychology. In S. N. Gold (Ed.), *APA handbook of trauma psychology* (pp. 501–526). American Psychological Association.

Carlisle, J., & McGuire, F. (2020). *Mersey Care NHS Foundation Trust - systemic factors and trauma informed care: Cultural change & managing trauma.* Paper presented at Trauma Informed Care in Forensic Settings Conference, March 2020.

Cattan, S, Conti, G. Farquarson, C., & Ginja, R. (2019). *The health effects of sure start.* Institute for Fiscal Studies.

Dell'Osso, L. Cremone, I., Carpita, B., Fagiolini, A., Massimetti, G., Bossini, L., … & Gesi, C. (2018). Correlates of autistic traits among patients with borderline personality disorder. *Comprehensive Psychiatry, 83*, 7–11. doi:10.1016/j.comppsych.2018.01.002

Ellis, S. (2021). *The racial history of forensic psychology in Britain and in its former colonies: An archival analysis.* Presentation at the Division of Forensic Psychology Conference, Online 16 June 2021.

Francis, R. (2013). *Report of the Mid Staffordshire NHS Foundation Trust Public Inquiry.* The Stationery Office.

Graziano, J. N., & Wagner, E. F. (2016). Trauma among lesbians and bisexual girls in the juvenile justice system. *Traumatology, 17*(2), 45–55. doi:10.1177/1534765610391817

Heilbron, J. L. (2005). Censorship of astronomy in Italy after Galileo. In McMullin, E (Ed.). *The church and Galileo* (pp. 279–322). University of Notre Dame Press.

Hinshelwood, R.D. (1987). *What happens in groups? Psychoanalysis, the individual and the community.* Free Association Books.

Hobfoll, S. E., Halbesleben, J., Neveu, J. P., & Westman, M. (2018). Conservation of resources in the organizational context: The reality of resources and their consequences. *Annual Review of Organizational Psychology and Organizational Behavior, 5*, 103–128. doi:10.1146/annurev-orgpsych-032117-104640

Javier, R. A., Owen, E. A., & Maddux, J. A. (2020). *Assessing trauma in forensic contexts.* Springer.

Johnstone, L. & Boyle, M. with Cromby, J., Dillon, J., Harper, D., Kinderman, P., Longden, E., Pilgrim, D., & Read, J. (2018). *The power threat meaning framework: Towards the identification of patterns in emotional distress, unusual experiences and troubled or troubling behaviour, as an alternative to functional psychiatric diagnosis.* British Psychological Society.

Jones, L. F. (2007). Iatrogenic interventions with personality disordered offenders. *Psychology, Crime & Law, 13*(1), 69–79. doi:10.1080/10683160600869809

Jones, L.F. (2015). The Peaks unit: from a pilot for 'untreatable' psychopaths to trauma-informed milieu therapy. *Prison Service Journal, 218*, 17–23.

Kerig, P. K., & Becker, S. P. (2010). From internalizing to externalizing: Theoretical models of the processes linking PTSD to juvenile delinquency. In S. J. Egan (Ed.), *Posttraumatic stress disorder (PTSD): Causes, symptoms and treatment* (pp. 33–78). Nova Science.

Kurtz, A. (2020). *How to run reflective practice groups: A guide for healthcare professionals.* Routledge.

Layne, C. M., & Hobfoll, S. (2020). Understanding post-traumatic adjustment trajectories in school-age youth: Supporting stress resistance, resilient recovery, and growth. In E. Rossen (Ed.), *Supporting and educating traumatized students: A guide for school-based professionals* (pp. 75–97). Oxford University Press.

Ministry of Justice. (2020). *Costs per place and costs per prisoner by individual prison.* Ministry of Justice.

Montalbano, W. (1992, November 1). Vatican finds Galileo "not guilty". *Washington Post.* Retrieved from www.washingtonpost.com/

Pearson, A., Rees, J., Rose, K., & Forster, S. (2020). *"This was just how this friendship worked": Experiences of interpersonal victimisation in autistic adults.* OSF Preprints. Retrieved from https://osf.io/amn6k/ 23rd August, 2021.

Quiros, L., Varghese, R., & Vanidestine, T. (2020). Disrupting the single story: Challenging dominant trauma narratives through a critical race lens. *Traumatology, 26*(2), 160–168 doi:10.1037/trm0000223

Rumball, F., Happé, F., & Grey, N. (2020). Experience of trauma and PTSD symptoms in autistic adults: Risk of PTSD development following DSM-5 and non-DSM-5 traumatic life events. *Autism Research, 13* (12), 2122–2132. doi:10.1002/aur.2306

Sue, D. W. (2010). *Microaggressions in everyday life: Race, gender, and sexual orientation.* John Wiley & Sons.

Westphal, A. (2016). Trauma and violence in autism. *Journal of the American Academy of Psychiatry and the Law, 44*(2), 198–199.

Yalom, I. D. (2011). *Staring at the Sun: Being at peace with your own mortality.* Hachette.

INDEX

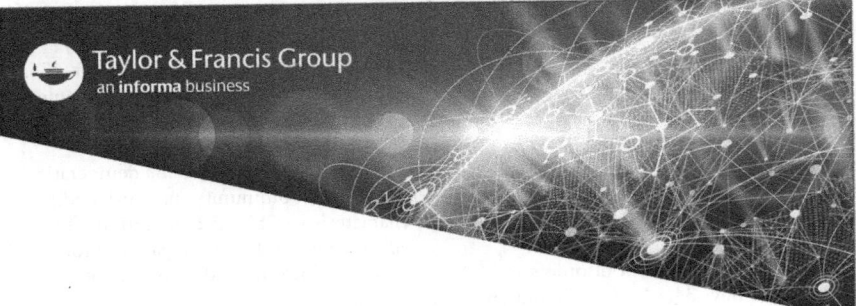
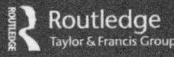
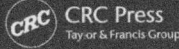